The PICU

MW00835572

Edited by

Ranna A. Rozenfeld, MD
Professor of Pediatrics
The Warren Alpert Medical School of Brown University
Attending Physician, Division of Critical Care Medicine,
Hasbro Children's Hospital
Providence, Rhode Island

New York   Chicago   San Francisco   Athens   London   Madrid
Mexico City   Milan   New Delhi   Singapore   Sydney   Toronto

The PICU Handbook

Copyright © 2018 by McGraw-Hill Education, Inc. All rights reserved. Except as permitted under the United States Copyright Act of 1976, no part of this publication may be reproduced or distributed in any form or by any means, or stored in a data base or retrieval system, with-out the prior written permission of the publisher.

1 2 3 4 5 6 7 8 9 LCR 23 22 21 20 19 18

ISBN: 978-1-259-83437-0
MHID: 1-259-83437-9

Notice

Medicine is an ever-changing science. As new research and clinical experience broaden our knowledge, changes in treatment and drug therapy are required. The authors and the publisher of this work have checked with sources believed to be reliable in their efforts to provide information that is complete and generally in accord with the standards accepted at the time of publication. However, in view of the possibility of human error or changes in medical sciences, neither the authors nor the publisher nor any other party who has been involved in the preparation or publication of this work warrants that the information contained herein is in every respect accurate or complete, and they disclaim all responsi-bility for any errors or omissions or for the results obtained from use of the information contained in this work. Readers are encouraged to confirm the information contained herein with other sources. For example and in particular, readers are advised to check the product information sheet included in the package of each drug they plan to administer to be certain that the information contained in this work is accurate and that changes have not been made in the recommended dose or in the contraindications for administration. This recommendation is of particular importance in connection with new or infre-quently used medications.

This book was set in Minionpro-Regular by MPS Limited.

The editors were Andrew Moyer and Regina Y. Brown.
The production supervisor was Rick Ruzycka.
Project management was provided by Nikhil, MPS Limted.
The cover designer was Randomatrix.

Library of Congress Cataloging-in-Publication Data

Names: Rozenfeld, Ranna, editor.
Title: The PICU handbook / editor, Ranna A. Rozenfeld, MD, Professor of
    Pediatrics, The Warren Alpert Medical School of Brown University,
    Attending Physician, Division of Critical Care Medicine,
    Hasbro Children's Hospital, Providence, RI.
Description: New York : McGraw-Hill, [2018]
Identifiers: LCCN 2018003123 | ISBN 9781259834370 (paperback)
Subjects: LCSH: Pediatric intensive care—Handbooks, manuals, etc. |
    Pediatric emergencies—Handbooks, manuals, etc. | BISAC: MEDICAL /
    Pediatrics.
Classification: LCC RJ370 .P58 2018 | DDC 618.92/0028--dc23 LC record available at https://na01.safelinks.
protection.outlook.com/?url=https%3A%2F%2Flccn.loc.gov%2F2018003123&data=01%7C01%7Cleah.
carton%40mheducation.com%7C619a5e8fe8c74e6aceef08d5672a28b3%7Cf919b1efc0c347358fca0928ec39d8d
5%7C0&sdata=hFwyciIyxKopoZ%2BKnM3uNsqQTQnSKmRvb3MIn0y6nJo%3D&reserved=0

McGraw-Hill Education books are available at special quantity discounts to use as premiums and sales pro-motions, or for use in corporate training programs. To contact a representative, please visit the Contact Us pages at www.mhprofessional.com.

Contents

Contents

I would like to dedicate this book to the patients and families that I have had the privilege of caring for in the PICU. I would also like to thank Noah, Rebecca, Ilana, Eli and Shane for their love and support.

Contributors

Tord D. Alden, MD, Associate Professor of Neurological Surgery, Department of Neurological Surgery, Ann & Robert H. Lurie Children's Hospital of Chicago, Chicago, Illinois

Kiona Y. Allen, MD, Assistant Professor of Pediatrics, Northwestern University Feinberg School of Medicine, Ann & Robert H. Lurie Children's Hospital of Chicago, Department of Pediatrics, Division of Critical Care Medicine & Division of Cardiology, Chicago, Illinois

Lauren M. Baumann, MD, MHS, Resident, General Surgery, University of Cincinnati, Research Fellow, Pediatric Surgery, Ann & Robert H. Lurie Children's Hospital of Chicago

Amy Bobrowski, MD, Assistant Professor of Pediatrics, Feinberg School of Medicine, Northwestern University, Attending Physician, Division of Kidney Diseases, Ann & Robert H. Lurie Children's Hospital of Chicago, Chicago, Illinois

Meredith Bone, MD, MSCI, Assistant Professor of Pediatrics Feinberg School of Medicine, Northwestern University, Pediatric Critical Care Medicine, Ann & Robert H. Lurie Children's Hospital of Chicago, Chicago, Illinois

Ryan K. Breuer, MD, Assistant Professor, Department of Pediatrics, University at Buffalo Jacobs School of Medicine and Biomedical Sciences, Attending Physician in Pediatric Critical Care, Women and Children's Hospital of Buffalo, Buffalo, New York

Jillian Bybee, MD, Clinical Assistant Professor, Michigan State University. Attending Physician, Pediatric Critical Care Medicine, Helen DeVos Children's Hospital, Grand Rapids, Michigan

A. Sami Chaouki, MD, PhD, Assistant Professor of Pediatrics, Northwestern University Feinberg School of Medicine, Ann & Robert H. Lurie Children's Hospital of Chicago, Department of Pediatrics, Division of Cardiology, Chicago, Illinois

Lynn Chlebanowski, Clinical Educator in Respiratory Therapy, Ann & Robert H. Lurie Children's Hospital of Chicago, Chicago, Illinois

Anne G. Ciriello, MSN, CPNP-AC, CCRN, Children's National Health System, Washington, DC

Bria M. Coates, MD, Assistant Professor of Pediatrics, Northwestern University Feinberg School of Medicine, Attending Physician, Division of Pediatric Critical Care Medicine, Ann & Robert H. Lurie Children's Hospital of Chicago, Chicago, Illinois

Danielle D. DeCourcey, MD, MPH, Department of Medicine, Division of Medicine Critical Care, Boston Children's Hospital, Assistant Professor of Pediatrics, Harvard Medical School, Boston, Massachusetts

Sabrina F. Derrington, MD, Assistant Professor of Clinical Pediatrics, Northwestern University Feinberg School of Medicine, Attending Physician in Critical Care and Palliative Care, Ann and Robert H. Lurie Children's Hospital of Chicago, Chicago, Illinois

Conrad L. Epting, MD, FAAP, Associate Professor of Pediatrics and Pathology, Northwestern University School of Medicine, Staff Physician, Pediatric and Cardiac Critical Care, Ann & Robert H. Lurie Children's Hospital of Chicago, Chicago, Illinois

Michael Gart, MD, Fellow, Hand & Upper Extremity Surgery, OrthoCarolina Hand Center, Charlotte, North Carolina

Katherine A. Gregersen, DO, Assistant Professor of Pediatrics, Loma Linda University School of Medicine, Pediatric Intensivist, Loma Linda University Children's Hospital, Loma Linda, California

Vishal Gunnala, MD, Assistant Professor of Pediatrics, University of Arizona College of Medicine – Phoenix, Attending Physician PICU, Division of Critical Care Medicine, Phoenix Children's Hospital, Phoenix, Arizona

Z. Leah Harris, MD, Posy and John Krehbiel Professor of Critical Care Medicine, Professor of Pediatrics, Department of Pediatrics, Northwestern University Feinberg School of Medicine, Ann & Robert H. Lurie Children's Hospital of Chicago, Chicago, Illinois

Amanda B. Hassinger, MD, MS, Assistant Professor, Department of Pediatrics, University at Buffalo Jacobs School of Medicine and Biomedical Sciences, Attending Physician in Pediatric Critical Care, Women and Children's Hospital of Buffalo, Buffalo, New York

Sue J. Hong, MD, Assistant Professor of Pediatrics, Northwestern University Feinberg School of Medicine, Attending Physician, Department of Pediatrics, Division of Critical Care Medicine, Division of Neurology, Ann & Robert H. Lurie Children's Hospital of Chicago, Chicago, Illinois

Russ Horowitz, MD, RDMS, Assistant Professor of Pediatrics, Northwestern University Feinberg School of Medicine, Attending Physician, Director, Emergency and Critical Care Ultrasound, Ann & Robert H. Lurie Children's Hospital of Chicago, Chicago, Illinois

Jonathan B. Ida, MD, MA, FACS, FAAP, Assistant Professor, Department of Otolaryngology/Head and Neck Surgery, Northwestern-Feinberg School of Medicine, Clinical Faculty, Division of Pediatric Otolaryngology, Department of Surgery, Ann & Robert H. Lurie Children's Hospital of Chicago, Chicago, Illinois

Daniel Kelly, MD, Division of Medicine Critical Care, Boston Children's Hospital, Instructor of Pediatrics, Harvard Medical School, Boston, Massachusetts

Elizabeth W. J. Kerris, MD, Children's National Medical Center, Washington, DC

Jonathan E. Kurz, MD, PhD, Ruth D. & Ken M. Davee Pediatric Neurocritical Care Program, Department of Pediatrics, Ann & Robert H. Lurie Children's Hospital of Chicago, Northwestern University Feinberg School of Medicine, Chicago, Illinois

Timothy B. Lautz, MD, Assistant Professor of Surgery, Northwestern University, Feinberg School of Medicine, Pediatric Surgeon, Ann & Robert H. Lurie Children's Hospital of Chicago, Chicago, Illinois

Steven O. Lestrud, MD, Attending Physician, Division of Critical Care Medicine and Division of Pulmonary Medicine, Northwestern University Feinberg School of Medicine, Ann & Robert H. Lurie Children's Hospital of Chicago, Chicago, Illinois

Amanda Levin, MD, Assistant Professor, The George Washington University, Attending Physician, Pediatric Critical Care Medicine, Children's National Health System, Washington, DC

Lauren Marsillio, MD, Assistant Professor of Pediatrics, Northwestern University Feinberg School of Medicine, Attending Physician, Division of Pediatric Critical Care Medicine, Ann & Robert H. Lurie Children's Hospital of Chicago, Chicago, Illinois

Mjaye L. Mazwi, MBChB, Staff Physician Critical Care Medicine, Director, Clinical Translational Engineering, The Hospital for Sick Children, Toronto, Ontario, Canada

Maureen McCarthy-Kowols, MSN, BSN, CCRN, Clinical Educator, Ann & Robert H. Lurie Children's Hospital of Chicago, Chicago, Illinois

Kelly Michelson, MD, MPH, FCCM, FAAP, Associate Professor of Pediatrics and Julia and David Uihlein Professor in Bioethics and Medical Humanities, Northwestern University Feinberg School of Medicine, Director, Center for Bioethics and Medical Humanities, Northwestern University Feinberg School of Medicine, Attending Physician, Ann & Robert H. Lurie Children's Hospital of Chicago, Chicago, Illinois

Thomas Moran, PharmD, MS, BCPS, Ann & Robert H. Lurie Children's Hospital of Chicago Department of Pharmacy, Chicago, Illinois

Lindsey A. Morgan, MD, Department of Neurology, Seattle Children's Hospital, University of Washington, Seattle, Washington

Zehava L. Noah, MD, Associate Professor of Pediatrics, Northwestern University Feinberg School of Medicine, Ann & Robert H. Lurie Children's Hospital of Chicago, Chicago, Illinois

Russell Jason Orr, PharmD, MBA, University of Chicago Hospitals, Department of Pharmacy, Chicago, Illinois

Vickie Papageorge, RPh, Ann & Robert H. Lurie Children's Hospital of Chicago Department of Pharmacy, Chicago, Illinois

Erin Talati Paquette, MD, JD, MBe, FCCM, FAAP, Assistant Professor of Pediatrics, Northwestern University Feinberg School of Medicine, Attending Physician, Ann & Robert H. Lurie Children's Hospital of Chicago, Northwestern University Feinberg School of Medicine, Chicago, Illinois

Rupal Patel, PharmD, BCPPS, Pediatric Antimicrobial Stewardship Coordinator, Levine Children's Hospital, Carolinas HealthCare System, Charlotte, North Carolina

Sameer Patel, MD, MPH, Associate Professor of Pediatrics, Northwestern University Feinberg School of Medicine, Attending Physician, Pediatric Infectious Disease, Director of Antimicrobial Stewardship, Ann & Robert H. Lurie Children's Hospital of Chicago, Chicago Illinois

Vamshi K. Rao, MD, Assistant Professor of Pediatrics, Northwestern University Feinberg School of Medicine, Attending Physician, Department of Pediatrics, Division of Neurology, Ann & Robert H. Lurie Children's Hospital of Chicago, Chicago, Illinois

Charles Baron Rothschild, MD, Palliative Care Fellow, Seattle Children's Hospital, Seattle, Washington

Ranna A. Rozenfeld, MD, Professor of Pediatrics, The Warren Alpert Medical School of Brown University, Attending Physician, Division of Critical Care Medicine, Hasbro Children's Hospital, Providence, Rhode Island

Laura Russo, RD, CSP, LDN, Department of Clinical Nutrition, Registered Dietitian, Ann & Robert H. Lurie Children's Hospital of Chicago, Chicago, Illinois

Christopher Schneller, MD, Assistant Professor of Pediatrics, The University of Texas at Austin Dell Medical School, Pediatric Critical Care Medicine, Dell Children's Medical Center of Central Texas, Austin, Texas

Astha Khanna Sharma, MD, FAAP, Assistant Professor of Pediatrics, Attending Physician – Pediatric Critical Care Medicine, Ronald McDonald Children's Hospital, Loyola University Medical Center, Maywood, Illinois

Ashley Siems, MD, Children's National Health System, Assistant Professor of Pediatric Critical Care Medicine, George Washington University, Washington, DC

Craig M. Smith, MD, Assistant Professor of Pediatrics, Northwestern University Feinberg School of Medicine, Pediatric Critical Care Medicine, Pediatric Neurocritical Care, Ann & Robert H. Lurie Children's Hospital of Chicago, Chicago, Illinois

Lauren Sorce, RN, PhD(c), MSN, CPNP-AC/PC, FCCM, Pediatric Critical Care Nurse Practitioner, Manager, Associate Director, Nursing Research, Ann & Robert H. Lurie Children's Hospital of Chicago, Chicago, Illinois

Carolyn Stickney, MD, Department of Medicine, Division of Medicine Critical Care, Boston Children's Hospital, Instructor of Pediatrics, Harvard Medical School, Boston, Massachusetts

Mark S. Wainwright, MD, PhD, Herman and Faye Sarkowsky Endowed Chair Head, Division of Pediatric Neurology, Professor of Neurology, University of Washington, Seattle Children's Hospital, Seattle, Washington

Eric L. Wald MD, MSCI, Associate Professor of Pediatrics, Northwestern University's Feinberg School of Medicine, Attending Physician PICU and CICU, Divisions of Critical Care Medicine and Cardiology, Ann & Robert H. Lurie Children's Hospital of Chicago, Chicago, Illinois

Laura Westley, BSN, MSM, RN, C-NPT, Ann & Robert H. Lurie Children's Hospital of Chicago, Senior Director: Emergency Services, Interfacility Transport, and Patient Access Center, Chicago, Illinois

Katie K. Wolfe, MD, Instructor of Pediatrics, Northwestern University Feinberg School of Medicine, Attending Physician, Division of Pediatric Critical Care Medicine, Ann & Robert H. Lurie Children's Hospital of Chicago, Chicago, Illinois

Preface

This book was inspired by my interest in medical education. I first began writing an internal handbook for the pediatric residents at Children's Memorial Hospital in 2005. That book grew and inspired what is now this PICU handbook. I would like to acknowledge the pediatric residents and pediatric critical care fellows who gave feedback on the internal book over the past 10 years. It was their interest in having a resource that inspired me to create and refine the handbook and now to publish the book for medical students, residents, fellows, and advanced practice nurses at any institution.

The handbook is meant to be an easy reference guide. It is separated into Part I: General Pediatric Critical Care, which includes resuscitation and stabilization, critical care procedures, and pharmacology, and then Part II: Organ Systems, which includes sections on respiratory, cardiovascular, neurology, renal/fluids and electrolytes, hematology/oncology, endocrine, gastroenterology/nutrition/hepatology, environmental/toxicology emergencies, and allergy/immunology/genetics.

The intent is for this to be a pocket handbook that can be carried around and easily accessed for those working in the pediatric intensive care unit. This is intended to be a reference for pediatric residents, family medicine residents, emergency medicine residents, pediatric critical care fellows, emergency medicine fellows, surgical critical care fellows, pediatric hospitalists, pediatric nurse practitioners, and medical students.

I would like to thank the nurses, nurse practitioners, respiratory therapists, pharmacists, and nutritionists who taught me about the true multidisciplinary approach to pediatric critical care medicine. This book has authors from all these disciplines contributing to a truly multidisciplinary handbook.

The various contributors to this handbook also deserve thanks. Several contributors were former pediatric critical care fellows who worked with me on the internal handbooks throughout the years. These individuals shared an interest and passion in medical education.

I would like to thank the production staff at McGraw-Hill Education, especially Andrew Moyer, Senior Editor, who has guided me through the process.

Finally, I would like to thank Eli, Ilana, Rebecca, Noah and Shane, for all their support and for allowing me the time to work on this book. I also thank my children for contributing artwork to the internal editions of this book over the years. Lastly, I thank my parents, Dr. Irving and Betty Rozenfeld, for their unwavering support throughout my career.

PART 1

General Pediatric Critical Care

1

General

1   Common Formulas, Normal Values and Vital Signs

Normal Pediatric Vital Signs

Age	Heart Rate (per min)	Respiratory Rate (per min)	Blood Pressure Systolic/Diastolic (MAP)	Circulating Blood Volume (mL/kg)
0–2 months	100–180	30–80	60–90/30–60 (40 s–50 s)	85–90
2–12 months	100–160	30–60	87–105/53–66 (50 s)	75–80
1–3 years	80–110	24–40	95–105/53–66 (60–65)	75–80
3–5 years	70–110	22–34	96–108/55–67 (65–69)	75–80
5–12 years	65–110	18–30	97–112/57–71 (70–77)	70–75
13 years+	60–90	12–16	112–128/66–80 (77–80 s)	65–70

MAP: mean arterial pressure

METRIC CONVERSIONS

Pounds to kilograms: 2.2 lb = 1 kg
Inches to centimeters: 1 in = 2.54 cm
Fahrenheit temperature to Celsius:

$\quad$ 98.6 = 37.0
$\quad$ 100.0 = 37.8
$\quad$ 101.0 = 38.3
$\quad$ 101.3 = 38.5
$\quad$ 102.2 = 39.0
$\quad$ 103.1 = 39.5
$\quad$ 104.0 = 40.0
$\quad$ 105.8 = 41.0

CALCULATING MAINTENANCE FLUID REQUIREMENTS IN CHILDREN

DAILY MAINTENANCE FORMULA

0–10 kg	100 mL/kg
11–20 kg	1000 mL for first 10 kg + 50 mL/kg for 11–20 kg
21+ kg	1500 mL for first 20 kg + 25 mL/kg for 21+ kg

HOURLY MAINTENANCE FORMULA

0–10 kg	4 mL/kg/hr
11–20 kg	40 mL/hr for first 10 kg + 2 mL/kg/hr for 11–20 kg
21+ kg	60 mL/hr for first 20 kg + 1 mL/kg/hr for 21+ kg
Adult maintenance	80–120 mL/hr
Insensible fluid rate	300–400 mL/m²/day, divide by 24 for rate/hr

BODY SURFACE AREA (BSA)

$$BSA(m^2) = ([Height(cm) \times Weight(kg)] / 3600)^{1/2}$$

A rough estimate of BSA may be made by: $[(wt\ in\ kg \times 4) + 7]/[90 + wt\ in\ kg]$

GLOMERULAR FILTRATION RATE (GFR)

GFR (Schwartz Equation) = k × Height (cm) / (Scr in g/dL) mL/min/1.73 m²
K value　　　　　　　 = 0.33 < 40 Gest Age
　　　　　　　　　　 = 0.45 40 wk – 1 yr
　　　　　　　　　　 = 0.55 1 yr – 13 yr males, > 1 yr females
　　　　　　　　　　 = 0.65 > 13 yr males

S_{cr}: serum creatinine

$$Creatinine\ Clearance(mL/min): CrCl = \frac{(Urine\ Cr)(Urine\ volume)}{(Plasma\ Cr)(Time\ in\ Min)}$$

Corrected for BSA: CrCl * 1.73 / BSA in m²

FRACTIONAL EXCRETION OF SODIUM (FENA)

$FeNa = (U_{Na}/P_{Na})/(U_{Cr}/P_{Cr}) \times 100\%$
　U_{Na} – Urine sodium
　P_{Na} – Plasma sodium
　U_{Cr} – Urine creatinine
　P_{Cr} – Plasma creatinine

Calculated Serum Osmolality = 2*(Na) + Glu/18 + BUN/2.8
　Na – Serum sodium
　Glu – Serum glucose in mg/dL
　BUN – Blood urea nitrogen

Osmolal Gap: Osm (measured) – Osm (calculated)
　Normal osmolal gap < 10 mOsm

Anion Gap = $Na^+ - [(Cl^-) + (HCO_3^-)]$
　Normal anion gap 8–12 mEq/L

SUGGESTED READINGS

de Caen AR, Berg MD, Chameides L, et al. Part 12: Pediatric advanced life support: 2015 American Heart Association guidelines update for cardiopulmonary resuscitation and emergency cardiovascular care. *Circulation*. 2015;132:S526-S542.

Holliday MA, Segar WE. The maintenance need for water in parenteral fluid therapy. *Pediatrics*. 1957;19(5):823-832.

Mistovich JJ, Karren KJ, Hafen B. *Prehospital Emergency Care*. 10th ed. Pearson, Upper Saddle River, NJ. 2014.

2 Pediatric Neonatal Specialty Transport Teams

TEAM COMPOSITION

- Pediatric neonatal specialty transport teams can have various team compositions.
- The optimal team makeup is best determined by the needs of the patient.
- Transport team personnel include physicians (MD/DO), advance practice nurses (APN), nurses (RN), respiratory care practitioners (RCP), paramedics (EMT-P), and emergency medical technicians (EMT).
- Examples of various team compositions:
  - RN-RCP
  - RN-RN
  - RN-MD/DO/APN
  - RN-EMT-P
  - RN-RCP-MD/DO/APN
  - Some teams routinely take a physician or APN; other teams take them as needed
- Importance of the decision
  - The team composition should support the team's scope of care.
  - Team members should be able to initiate the desired level of care on arrival to the referring hospital.
- Team members must hold certifications to support the scope of practice to care for the patients transported. Examples include:
  - PALS
  - ACLS
  - NRP
  - PEPP
  - C-NPT

MODE OF TRANSPORT

- Various modes of transport are utilized by pediatric neonatal specialty teams
  - Ground transport (ambulance)
  - Rotor wing aircraft (helicopter)
  - Fixed wing aircraft
- Some teams have all three modes available to them; other teams only utilize one or two modes and may contract out for the other modes
- Many teams utilize guidelines to help frame the decision on which mode to utilize for a specific patient
- Decision is based on:
  - Patient acuity
  - Time-sensitive nature of illness or injury
  - Distance
  - Travel time

ROLE OF MEDICAL CONTROL PHYSICIAN

- The medical control physician has multiple responsibilities
  - Acceptance of patient to the organization
  - Assure bed and specialty care are available

- ○ Determine necessary level of care
- ○ Determine mode of transport (must be familiar with various modes)
- ○ Medical decision making during transport
- ○ Must be familiar with transport topics such as altitude physiology
  - ▪ Patients with recent surgical procedures may have retained air, which can have a severe impact during flight at higher altitudes
  - ▪ Considerations must be given to air-filled endotracheal tube (ETT) cuffs or balloons in Foley catheters
- ○ Documentation by medical control physician
- ○ Recommendations given to referring hospital (see Figure 2-1)
- ○ Medical decision making with transport team throughout transport
- ○ Signing of any orders given to transport team

MEDICAL CONTROL TRANSPORT CALL RECORD

Patient Name _____ Age/Weight _____ MR# _____

Referring Hospital _____ Referring MD _____ Phone# _____

Allergies _____

Vitals Signs:

Time	Temp	HR	RR	BP	Pulse Ox	Cap Refill	GCS

Past Medical History:

_____

_____

HPI: _____

_____

Labs:

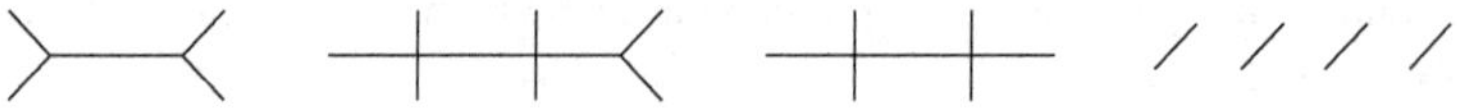

Medications: _____

Access: _____ **Imaging:** _____

Interventions: _____

Recommendations: _____

FIGURE 2-1 **Example of a transport call record for a medical control physician.**

PROTOCOLS AND CLINICAL GUIDELINES

- Protocols allow nonphysician teams to provide patient care within the team's scope under the authority of the medical director
- Teams may have multiple protocols depending on the scope of care. Examples include:
  - Neonatal protocols, including the care of the surgical neonate and neonates with congenital heart disease
  - Pediatric protocols
  - Trauma protocols
- Protocols require initial review with legal/risk management team
  - In many states protocols are legally necessary to allow hospital-based, nonphysician team members to provide critical care outside the hospital
- Protocols require annual review to assure they reflect current practice

DISPATCH AND COMMUNICATION

- Dispatch and communication centers can be located on site or at a central facility
- They are often staffed by nurses or paramedics
- Responsibilities include:
  - Intake phone call with demographics and clinical information
  - Communication between referring facility and medical control physician
  - Bed placement at receiving hospital
  - Arranging mode of transport once mode is determined
  - Ongoing team communication
  - Ongoing team tracking
- All communications should take place via a recorded line
  - Quality control
  - Documentation of recommendations made to referring facility

TEAM RESOURCES

- Equipment and supplies
  - Factors that determine the appropriate equipment for the transport environment:
    - Size
    - Weight
    - Battery life
    - Ability to secure
  - Strict compliance with hospital, local, state, federal, and Federal Aviation Administration guidelines is necessary
  - Equipment and supplies necessary to support scope of care
  - The population served by each team will determine the type of equipment and the variety of sizes they are required to have available
  - Typical equipment carried: see Tables 2-1 and 2-2
  - Departure checklists are recommended for daily operations
- Medications
  - Checked daily and after transport to assure availability
  - Checked monthly to assure medications used within expiration date
  - Narcotics and other controlled substances are carried by many teams; safe storage, oversight, and administration are vital to safe practice

TABLE 2-1	Equipment for Transport
Type of Equipment	**Examples of Equipment**
Monitoring Equipment	Monitor, electrocardiogram (ECG) leads, ECG cables, pulse oximeter probes, pulse oximeter cable, stethoscope, thermometer, pen light, blood pressure cuff in various sizes
Resuscitation Equipment	Defibrillator, defibrillator pads, gel
Intravenous/Interosseous Equipment	Angiocatheters, intraosseous needles, arm boards, tape, tourniquet, bandages, Tegaderm, gauze, T-connector, umbilical venous and arterial catheters
Nasogastric/Foley Equipment	Replogle tubes, Anderson tubes, feeding tubes, Foley catheters, syringes
Suction Equipment	Suction catheters, Yankauer tips, suction apparatus
Chest Tube/Needle Aspiration Equipment	Chest tubes, pleurovacs, angiocatheters, butterfly catheters, syringes, stopcocks, Vaseline gauze, Tegaderm
Communication Devices	Cellular telephones, two-way radios
Charting Devices	Laptop computer or tablet, clipboard and paper chart
Miscellaneous	Cervical collars, syringes, needles, survival kit, rescue blanket

TABLE 2-2	Respiratory Equipment for Transport
Type of Equipment	**Examples of Equipment**
Intubation Equipment	Endotracheal tubes, end-tidal carbon dioxide detector device (easy cap or capnometry), Magill forceps, oropharyngeal and nasopharyngeal airways, tape, skin prep, stylets, laryngeal mask airways
Laryngoscopy Equipment	Laryngoscope handles and blades, bulbs, batteries, video laryngoscope
Masks	Simple masks, Ventimasks, nonrebreather masks, resuscitation masks
Bags	Flow inflating bags, self-inflating bags
Oxygen Delivery Devices	Nasal cannula, oxygen tubing, head hood, flowmeter, humidifier for high-flow system, oxygen tanks
Aerosol Delivery Devices	Aerosol mask, nebulizer kit, diluent
Tracheostomy Supplies	Tracheostomy tubes, trach collars, artificial nose

  ○ Medications requiring refrigeration can be safely carried in an insulated pack for transport
  ○ Types of medications carried: see Table 2-3
• Handoff tool
  ○ Handoff should be standardized
  ○ Reference cards are helpful to assure consistent content (see Figure 2-2)
• Risk assessment tool
  ○ To help determine safety of transport and risk avoidance

TABLE 2-3 Medications for Transport	
Type of Medications	**Examples of Specific Medications**
Resuscitation Medications	Epinephrine, atropine, calcium chloride
Intubation Medications	
Sedative Hypnotics	Midazolam, ketamine, etomidate
Analgesics	Fentanyl, morphine
Neuromuscular Blocking Agents	Rocuronium, succinylcholine
Antiarrythmic Agents	Adenosine, amiodarone, lidocaine, procainamide, magnesium sulfate
Antiepileptic Agents	Lorazepam, fosphenytoin, phenobarbital, diazepam, levetiracetam
Antihypertensive Agents	Enalaprilet, labetalol, nicardipine
Antimicrobial Agents	Ampicillin, gentamicin, ceftriaxone, acyclovir
Bronchodilators/Asthma Therapy	Albuterol, ipratropium, terbutaline, methylprednisolone
Anaphylaxis Therapy	Epinephrine, diphenhydramine
Reversal Agents	Flumazenil, naloxone
Continuous Infusion Medications	Dopamine, epinephrine, norephinephrine, prostaglandin E1, terbutaline, insulin, lidocaine
Intravenous Fluids	Normal saline (NS), lactated Ringer's, D5/0.9NS, D5/0.45NS
Miscellaneous	Acetaminophen, activated charcoal, calcium gluconate, dantrolene, dextrose, furosemide, heparin, hydrocortisone, mannitol, sodium bicarbonate, surfactant

Transport Team Handoff	
▪ Demographics	**▪ Current Clinical Status**
o Patient Name	o Current Vital Signs
o DOB/Age	o Head to Toe assessment
o ID/location of band	o Line Access/Fluids Running
o Weight	o Drips: Concentration/Dose/Rate
	o Medications given on Transport &
▪ History	Response to medications
o Chief Complaint, HPI	o Procedures and interventions &
o Prenatal/Birth History	Response to interventions
o PMH	o Current airway/oxygen
o Isolation Status	requirements/ventilator settings
o Allergies	o Labs, Imaging, & Test results
o Immunization status	o How Transport was tolerated
o Home Medications	o Parent Contact Information
o NPO status	o Chart and imaging from OSH left at
o Interventions at OSH	bedside

FIGURE 2-2 **Example of a handoff tool.**

- Items include:
  - Weather conditions
  - Road conditions and flight conditions
  - Crew experience
  - Crew member fatigue
  - Time of day

DOCUMENTATION

- Request for transport form/intake form/call record
  - Referring facility information
  - Patient demographics
  - Clinical description of patient, care rendered, and medications given by referring facility
- The transport record
  - Initial assessment, care rendered, and medications given by transport team; patient response to therapies
  - All entries should be dated and timed
  - Transport record can be a paper record that is then scanned into the electronic health record (EHR) or an electronic record if compatible with the EHR of the receiving facility
- The information obtained on the initial request form as well as the transport record becomes part of the patient's permanent medical record

TEAM TRAINING

- Orientation for new team members should be standardized
- Ongoing team education should occur on a regular basis
- Topics include:
  - Patient medical management
  - Crew resource management
  - Transport-specific topics such as altitude physiology
  - Compliance issues and regulations
  - EMS radio communications
  - Infection prevention and control
- Team competencies
  - Device competency: Each team has to decide which devices it will bring on transport; teams need to maintain competencies for devices utilized
    - Monitor
    - Ventilators
      - Neonatal ventilator typically built into isolette
      - Conventional mechanical ventilator
      - Noninvasive positive pressure ventilator
      - High-frequency ventilator
    - Gases
      - Oxygen
      - Air
      - Nitric oxide
    - Isolette
    - Defibrillator
    - Head cooling or total body cooling devices

- Procedure competency: Each team has to decide which procedures it will perform on transport; teams need to maintain competencies in procedures that are performed
  - Intubation
  - Peripheral IV placement
  - Arterial or venous puncture
  - Central venous catheter placement
  - Interosseous placement
  - Needle decompression of pneumothorax
  - Chest tube placement
  - Umbilical arterial catheter placement
  - Umbilical venous catheter placement

SAFETY

- Vehicle safety
  - Crews must be familiar with all vehicles used for transport.
  - Policies are necessary to direct securement of crew members and equipment at all times.
  - Regular maintenance per manufacturer recommendations is vital to avoid unnecessary delays during patient transport.
  - Risk assessment tools consider weather, crew experience, road conditions, and time of day to assist in risk avoidance.
  - Teams should not be pressured to proceed in unsafe driving or flying conditions due to patient acuity.
  - Lights and siren usage should be monitored and used based upon patient acuity rather than as routine practice.
  - Protocols for restraint use should guide crew members to be restrained at all times unless engaged in emergent patient care.
  - Patients should be restrained at all times.
- Crew safety
  - Crew uniforms should include protective clothing and footwear
    - Flame-retardant materials and helmets for flight
    - Sturdy pants and shirts for ground
    - Appropriate for environment and weather in all modes of transport
  - Personal protective equipment in the transport environment should be consistent with standard recommendations.
  - Post-transport debriefs are important to identify safety-related issues and concerns.

TRANSPORT LEGAL ISSUES

- Consent
  - A consent to transport form must be signed prior to transport.
  - If parents are unavailable or unable to make decisions, laws are supportive of physicians and care providers acting on a child's behalf.
  - Required emergency care should never be withheld pending consent.
- Liability
  - Transport team members must always function within their scope of practice/licensure.
  - If providers function beyond this scope, they are open to medical liability.
  - Medical practice acts vary from state to state.
  - There is shared liability between the referring facility and the receiving facility as the call is taken and any recommendations are given.

- Emergency Medical Treatment and Labor Act (EMTALA)
  - Law enacted to prevent hospitals from refusing to treat patients because of their type of insurance.
  - EMTALA requires hospitals with emergency departments (ED) to provide emergency medical care to everyone who needs it, regardless of ability to pay or insurance status.
  - Hospitals are required to provide a medical screening examination to determine the presence of an emergency medical condition for all patients who request care.
  - Only ED patients with unstable medical conditions fall under EMTALA.
  - Patients in unstable conditions may be transferred under EMTALA under certain conditions.
- EMTALA and liability
  - The transferring physician has the legal responsibility to select the appropriate mode of transport. This includes deciding upon the optimal personnel and equipment.
  - The transferring physician maintains responsibility for patient care until the patient arrives at the receiving facility.
  - Although EMTALA states that the referring physician has responsibility, transport services clearly assume some liability once they begin rendering care.
  - Medical direction during the transport of the transferred patient is a shared responsibility.
- Insurance coverage for transport teams should be evaluated annually to assure adequate coverage.

ACCREDITATION

- Transport team accreditation is voluntary
- Two organizations provide accreditation:
  - Commission on Accreditation of Medical Transport Services (CAMTS)
  - Commission on Accreditation of Ambulance Services (CAAS)
- The accreditation process focuses on two areas:
  - Quality
  - Safety

USEFUL RESOURCES

1. The Association of Critical Care Transport (ACCT): www.acctforpatients.org
2. Association of Air Medical Services (AAMS): www.aams.org
3. American Academy of Pediatrics Section on Transport Medicine (AAP SOTM): https://www.aap.org/en-us/about-the-aap/Committees-Councils-Sections/section-transport-medicine/Pages/default.aspx
4. Commission on Accreditation of Medical Transport Systems (CAMTS): www.camts.org
5. Commission on Accreditation of Ambulance Services (CAAS): www.caas.org

SUGGESTED READINGS

Blumen IJ, ed. *Principles and Direction of Air Medical Transport. Advancing Air and Ground Critical Care Transport Medicine*. 2nd ed. Air Medical Physician Association, Salt Lake City, UT. 2015.

CAMTS Accreditation Standards. 10th ed. Commission on Accreditation of Medical Transport Systems, Anderson, SC. 2015.

Horowitz R, Rozenfeld RA. Pediatric critical care interfacility transport. *Clin Pediatr Emerg Med*. 2007;8:190-202.

Insoft R, ed. *Guidelines for Air and Ground Transport of Neonatal and Pediatric Patients*. 4th ed. American Academy of Pediatrics, Elk Grove Village, IL. 2016.

McCloskey K, Orr R. *Pediatric Transport Medicine*. Mosby, St Louis, MO; 1995.

Communication with Families

COMMUNICATION WITH FAMILIES

GENERAL PRINCIPLES FOR COMMUNICATION WITH PARENTS

- Establishing the Relationship
  - In introducing yourself to the family/child, identify key caretakers and decision makers.
  - Endeavor to understand parent preferences regarding communication; for example:
    - Some parents may expect frequent updates with a high level of detail.
    - Other parents may prefer a less detailed summary with updates only for big changes.
  - Endeavor to understand parent framework for medical decision making.
    - Some parents rely almost exclusively on physician recommendations.
    - Other parents are quite autonomous and prefer to receive all of the information and make decisions independently when the clinical situation allows.
  - Provide a framework for expectations that parents can have around communication.
    - Reassure parents that someone is always available to answer urgent questions and concerns.
- Considerations in Communicating During an ICU Stay
  - Be sensitive to where the parent may wish to have medical conversations (i.e., in the presence of the child or not).
  - When communicating new information, always allow time for parents to process information and reflect on it and/or ask questions.
  - Family-centered rounds are often insufficient to meet daily communication needs for families of critically ill children.
  - Involve existing outpatient/inpatient providers in discussions with parents when appropriate, particularly in family meetings (see later) or for difficult, big-picture conversations.

FAMILY-CENTERED ROUNDS IN THE PICU

- Parental Preparation Prior to Rounds
  - *Orientation*
    - Have a designated provider (RN or MD) discuss timing, structure, and goals of family-centered rounds **prior to** first morning rounds.
    - Clarify the role of the parent in morning rounds based on your unit preferences.
  - *Invitation:*
    - Extend a neutral invitation to rounds, and assess parent preference regarding participation.
    - It can be helpful to note that rounds are only one of several options for communicating with MDs in the PICU.
- Team Preparation for Rounds
  - Identify all relevant participants—besides parents—for rounds and ensure their presence at the appointed time.
    - Consider primary subspecialists (e.g., oncologists, primary surgeon), respiratory therapist, social worker, nutritionist, etc.
  - On occasion, it may be necessary to "pre-round" as a team to discuss sensitive issues or challenging management decisions prior to presentation to the family.
    - Attempt to incorporate bedside RN and other relevant rounds participants into this "pre-round" if possible.

- Conducting Family-Centered Rounds
  - *Introduction of Team/Rounds*
    - Presenting provider should introduce himself or herself to the family member(s).
    - It can be helpful to reiterate a short overview of the format of rounds, for example, "I'll be talking about what brought Susie into the hospital, what we have done for her, and what our plans for today will be."
    - It may be appropriate to encourage parents to clarify details of the history or interval events.
  - *Patient Presentation*
    - Be familiar with the preferred practice of your PICU with regard to use of lay language during presentations.
      - Some PICUs will use exclusively medical terminology and provide a lay summary of the assessment and plan for the parent at the conclusion of the presentation.
      - Other PICUs encourage the use of lay terminology throughout the presentation.
    - Recognize that parents want the opportunity to advocate for their children, especially as a plan for the day is being generated.
  - *Teaching During Family-Centered Rounds*
    - With sensitivity to the particular patient and his or her family and circumstances, pauses for teaching should be encouraged.
    - Clarify educational moments for parents: knowing that the team is not specifically discussing their child may decrease the potential for misunderstanding or anxiety.
  - *Concluding Rounds*
    - It is generally appropriate to ask the parent if they have any questions about the information and plan that have been presented.
    - If a parent has several questions or concerns, a member of the team should specify a time after rounds at which they will return to address them.

FAMILY MEETINGS IN THE PICU

- Preparation Prior to the Meeting
  - Establish an Agenda
    - *Invitations*: Decide who should be present. In addition to the parents and child (if applicable), this may include extended family, primary nurses, primary PICU physician, key consultants, social worker, discharge planning coordinator, spiritual leader, and an interpreter.
    - *Medical Facts and Meeting Goals*: The team should agree on the current patient assessment and management options, as well as the meeting goals, prior to meeting with the family. This may require a "team meeting" in advance. The group should also decide which clinician will lead the discussion and facilitate the meeting.
  - Setting
    - Find an appropriate location where you can assure comfort, privacy, and the absence of interruptions such as pagers or phones.
    - Ensure sufficient seating and bring tissues.
- Set the Stage by Introducing the Purpose and Structure of the Meeting
  - Identify who will be leading the meeting, and give everyone an opportunity to introduce themselves.
  - Set "ground rules" regarding confidentiality, courtesy, interruptions, etc.
  - State the specific issues to be addressed or necessary decisions to be made.
    - Provide time frame allotted for the meeting

- Align with the Family by Assessing Illness Understanding and Preferred Communication Style
  - Align with the family.
    - Establish trust and alliance around an appreciation of the child as a person and family member.
  - Assess the family's understanding of the patient's medical condition, for example:
    - "Before we begin, let's make sure we are all on the same page."
    - "What is your understanding of your child's medical condition right now?"
  - Assess preferences for information sharing.
    - "Some families prefer to hear about the small details, whereas others prefer to only hear the big picture. Which do you prefer?"
- Summarize the Child's Medical Condition and Any Critical Clinical Decisions
  - Be brief, limiting key messages to a few sentences.
    - Give plain, jargon-free information
    - Tailor information to family preferences
    - Grade exposure to upsetting information
  - Address issues that appear unclear to the family.
  - Discuss best- and worst-case scenarios.
    - Convey uncertainty
    - Maintain hope but avoid any false reassurances
  - Let the family ask questions and absorb information at their own pace.
    - Note any family dynamics, conflicts
- Explore and Address Family Concerns or Questions
  - Listen for and respond to concerns and emotions, for example:
    - "Tell me how you are feeling about the information we have shared today."
  - If appropriate, deepen the encounter:
    - "What are your biggest fears and worries about your child's health?"
    - "What are you hoping for?"
    - "If your child's health worsens, what are your most important goals?"
  - Tolerate silence.
  - Encourage questions and clarify when appropriate.
  - Provide psychosocial and spiritual support.
  - Consider culture and religion.
- Frame Recommendations
  - Frame recommendations based upon patient's and family's goals and values, as well as what is known about the child's medical condition.
  - Identify milestones and clinical events to define success or failure of any interventions with a reasonable time frame for reassessment.
- Offer Next Steps
  - Make a plan for further information sharing, for example
    - "Let's meet again in 48 hours when we have a sense of how this treatment is working."
  - Provide support and assure accessibility of the team.
    - "We have shared a lot of information today; here is my contact information if you have questions."
- Reflect and Document
  - Reflect with the team about the challenges encountered and next steps.
  - Document key decisions made during the family meeting in the medical record.
    - Communicate information to stakeholders who were not present

SUGGESTED READINGS

Billings JA, Block SD. Part III: a guide for structured discussions. *J Pall Med.* 2011;14(9):1058-1064.

Davidson JE, Aslakson RA, Long AC. Guidelines for family-centered care in the neonatal, pediatric and adult ICU. *Crit Care Med.* 2017;45(1):103-128.

Feudtner C. Collaborative communication in pediatric palliative care: a foundation for problem-solving and decision-making. *Pediatric Clin North Am.* 2007;54(5):583-607.

Levetown M. Communicating with children and families: from everyday interactions to skill in conveying distressing information. *Pediatrics.* 2008;121(5):e1441-e1460.

Mittal V. Family-centered rounds. *Pediatr Clin N Am.* 2014;61:663-670.

Nelson JE, Walker AS, Luhrs CA, et al. Family meetings made simpler: a toolkit for the intensive care unit. *J Crit Care.* 2009;24(4):626.e7-626.e14.

Stickney CA, Ziniel SI, Brett MS, et al. Family participation during intensive care unit rounds: goals and expectations of parents and health care providers in a tertiary pediatric intensive care unit. *J Pediatr.* 2014;165(6):1245-1251.

4 Palliative Care

INTEGRATING PALLIATIVE CARE INTO THE PICU

PALLIATIVE CARE PRINCIPLES

These principles can and should be integrated into every intensive care provider's practice.

- Prevent and minimize suffering:
  - Suffering includes physical pain and other uncomfortable symptoms, as well as emotional distress and spiritual isolation.
  - Suffering is experienced by the patient but also by family members or other significant relationships.
  - Every critically ill patient and their loved ones are at risk for substantial suffering.
  - Suffering should be addressed, regardless of the clinical situation, the treatment plan, or whether the choices of the family align with the preferences of the care team.
- Enhance and support quality of life:
  - What constitutes an acceptable "quality of life" is subjective and quite variable among individuals and families.
  - Supporting quality of life means making each day as good as it can be and, in particular, supporting important relationships for the patient and their family.
  - In the PICU, this might look like facilitating a sibling visit, encouraging parents to hold their child or participate in bathing, or simply taking the time to look at family pictures and listen to cherished stories.
- Understand and advocate for patient/family goals of care:
  - The goals of care should always be discussed openly so that a shared understanding is reached between the patient, family, and medical team.
  - Goals of care are constrained by what is possible; thus, the medical team should be clear with the family about what can or cannot be reasonably hoped for.
  - However, goals of care are primarily informed by what is most important to patients and families—their values and priorities.
  - Patients and families may hold many different kinds of hope, often simultaneously. For many, the hope of complete healing never goes completely away, yet they may also be able to focus on more achievable goals like relieving pain, being with loved ones, or celebrating a milestone like a birthday.
- Facilitate medical decision making:
  - In the ideal form of shared decision making, the patient/family shares information about the patient's values, goals, and preferences relevant to the decision at hand. Clinicians share information about the relevant treatment options and their risks and benefits. Clinicians and patients/families then work together to determine which option is most appropriate for the patient.
  - Facilitating authentic decision making means ensuring that patients/families have all the information they need about the various treatment options and providing whatever kind of support they need to consider these options in light of their values, hopes, and needs.

PALLIATIVE CARE SUPPORT

Sometimes additional specialty-level support is needed.

- Inpatient palliative care consultation: A growing number of hospitals offer an inpatient consult service for palliative care. Most pediatric palliative care teams are multidisciplinary and may include physicians, advanced practice nurses, chaplains, social workers, and nurse case managers, as well as supportive therapies such as child life, music therapy, and art therapy. When a child has a life-threatening or life-limiting (likely to cause death before adulthood) diagnosis, palliative care consultation is appropriate for any of the following reasons:

- ○ *Symptom management:* The patient has a high degree of pain or other uncomfortable symptoms, including nausea, spasticity, dyspnea, anxiety/depression, and fatigue.
- ○ *Assessing goals of care:* Specialty-level expertise (and/or significant time) is needed to evaluate the patient's/family's goals of care.
- ○ *Extra support:* The patient and/or family exhibit signs of significant emotional or spiritual distress and would benefit from an extra layer of support.
- ○ *Long-term management:* The patient is likely to survive the current PICU stay but has a life-limiting diagnosis and would benefit from longitudinal palliative care support.
- • In-home palliative care (and hospice): Specialized teams of nurses, social workers, chaplains, child life specialists, and other therapists provide in-home palliative care or hospice support for children with life-limiting illness.
- ○ In palliative care, the child continues to receive at least some disease-directed therapies and may not have any limitations in place regarding resuscitation. Disease-directed care and equipment continue to be billed through their insurance company while the palliative care team provides weekly to monthly (depending on the needs of the patient/family) visits to help manage symptoms and enhance quality of life.
- ○ In hospice, the patient/family has usually made a decision not to return to the hospital and to focus on staying at home and maintaining comfort until death. Typically (though not always—and not required) the patient has a do not attempt resuscitation (DNAR) order. The palliative care team visits as often as necessary in order to deal with escalating symptoms and to help support the family through the process of their child's decline and eventual death. All medication and equipment come through the hospice company and can usually be delivered to the family.

END-OF-LIFE CARE FOR THE CRITICALLY ILL CHILD

- • The dying process: The timing of a child's dying process will depend on whether or not the child is currently being supported by mechanical ventilation and inotropes and whether he or she dies in spite of that support or because that support is withdrawn. In general, as death approaches, children may experience
- ○ Decreased level of consciousness
- ○ Confusion and anxiety
- ○ Pain and discomfort
- ○ Labored breathing (gasping, gurgling, respiratory pauses)
- ○ Swings in heart rate, eventually slowing to a stop
- ○ Changes in skin color (cyanosis, mottling) and temperature (cold)
- • Providing comfort, relieving distress: Our job is to do everything possible to keep the child comfortable and to relieve the family's distress. Our primary tools include opiates (morphine, fentanyl, etc.), benzodiazepines (lorazepam, midazolam), and oxygen for symptom management, and compassionate reassurance and management of the environment for the family.
- ○ Morphine or other opioid medications can effectively relieve pain and air hunger. In order to do so, especially for children who have been receiving these medications previously and have developed tolerance, the dose may need to be increased—sometimes multiple times or to very high levels.

- Benzodiazepines like lorazepam or midazolam may be used to treat anxiety and provide relaxation. These medications often drop the blood pressure and are used with caution in patients in whom we are still trying to prevent death. For a patient who is actively dying, however, the decrease in blood pressure is seen as acceptable in order to provide comfort.
- Oxygen may be given to ease dyspnea and air hunger of a dying patient who is not already intubated. Titrate to patient comfort, not to a specific SpO_2.
- Glycopyrrolate or atropine, fluid restriction, and suctioning may help with the pooling of secretions that cause the gurgling noise often called "the death rattle."
- Parents should be reassured that we will do everything possible to keep their child comfortable. If the parents perceive that their child is in pain, we should take their concerns seriously and do something to address the discomfort.
- It may help to explain that changes in the breathing pattern and in the color and temperature of the child are a normal part of the dying process.
- When the oxygen saturation and heart rate begin to steadily decline, the alarms should be silenced and the monitors should be dimmed so that they do not disturb the family. Unless asked to do so by the attending physician, do not turn the monitor all the way off so that the vital signs can still be recorded at the central station.
- When a child has been in the ICU, often their parents have been unable to hold them for quite some time. During the dying process we should offer the opportunity to hold their child to the parents and do everything possible to facilitate that opportunity. This may include allowing the parent to climb in bed with their child or placing a chair close to the ventilator and IV pole so that the parent can hold the child on their lap without disconnecting support.

- **Withdrawing support:**
  - When a family decides to withdraw measures that are artificially supporting the child's body, death may come very quickly or may take hours or even days. The same principles of comfort care described earlier apply in these situations (opioids, oxygen, etc.). When a child is expected to die quickly, the physician, nurse, and respiratory therapist should work together to remove artificial measures in a way that allows the parents to hold their child (if that is their wish) as he or she dies. Again, alarms should be silenced and monitors dimmed to allow for as peaceful an environment as possible.

- **Death after a code:**
  - Some children die despite aggressive resuscitation efforts. These deaths can be particularly devastating for parents—and for staff. However, it is extremely important that parents be allowed to witness the code, unless they do not want to be present, and as long as they are not interfering with the team's efforts. Being present for the code and at the time of their child's death can allow parents to know "we did everything possible" and may help them achieve some closure. It is important to have a social worker, nurse, or physician who can stay with the parents, explaining what is happening and comforting them during the process. After the attending physician calls an end to the code, the parents should be allowed to be with and hold their child. It is usually appropriate to remove ECG leads, IV tubing, and the endotracheal tube at this time (exceptions include medical examiner's/coroner's cases and unexpected deaths with unclear causes—ask the attending physician if unsure).

- **After death:**
  - Many families want to spend time with the child's body, and we should make every effort to accommodate their needs. During this time, we allow additional visitors. It is nice to provide water or juice for them.
  - Before the parents leave, the attending physician or fellow needs to discuss the option of autopsy and have them sign the release of body form.

- ○ Some parents will want to help wash and clean the body. It is also an option to create mementos during this time, including handprints or footprints.
- ○ Eventually the body needs to be transported to the morgue. It is very important that the completed death certificate (unless an autopsy will be performed), as well as the release of body form, accompany the body.
- Processing and personal recovery:
  - ○ Recognize that you have just been through a difficult and perhaps traumatic experience. Give yourself time to recover. It is not unusual to feel angry, sad, or tired, sometimes for days afterwards.
  - ○ Debriefing with the medical team after a patient death is important. It allows the team to review the clinical issues but also acknowledge the emotional impact of the event. Some debriefings may include a moment of silence to honor the life of the child. If you haven't heard about a debriefing for your patient, feel free to ask.
  - ○ Talk to others! Reach out to the physicians and nurses involved with your patient. Talking about the death—what went well, what you were unsure about, how you feel afterward—is a crucial part of helping you process the experience.

SUGGESTED READINGS

Boss R, Nelson J, Weissman D, et al. Integrating palliative care into the PICU: a report from the Improving Palliative Care in the ICU Advisory Board. *Pediatr Crit Care Med.* 2014;15(8):762-767.

Carter B, Craig F. Intensive-care units. In: Goldman A, Hain R, Liben S, eds. *Oxford Textbook of Palliative Care for Children.* 2nd ed. New York City, NY: Oxford University Press; 2012:401-409.

Kon AA, Davidson JE, Morrison W, Danis M, White DB. Shared decision-making in intensive care units. Executive summary of the American College of Critical Care Medicine and American Thoracic Society policy statement. *Amer J Resp Crit Care Med.* 2016;193(12):1334-1336.

5

Ethics

FOUNDATIONAL APPROACHES/THEORY

Two approaches have dominated Western thinking about medical ethics: consequentialism and deontology.[1]

CONSEQUENTIALISM

A philosophical approach that judges the correctness of an action based on the effect it will likely have. The focus is on the consequences of an action. Advocates, including utilitarian philosophers, argue for actions that seek the greatest happiness for the greatest number of people.

DEONTOLOGY

A philosophical approach that argues that actions have intrinsic moral worth. Supporters purport that certain universal truths and rules should be followed, regardless of their consequence.

FOUR PRINCIPLES

Most people feel that four principles should guide approaches to care and decision making:

- Beneficence: Provide care that benefits the patient
- Maleficence: Avoid causing harm
- Autonomy: When possible, individuals should decide for themselves what is in their best interests
- Justice: Relates to fairly distributing services and resources

DECISION MAKING

DECISION MAKERS

The legally authorized decision maker is determined by the patient's age and the capacity for an individual to make a decision.

- Adult patients: Patients >18 years old can make decisions for themselves if they have decision-making capacity. An adult can identify a decision maker in the event he or she does not have decision-making capacity. Surrogate decision makers should make decisions based on substituted judgment when possible.
  - *Decision-making capacity*: A clinical determination that an individual can 1) understand and communicate about the medical situation; 2) manipulate information about the situation and consider the consequences of alternatives; 3) make a choice among the alternatives
  - *Competence*: Typically considered a legal term reflecting the ability of an individual to make a decision
  - *Power of attorney*: A legal document giving decision-making authority for the patient to an individual
  - *Legal surrogate*: A person legally charged with acting on behalf of another person
  - *Substituted judgment*: A decision made on behalf of another person based on knowledge about what the person would decide if he or she could speak for himself or herself

- Pediatric patients: For patients <18 years old, parents or the patient's legal guardian is the legal decision maker and should make decisions based on the best interest standard. However, the state can intervene when parents make decisions that place the child's health, well-being, or life in jeopardy. The American Academy of Pediatrics supports involving developmentally appropriate patients in clinical decision making, provided that his or her views will be considered.[2]
  - Best interest standard: The decision pursued should be the one most favorable for the child.[3]
  - Exceptions: In certain state-determined clinical situations (e.g., issues related to sexually transmitted infections or pregnancy), the patient can make his or her own decisions. States also have unique laws that determine who is eligible to be an emancipated or mature minor and therefore make his or her own medical decisions.
  - Patient assent: Patient approval or agreement about decisions.

SHARED DECISION MAKING

Although the patient or his or her family member may be the legal decision maker, experts advocate using a process of shared decision making, particularly for value-laden decisions. Shared decision making seeks to arrive at appropriate choices for patients and families through consideration of available options and the patient's and family's values. In shared decision making, communication exchange is bidirectional and comprehensive. Clinicians share medical information with families, and families share their values, attitudes, and preferences with the health care team. With shared decision making, patients and the family determine their role in decisions; that is, some people may choose to make decisions without guidance from clinicians, whereas others may request the clinicians make the final choice based on knowledge of the patient's and family's values and goals.[4]

DO NOT ATTEMPT RESUSCITATION (DNAR) AND FUTILITY

DO NOT ATTEMPT RESUSCITATION (DNAR)

There is a presumed desire for resuscitation, including cardiopulmonary resuscitation.[5] Absent an order not to attempt resuscitation, it should be attempted in all patients. Competent adults and their surrogates (e.g., parents of pediatric patients) may refuse medical care, including resuscitation.

- Bilateral DNAR: The medical team and patient and family both agree that treatment limitation is appropriate.
- Unilateral DNAR: An order placed based on the direction of the medical team. Only some states have laws supporting this controversial approach.

FUTILITY

Futility is sometimes used as a justification not to offer potential treatments felt not to be in the patient's interests.[6] There are variable ways to define futility:

- Futility by condition: Treatment for a particular diagnosis is felt to never be successful
- Qualitative futility: Treatment preserves a patient in a state that by some would be considered unalterable; dependence on intensive medical care will never cease
- Quantitative futility: In the last "X" years, treatment for a given condition has been unsuccessful
- Physiologic futility: Proposed treatment is not able to meet intended physiologic goals

Because of the many definitions of futility and the need to consider every intervention in terms of the goals of the patient and family, there is movement away from using the concept of futility to support decisions about the use of potentially inappropriate care.[7]

WITHDRAWAL OF OR WITHHOLDING LIFE-SUSTAINING THERAPIES AND END-OF-LIFE CARE

Although the goal of most medical therapy is to preserve life, there are circumstances in which the burdens of care outweigh the potential benefits. In those cases, withdrawal or withholding of life-sustaining therapies may be warranted. There is strong ethical and legal consensus that both withdrawal and withholding of life-sustaining therapies may be acceptable options.[8] In all end-of-life care situations, clinicians should give attention to the ethics of pain and symptom management.

LIFE-SUSTAINING THERAPIES

Life-sustaining therapies refer to interventions that may prolong the life of a patient.

• Examples of life-sustaining therapies: Include mechanical interventions like ventilators or kidney dialysis, surgical interventions like transplantation, or medical interventions like administration of chemotherapy or antibiotics.[9]

DOCTRINE OF DOUBLE EFFECT

This doctrine argues that it is ethically acceptable to do something that may have a bad side effect if the goal is to do something morally good. For example, it is ethically acceptable to give medication to ensure patient comfort at the end of life even if there is a risk that giving such medication might hasten death. Five conditions are required: 1) the action intended is morally good; 2) the good effect is intended; 3) the bad effect is not guaranteed; 4) the good effect is not achieved as a result of the bad effect; and 5) achieving the good effect outweighs the bad effect.

USE OF NEUROMUSCULAR BLOCKADE IN END-OF-LIFE CARE

Most experts discourage the use of neuromuscular blockade during end-of-life care, including during withdrawal of mechanical ventilation. Arguments against using neuromuscular blockage in these situations include the following: 1) it masks signs of air hunger and thus limits the clinician's ability to provide adequate sedation; 2) it does not allow for the possibility that the patient might survive after withdrawal of life-sustaining therapies; and 3) it does not allow meaningful interactions between the patient and family at the end of life.

WITHHOLDING OF FLUIDS AND NUTRITION

Although the provision of fluids and nutrition holds significant emotional, cultural, and sometimes religious significance, many argue that it is ethically justifiable, in certain circumstances, to withhold fluids and nutrition. As with all decisions, families and staff need to have full understanding of the indications and rationale for withholding fluids and nutrition and of the likely outcome of taking such an approach.

ETHICS OF DEFINING DEATH AND ORGAN DONATION

DEFINING DEATH

Death is defined by the Uniform Determination of Death Act. An individual must meet certain criteria for either brain death or circulatory death to be considered dead.[10]

There are ethical challenges to defining death either by neurologic or circulatory criteria; however, no changes to the legal definition of death or organ donation by these criteria have been made.

- Death by neurologic criteria: Irreversible cessation of all functions of the brain, including the brainstem (see chapter 47 for how to determine brain death)
- Death by circulatory criteria: Cessation of circulatory and respiratory functions

DEAD DONOR RULE

The dead donor rule requires providers caring for a patient to ensure that the patient meets criteria for death prior to organ procurement.[10]

- Heart-beating brain-dead donors: Individuals who donate organs based on death by neurologic criteria.
- Non–heart-beating donors: Individuals who donate organs based on death by circulatory criteria. Organ donation in this setting is called donation after circulatory determination of death (DCDD) or donation after circulatory/cardiac death (DCD).

ORGAN PROCUREMENT AGENCIES

- Organ Procurement Organizations (OPOs): Federally designated regional agencies for organ procurement throughout the United States
- Organ Procurement and Transplantation Network (OPTN): A network of all organ procurement agencies to match organs to recipients
- United Network for Organ Sharing (UNOS): A private organization that contracts with the government to manage the OPTN

PROFESSIONAL ISSUES

MORAL DISTRESS

Moral distress arises when the provider has a strong personal sense of what the morally "correct" action is but is asked or required to act otherwise.[11] It often comes up in situations where there are disagreements over the direction of care for a patient. Moral distress can be encountered by any member of the health care team and can build over time, leading to residual distress after a situation is resolved.

CONSCIENTIOUS OBJECTION

Conscientious objection refers to refraining from providing actions that the provider morally opposes.[12] Individual states may either have laws that *permit refusal* based on ethical, moral, or religious grounds or that *require* health care workers to provide services to which they might have ethical, moral, or religious objections.

RESEARCH ETHICS

RESEARCH VERSUS PRACTICE OR INNOVATION

There are differences between clinical practice, research, and innovation.[13]

- Practice: Interventions designed to enhance well-being of individual patient(s); provide diagnosis or treatments to specific individuals.
- Research: Activities designed to contribute to generalizable knowledge.
- Innovative procedures: Novel procedures not always introduced as research; depends on what their purpose is and how they are judged by the medical community.

ETHICAL RESEARCH AND INFORMED CONSENT

The Belmont Report outlines principles for ethical research. Similar to principles for clinical ethics, the principles described in the Belmont report include respect for persons (treating individuals with autonomy), beneficence and justice. Informed consent is an important component of ethical research. Informed consent generally requires three elements: information disclosure, comprehension, and voluntariness.[13]

- Information Disclosure: Potential participants should understand research procedures, risks/benefits, and alternative procedures (when available) and have the opportunity to ask questions. Everyone should be informed that they can withdraw participation at any time.
- Comprehension: Information must be adapted to meet the capacity of the individual from whom consent is sought. For those without capacity (e.g., infants, cognitively impaired individuals, comatose patients), third-party permission is sought. Individuals should be given the opportunity to choose to the extent able.
- Voluntariness: Consent should be given free of coercion or undue influence.

EQUIPOISE

Equipoise refers to true uncertainty about the superiority of either arm in a trial. Equipoise is lost when it becomes clear that one treatment/arm is superior to another.[14]

REFERENCES

1. Frader J, Michelson K. Ethics in pediatric intensive care. In: Fuhrman P, Zimmerman J, Carcillo J, et al., eds. *Pediatric Critical Care*. 4th ed. Philadelphia, PA: Elsevier Sanders; 2011:102-109.
2. Committee on Bioethics, American Academy of Pediatrics. Informed consent, parental permission, and assent in pediatric practice. *Pediatrics*. 1995;95(2):314-317.
3. Diekema DS. Revisiting the best interest standard: uses and misuses. *J Clin Ethics*. 2011;22(2):128-133.
4. Makoul G, Clayman ML. An integrative model of shared decision making in medical encounters. *Patient Educ Couns*. 2006;60(3):301-312.
5. Burns JP, Edwards J, Johnson J, Cassem NH, Truog RD. Do-not-resuscitate order after 25 years. *Crit Care Med*. 2003;31(5):1543-1550.
6. Burns JP, Truog RD. Ethical controversies in pediatric critical care. *New Horiz*. 1997;5(1):72-84.
7. Bosslet GT, Pope TM, Rubenfeld GD, et al. An official ATS/AACN/ACCP/ESICM/SCCM Policy statement: responding to requests for potentially inappropriate treatments in intensive care units. *Am J Respir Crit Care Med*. 2015;191(11):1318-1330.
8. Frost N. Ethical issues in death and dying. In: Fuhrman P, Zimmerman J, Carcillo J, et al., eds. *Pediatric Critical Care*. 4th ed. Philadelphia, PA: Elsevier Sanders; 2011:110-114.
9. American Academy of Pediatrics Committee on Bioethics. Guidelines on foregoing life-sustaining medical treatment. *Pediatrics*. 1994;93(3):532-536.
10. Paquette E, Frader J. Controlled donation after cardiac death in pediatrics. In: Greenberg R, Goldberg A, Rodriguez-Arias D, eds. *Ethical Issues in Pediatric Organ Transplantation*. Switzerland: Springer International Publishing; 2015:340.
11. Hamric AB. Empirical research on moral distress: issues, challenges, and opportunities. *HEC Forum*. 2012;24(1):39-49.
12. Lynch HF. *Conflicts of Conscience in Health Care: An Institutional Compromise*. Cambridge, MA: MIT Press; 2008.

13. National Commission for the Protection of Human Subjects of Biomedical and Behavioral Research. *The Belmont Report: Ethical Principles and Guidelines for the Protection of Human Subjects Of Research*. Bethesda, MD: U.S. Government Printing Office; 1978.
14. Freedman B. Equipoise and the ethics of clinical research. *N Engl J Med*. 1987;317(3):141-145.

2

Resuscitation & Stabilization

6 Endotracheal Intubation

INDICATIONS

- Respiratory
  - Apnea
  - Hypoventilation
  - Severe respiratory distress/respiratory muscle weakness
  - Acute respiratory failure (PaO_2 <50 mmHg in patient with FiO_2 >0.5 and $PaCO_2$ >55 mmHg acutely)
  - Need to control oxygen delivery (e.g., institution of positive end-expiratory pressure [PEEP], accurate delivery of FiO_2 >0.5)
  - Need to control ventilation (e.g., to decrease work of breathing, to control $PaCO_2$, to provide muscle relaxation)
- Neurologic
  - Inadequate chest wall function (e.g., in patient with Guillain-Barre syndrome, poliomyelitis)
  - Absence of protective airway reflexes (loss of cough, gag)
  - Glasgow Coma Score <8
- Airway
  - Upper airway obstruction
  - Infectious processes (epiglottis, croup)
  - Trauma to the airway
  - Burns (concern for airway edema)
- Cardiac
  - Cardiopulmonary failure/arrest
  - Low cardiac output states (reduced oxygen demand/consumption)
- Other
  - Transport of a patient with potential for respiratory failure

CONTRAINDICATIONS

- Absolute
  - Nasotracheal intubation is contraindicated in patients with nasal fractures or basilar skull fractures
- Relative
  - None

RISKS

- Bradycardia
- Hypoxemia/desaturation
- Hypotension
- Inability to intubate

EQUIPMENT-SEE FIGURES 6-1 AND 6-2

- Suction – source, catheters; should have a tonsil-tipped suction device or a large-bore suction catheter, as well as a suction catheter of appropriate size that fits into the endotracheal tube (ETT)

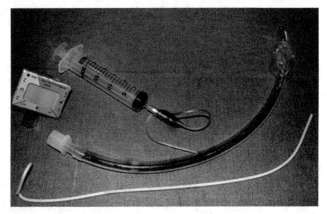

FIGURE 6-1 Intubation equipment.
Reproduced with permission from Chapter 27. Oral Endotracheal Intubation. In: Hanson C, III. eds. *Procedures in Critical Care* New York, NY: McGraw-Hill; 2009.

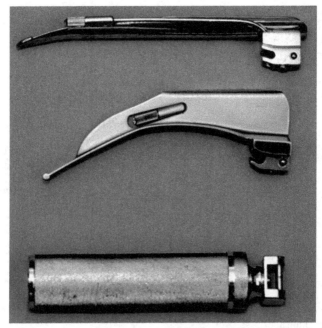

FIGURE 6-2 Laryngoscope blades and handle. Top: straight blade, middle: curved blade.
Reproduced with permission from Klock A, et al, Airway Management. In: Longnecker DE, et al, eds. *Anesthesiology, 3e* New York, NY: McGraw-Hill, 2018.

- Oxygen – source
- Ventilation bags – flow inflating bags and self-inflating bags
- Masks – appropriate sizes for ventilation
- Laryngoscope – blade (straight or curved), handle, bulb, battery
  - Handle with battery and blade with light source
  - Adult and pediatric handles fit all blades and differ only in handle diameter
- Video laryngoscope if available
- Endotracheal tubes – appropriate sizes, cuffed, uncuffed
- Forceps
- Oropharyngeal airway
- Tongue blade
- Bite block
- Tape – to secure tube or tube securement device
- Stylet – appropriate sizes
- CO_2 detector device – colorimetric detection device or capnography
- Syringe to inflate the endotracheal tube balloon on cuffed tubes
- Laryngeal mask airways (LMA) – appropriate sizes
- Medications (see medication section later)
- Normal saline or Lactated Ringer's for fluid resuscitation

GUIDELINES FOR LARYNGOSCOPE, ETT, SUCTION CATHETERS BASED ON AGE AND WEIGHT – SEE TABLE 6-1

- Historically, uncuffed tubes were recommended for children <8 years of age; however, current research shows that cuffed tubes are safe in all patients except in the newborn period.
- If a difficult intubation is anticipated due to altered supraglottic anatomy, absolutely no irreversible anesthetics or muscle relaxants should be administered.
- Such patients should generally be intubated awake or in the operating room with inhaled anesthetic.
- For difficult intubations, other techniques, such as fiber-optic intubation, may be used.

DISTINGUISHING FEATURES OF THE INFANT AND CHILD AIRWAY COMPARED WITH ADULTS

- The larynx is more cephalad.
- The epiglottis is omega shaped.
- In children younger than 8 years, the cricoid is the narrowest part of the airway.
- The infant larynx is one-third the size of the adult larynx.
- The vocal cords are short and concave.
- Aligning the mouth, pharynx, and glottis to create a visual field is difficult.
- The endotracheal tube size relates to the cricoid ring.
- In children, the lower airways are smaller, have less supporting cartilage, and may easily obstruct.
- A small reduction in diameter results in a large reduction in the cross-sectional area and therefore increased airway resistance.

PROCEDURE

Checklists are helpful to ensure all team members are prepared for the procedure.
  See Table 6-2

TABLE 6-1	Guidelines for Laryngoscope, ETT, and Suction Catheters Based on Age and Weight				
			ETT size internal diameter (mm)	**Distance lip to midtrachea (cm)**	**Suction cath (Fr)**
Age	**Wt (kg)**	**Laryngoscope**	$\dfrac{\text{Age (yrs)}}{4} + 4$	**3 × ETT size**	**2 × ETT size**
Preterm Infant	2	Miller 0	2.5, 3.0 uncuffed	8	5–6
Term Infant	4	Miller 0–1	3.0, 3.5 uncuffed	9–10	6–8
6 mo	8	Miller 1	3.5, 4.0 uncuffed 3.0, 3.5 cuffed	10.5–12	8
1 yr	10	Miller 1	4.0, 4.5 Uncuffed 3.5, 4.0 cuffed	12–13.5	8
2 yr	12–14	Miller 2 Macintosh 2	4.5 uncuffed 4.0 cuffed	13.5	8
4 yr	16–20	Miller 2 Macintosh 2	5.5 uncuffed 4.5 cuffed	15	10
6 yr	22–28	Miller 2 Macintosh 2	5.0, 5.5 uncuffed 5.0 cuffed	16.5	10
8–12 yr	28–45	Miller 2–3 Macintosh 2–3	6.0–7.0 cuffed	18–21	12
>14 yr	50+	Miller 3 Macintosh 3	7.0, 8.0 cuffed	21	12

PATIENT PREPARATION

- Preoxygenate with 100% FiO_2.
- In an older child, explain each step as it is done.

PATIENT POSITIONING

- A neutral "sniffing" position without hyperextension of the neck is usually appropriate for infants and toddlers.
- Avoid extreme hyperextension in infants, because it may produce airway obstruction.
- It is sometimes helpful to place a towel under the patient's shoulders.
- In patients with head or neck injuries, the neck must be maintained in a neutral position.

SET UP PRIOR TO INTUBATION

- Check the intubation equipment before beginning.
- Attach the blade to the handle and be sure that the bulb illuminates.
- Attach suction to a suction machine and be sure that suction is turned on.
- If using a stylet, insert the stylet into the endotracheal tube. The tip of the stylet should be 1 to 2 cm proximal to the distal end of the endotracheal tube, ensuring that the stylet does not go through the Murphy eye.

TABLE 6-2	Proposed Intubation Checklist Items
Declaration of Airway Emergency	Example: "Sats are coming down. The patient is not responding. We are going to have to intubate. Nurse, can you get all of our intubation supplies ready?"
Verbalization of Team Roles	1. Drawing up medications (nurse/pharmacist)
	2. Administering medications (nurse)
	3. Preparing airway equipment (respiratory therapist)
	4. Managing the airway (physician/advanced practice nurse)
Patient Information	Age and weight
	Allergies
	Last time patient has eaten
	Airway abnormalities
Intubation Equipment	Endotracheal tube (ETT) size: cuffed versus uncuffed
	Stylet
	Laryngoscope – blade and handle
	Bag and appropriate size mask attached to oxygen
	Suction
	Oropharyngeal airway
	Syringe (to inflate cuff)
	Tape (to secure tube) or tube securement device
Patient monitoring/ access	Reliable IV access
	Electrocardiogram (ECG) monitor
	Noninvasive blood pressure (NIBP) monitoring system
	Pulse oximeter (SpO$_2$)
	CO$_2$ detector device
Medication(s)	Medication generic and trade name(s)
	Medication dosage(s)

Used with permission from Rozenfeld RA, et al. Verbal communication during airway management and emergent endotracheal intubation: observations of team behavior among multi-institutional Pediatric Intensive Care Unit in-situ simulations. *J Patient Saf.* 2016 epub ahead of print.

• Prepare to monitor the patient's heart rate, oxygen saturation levels, and blood pressure.

INITIAL STEPS IN PROCEDURE

1. Preoxygenate with 100% oxygen
2. Administer atropine in certain situations.
   • Infants and children can exhibit bradycardia due to vagal nerve stimulation.
   • Atropine may not be indicated in patients with significant tachycardia.
3. Administer IV sedation (e.g. fentanyl, morphine, midazolam, etomidate, ketamine, propofol; see medication section later).
4. Apply cricoid pressure in certain situations if indicated.
   • The cricoid cartilage is the first tracheal ring, located by palpating the prominent horizontal band inferior to the thyroid cartilage and cricothyroid membrane.

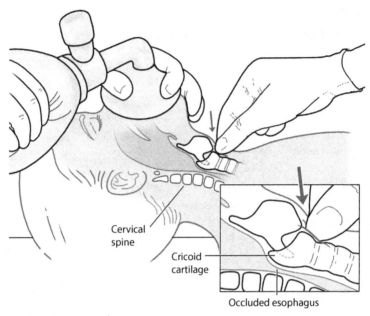

Cervical
spine

Cricoid
cartilage

Occluded esophagus

FIGURE 6-3 Cricoid pressure.
Reproduced with permission from Rozenfeld RA. Chapter 1. Bag-Mask Ventilation. In: Goodman DM, et al., eds. *Current Procedures: Pediatrics* New York, NY: McGraw-Hill; 2007.

- Cricoid pressure occludes the proximal esophagus by displacing the cricoid cartilage posteriorly. See Figure 6-3.
- The esophagus is compressed between the rigid cricoid ring and the cervical spine.
- Cricoid pressure can limit gastric distension in unconscious patients and may also prevent regurgitation and aspiration of gastric contents.
- Avoid excessive cricoid pressure because it may produce tracheal compression and obstruction or distortion of the upper airway anatomy.
- Use of cricoid pressure is controversial. There is insufficient evidence to recommend routine use.

5. Perform bag mask ventilation with 100% oxygen.
   - Bag mask ventilation gives the clinician time to prepare for more definitive airway management.
   - Good technique involves preserving good mask–face seal, inflating the chest with minimal required pressure, and maintaining the optimal patency of the upper airway through manipulation of the mandible and cervical spine.
   - The clinician should only use the force and tidal volume necessary to cause the chest to rise visibly.
   - The mask should extend from the bridge of the nose to the cleft of the chin, enveloping the nose and mouth but avoiding compression of the eyes.
   - The mask should provide an airtight seal.
   - The goal of ventilation with a bag and mask should be to approximate normal ventilation.

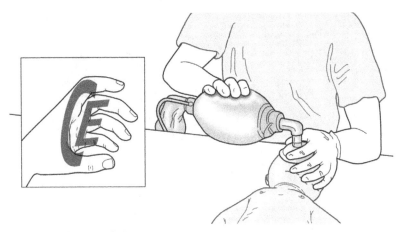

FIGURE 6-4 E-C clamp technique.
Reproduced with permission from Rozenfeld RA. Chapter 1. Bag-Mask Ventilation. In: Goodman DM, et al., eds. *Current Procedures: Pediatrics* New York, NY: McGraw-Hill, New York; 2007.

- Sequence for bag mask ventilation:
  1. Open the airway via chin lift/jaw thrust maneuver.
  2. Seal the mask to the face.
  3. Deliver a tidal volume that makes the chest rise.
- E-C clamp technique. See Figure 6-4.
  1. Tilt the head back and place a towel beneath the head.
  2. If head or neck injury is suspected, open the airway with the jaw thrust technique without tilting the head.
     ○ If a second person is present, have that person immobilize the spine.
  3. Apply the mask to the face.
  4. Lift the jaw, using the third, fourth, and fifth fingers from the left hand, under the angle of the mandible; this forms the "E."
  5. When lifting the jaw, the tongue is also lifted away from the posterior pharynx.
  6. Do not put pressure on the soft tissues under the jaw because this may compress the airway.
  7. Place the thumb and forefinger of the left hand in a "C" shape over the mask and exert downward pressure.
  8. Create a tight seal between the mask and the patient's face using the left hand and lifting the jaw.
  9. Compress the ventilation bag with the right hand.
  10. Be sure the chest rises visibly with each breath.
- If two people are present, then one person can hold the mask to the face, while the other person ventilates with the bag.
  1. One person uses both hands to open the airway and maintain a tight mask-to-face seal, while the second person compresses the ventilation bag. See Figure 6-5.
- If there is difficulty with bag mask ventilation, an oropharyngeal airway can be inserted. See Figure 6-6.
- Oropharyngeal airways provide a conduit for airflow through the mouth to the pharynx.

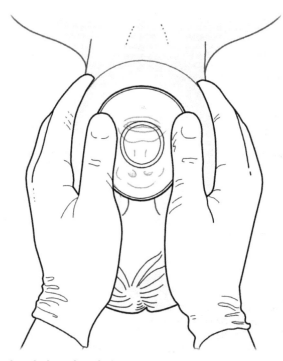

FIGURE 6-5 Two-handed mask technique.
Reproduced with permission from Rozenfeld RA. Chapter 1. Bag-Mask Ventilation. In: Goodman DM, et al., eds. *Current Procedures: Pediatrics* New York, NY: McGraw-Hill, New York; 2007.

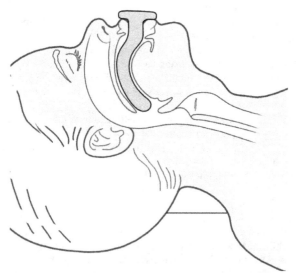

FIGURE 6-6 Sagittal view of oral airway in place.
Reproduced with permission from Rozenfeld RA. Chapter 2. Placement of Oropharyngeal Airway. In: Goodman DM, et al., eds. *Current Procedures: Pediatrics* New York, NY: McGraw-Hill, New York; 2007.

- Oropharyngeal airways prevent mandibular tissue from obstructing the posterior pharynx.
- Oropharyngeal airways may be used in the unconscious infant or child if procedures to open the airway (head tilt–chin lift, or jaw thrust) fail to provide and maintain a clear, unobstructed airway.
- An oropharyngeal airway should not be used in conscious or semiconscious patients because it may stimulate gagging and vomiting.
- Measure the distance from the central incisors to the angle of the mandible to approximate the correct size oral airway.

SEQUENCE FOR INTUBATION CONTINUED

6. Administer IV muscle relaxant (e.g. rocuronium, succinylcholine; see medication section later).
7. Never give patients a muscle relaxant until you are sure that you are able to bag-mask the patient and until a person capable of performing endotracheal intubation is present.
8. Open the mouth and insert the laryngoscope.

Laryngoscopes (see Figures 6-2 and 6-7):
- A straight blade provides greater displacement of the tongue into the floor of the mouth and visualization of a cephalad and anterior larynx.
- With a straight blade, the tip of the blade lifts the epiglottis directly.
- A curved blade may be used in the older child. The broader base and flange allow easier displacement of the tongue.
- With a curved blade, the tip of the blade is placed in the vallecula.
9. Avoid positioning the blade against the teeth, gums, or lips.
10. Visualize the glottic opening; see Figure 6-8.
11. Suction any secretions that may obscure visualization.
12. Insert the endotracheal tube, and observe the tube as it passes through the glottic opening.
13. Remove the stylet while holding the tube securely in place and ventilate the patient.
14. Secure the tube to the face.

CONFIRMING CORRECT POSITION OF ENDOTRACHEAL TUBE PLACEMENT

- Observe the ETT going through the glottic opening
- Auscultation for symmetrical breath sounds
- Good chest excursion
- Effective oxygenation
- Disposable colorimetric capnometer (color should change from purple to yellow if patient has a perfusing rhythm) or capnograph
- Obtain chest radiograph
- Absence of breath sounds over the upper abdomen
- If unilateral breath sounds are heard on the right, pull back the tube slowly while ventilating and listen for breath sounds on the left (probable intubation of right mainstem bronchus)

MEDICATIONS

Atropine – 0.02 mg/kg, IV (minimum dose 0.1 mg, maximum dose 0.5 mg) in certain circumstances

Sedation and analgesia medications should be given before the neuromuscular blocking medications

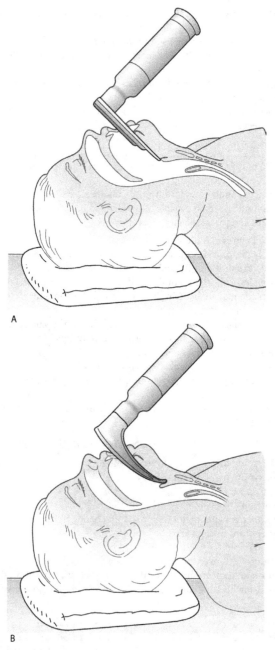

FIGURE 6-7 Sagittal view of laryngoscopes. A: Straight blade lifting epiglottis, B: Curved blade in vallecula.
Reproduced with permission from Rozenfeld RA. Chapter 4. Placement of Endotracheal Tube. In: Goodman DM, et al., eds. *Current Procedures: Pediatrics* New York, NY: McGraw-Hill, New York; 2007.

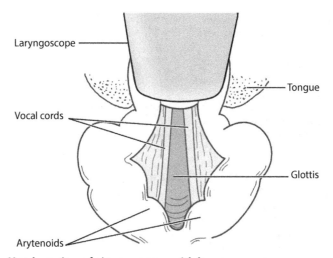

FIGURE 6-8 Head-on view of airway as seen with laryngoscope.
Reproduced with permission from Rozenfeld RA. Chapter 4. Placement of Endotracheal Tube. In: Goodman DM, et al., eds. *Current Procedures: Pediatrics* New York, NY: McGraw-Hill, New York; 2007.

Benzodiazepines
- Most commonly used medications
- Provide amnesia, not analgesia
- Examples include midazolam and lorazepam
- Flumazenil reverses the effects of benzodiazepines – dose: 0.01 mg/kg/dose, IV (maximum dose 0.2 mg/dose; may repeat every minute to cumulative dose of 0.05 mg/kg or 1 mg, whichever is lower)
- Flumazenil is contraindicated in patients with seizure disorder, tricyclic antidepressant ingestion, or long-term benzodiazepine use

1. Midazolam
   - Dose: 0.1 mg/kg, IV
   - Onset of action: within 3 to 5 minutes
   - Maximal depression may not be achieved for 5 to 7 minutes
   - Duration of effect: approximately 20 to 30 minutes
   - May cause apnea in some patients
   - Cautious use in patients with hepatic or kidney injury
2. Lorazepam
   - Dose: 0.05 to 0.1 mg/kg, IV
   - Onset of action: 15 to 30 minutes
   - Duration of effect: 8 to 12 hours
   - Metabolized in the liver to inactive compounds
   - Excreted in the urine
   - May not be optimal for intubation because of prolonged onset

Opioids
- Second most commonly used medications
- Provides analgesia, not amnesia
- Differences among drugs include chemical structure, half-life, potency, cardiovascular effects, and metabolic products

- Naloxone reverses the effects of opioids – dose: 0.01 to 0.1 mg/kg/dose, IV; up to maximum 2 mg/dose; may repeat every 3 to 5 minutes

1. Morphine
   - Dose: 0.1 mg/kg, IV
   - Onset of action: peak 20 minutes
   - Duration of effect: 3 to 5 hours
   - Metabolized in the liver to inactive and active compounds
   - Excreted in the urine
   - Cardiovascular effects: peripheral vasodilation
   - Respiratory depression may occur
2. Fentanyl
   - Dose: 2 to 3 mcg/kg, IV, maximum dose 100 mcg
   - Peak onset of respiratory depression is approximately 15 minutes
   - Onset of action: almost immediate
   - Duration of effect: 30 to 60 minutes
   - Respiratory depression may last longer than analgesia
   - May provide adequate anesthesia (and analgesia), especially in combination with other drugs and in patients with serious cardiovascular limitations
   - Unlike morphine, fentanyl rarely decreases blood pressure, even in patients with poor left ventricular function (no histamine release)
   - Incidence of chest wall rigidity from 0% to 100%; rigidity usually begins as patient is losing consciousness—succinylcholine reliably and rapidly terminates rigidity; rigidity is related to both dose and rate of infusion

Ketamine
   - Dose: 1 mg/kg, IV, maximum dose 100 mg
   - Onset of action: within 30 seconds
   - Duration of effect: 5 to 10 minutes
   - Recovery: 1 to 2 hours
   - Provides amnesia and analgesia
   - A "dissociative anesthetic"; may cause hallucinations in older children and adults, should pretreat with a benzodiazepine
   - Increases blood pressure and heart rate
   - Ventilation is maintained
   - Bronchial smooth muscle tone is relaxed
   - Preferred in patients with heart disease and may be the drug of choice in patients with asthma
   - Disadvantages include increased secretions (should always give a vagolytic agent, such as atropine), dysphoria, and increased skeletal muscle tone, often requiring muscle relaxation
   - Contraindications include elevated intracranial pressure, hypertension, and increased intraocular pressure

Etomidate
   - Dose: 0.1 to 0.4 mg/kg, IV, maximum dose 20 mg
   - Onset of action: 30 to 60 seconds
   - Duration of effect: 4 to 10 minutes
   - Nonbarbiturate, anesthetic agent
   - Decreases cerebral metabolic rate and intracranial pressure
   - Maintains cerebral perfusion pressure

- Minimal changes in mean arterial pressure, cardiac output, or systemic vascular resistance
- Disadvantages include pain on injection, myoclonus, nausea and vomiting, and adrenal suppression

Propofol
- Dose: 1.5 to 2 mg/kg, IV
- Onset of action: 30 to 40 seconds
- Duration of effect: 3 to 10 minutes
- Lipophilic sedative hypnotic
- May cause hypotension, vasodilatation, myocardial depression
- Metabolized in the liver to inactive metabolites
- Excreted in the urine
- Unsafe to use in patients with allergies to eggs or soybeans

Neuromuscular blocking agents
- No analgesic or amnestic properties
- Must be able to manage the airway

Depolarizing neuromuscular blocking agent
Succinylcholine

- Dose: 1 mg/kg, IV; can be given IM 3 mg/kg, maximum dose IV/IO/IM 100 mg
- Onset of action: 30 to 60 seconds
- Duration of effect: 4 to 6 minutes
- Major disadvantage is vagal stimulation; can result in bradycardia and cardiac arrest, especially after second dose
- Should always be preceded by atropine
- Metabolized by plasma pseudocholinesterase
- Contraindications include:
  ○ Traumatic and burn injuries (increased receptor density 24 hours to 6 months after injury; note: not contraindicated at time of injury)
  ○ Hyperkalemia
  ○ Neuromuscular disease (including muscular dystrophy but not cerebral palsy)
  ○ Renal failure
  ○ Severe intraabdominal infection
  ○ Raised intraocular pressure
  ○ Personal or family history of malignant hyperthermia

Nondepolarizing neuromuscular blocking agent
Rocuronium

- Dose: 0.6 to 1.2 mg/kg, IV, maximum dose 50 mg
- Dose for rapid sequence intubation: 1.2 mg/kg, IV
- Onset of action: 30 to 60 seconds
- Duration of effect: 30 to 60 minutes
- Excretion primarily biliary with some renal

MONITORING

- Continuous monitoring of oxygen saturation
- Continuous monitoring of capnography
- Continuous monitoring of heart rate

- Frequent monitoring of blood pressure
- The importance of monitoring is to make sure that the endotracheal tube remains in the correct position and is not obstructed

If an intubated patient's condition deteriorates, consider the following possibilities (DOPE):

- **D**isplacement of the tube from the trachea
- **O**bstruction of the tube
- **P**neumothorax
- **E**quipment failure

COMPLICATIONS

- Esophageal intubation
- Perforation of trachea, tracheal tear or rupture
- Intubation of right mainstem bronchus
- Aspiration
- Dental damage
- Laceration of lips or gums
- Injury to oropharynx
- Pneumothorax

SPECIAL CONSIDERATIONS

- If difficult intubation anticipated due to altered supraglottic anatomy, **NO PARALYTICS** should be given.
- **Intubate awake or in operating room with inhaled anesthetic.**
- Consider notifying anesthesia and/or otolaryngology if an airway is anticipated to be difficult.

RAPID SEQUENCE INTUBATION

- There is a risk of aspiration in patients who:
  - Have eaten less than 4 to 8 hours prior to intubation
  - Have undergone a traumatic event
  - Have gastroesophageal reflux
  - Have abdominal distention (ileus, ascites, pregnancy)
  - Are obese
- In these situations, patients should be intubated either awake (the patient may protect his or her own airway) or using a rapid sequence induction
  Rapid sequence induction
  1. Preoxygenation with 100% oxygen
  2. Administer atropine if indicated
  3. Apply cricoid pressure to prevent regurgitation
  4. Apply oxygen without active mask ventilation (apneic preoxygenation)
  5. Administer a rapid-acting anesthetic
  6. Administer a rapid-acting muscle relaxant

SUGGESTED READINGS

American Heart Association. *Dallas PALS Provider Manual.* TX: American Heart Association; 2015.

Bledsoe GH, Schexnayder SM. Pediatric rapid sequence intubation. *Pediatr Emerg Care.* 2004;20:339-344.

Hanson C III. *Procedures in Critical Care*; 2009 Available at: http://accessanesthesiology .mhmedical.com/content.aspx?sectionid=41840253&bookid=414&jumpsectionID= 41840677&Resultclick=2 Accessed: July 21, 2017.

Holinger LD, Lusk RP, Green CG, eds. *Pediatric Laryngology and Bronchoesophagology.* Philadelphia, PA: Lippincott-Raven Publishers; 1997.

Lexicomp Online: http://online.lexi.com, accessed 12/18/2017.

Longnecker DE, Brown DL, Newman MF, Zapol WM. *Anesthesiology.* 2nd ed. New York, NY: McGraw Hill; 2012.

Mondolfi AA, Grenier BM, Thompson JE, Bachur RG.. Comparison of self-inflating bags with anesthesia bags for bag-mask ventilation in the pediatric emergency department. *Pediatr Emerg Care.* 1997;13:312-316.

Phelps SJ, Hagemann TM, Lee KR, Thompson AJ. *Pediatric Injectable Drugs (The Teddy Bear Book).* 10th ed. American Society of Health-System Pharmacists, Inc. 2013, Bethesda.

Rozenfeld RA. Bag-mask ventilation: In: Goodman DG, Green TP, Unti SM, Powell EC, eds. *Current Procedures: Pediatrics.* McGraw Hill, New York; 2007:3-6.

Rozenfeld RA. Endotracheal intubation. In: Goodman DG, Green TP, Unti SM, Powell EC, eds. *Current Procedures: Pediatrics.* McGraw Hill, New York; 2007:12-19.

Rozenfeld RA, Nannicelli AP, Brown AR, et al. Verbal communication during airway management and emergent endotracheal intubation: observations of team behavior among multi-institutional Pediatric Intensive Care Unit in-situ simulations. *J Patient Saf.* 2016 epub ahead of print. PMID: 27811586.

Rozenfeld RA. Placement of oropharyngeal airway. In: Goodman DG, Green TP, Unti SM, Powell EC, eds. *Current Procedures: Pediatrics.* McGraw Hill, New York; 2007:7-8.

Sullivan KJ, Kissoon N. Securing the child's airway in the emergency department. *Pediatr Emerg Care.* 2002;18:108-121.

Cardiac Arrest

BACKGROUND

- Cardiac arrest is defined by a triad of derangements:
  - Pulselessness
  - Apnea
  - Unresponsiveness
- This state leads to progressive tissue ischemia and organ dysfunction, which, if not rapidly corrected, can result in irreversible deterioration of cardiac and neurologic function.
- Cardiac arrest occurs in 2% to 6% of pediatric patients who are admitted to the pediatric intensive care unit.
- Cardiac arrest occurs in approximately 16,000 children out of hospital in the United States each year.
- Because of the relative infrequency of out-of-hospital events, pediatric resuscitations are not common for providers outside of the pediatric intensive care unit.
- There continues to be a significant difference in outcomes (e.g., favorable vs. nonfavorable) between patients with in-hospital vs. out-of-hospital events.

ETIOLOGY

- In general, the cause of cardiac arrest falls into one of three categories:
  - Asphyxia
  - Ischemia
  - Arrhythmia
- Adults with cardiac arrest often have sudden, unexpected ventricular fibrillation and often have underlying coronary artery disease, which leads to myocardial ischemia.
- In contrast, pediatric cardiac arrest is rarely caused by a sudden coronary event or arrhythmia.
- Cardiac arrest in children is most often caused by progressive asphyxia from acute hypoxia or hypercarbia, which leads to acidosis and nutrient depletion.
- Ischemic events are the second most common etiology in pediatrics.
- Ischemic events occur secondary to inadequate myocardial oxygen delivery, which in children occurs most commonly in the setting of sepsis, hypovolemia, or myocardial dysfunction.
- Arrhythmias account for the smallest number of cardiac arrest events in pediatric patients, comprising only 10% of events.

PHASES OF CARDIAC ARREST

- Cardiac arrest can be broken down into four phases:
  - Prearrest
  - No flow (untreated cardiac arrest)
  - Low flow (cardiopulmonary resuscitation [CPR])
  - Postresuscitation

PREARREST

- Pediatric patients with in-hospital cardiac arrest may have physiologic changes in the hours leading up to their arrest.

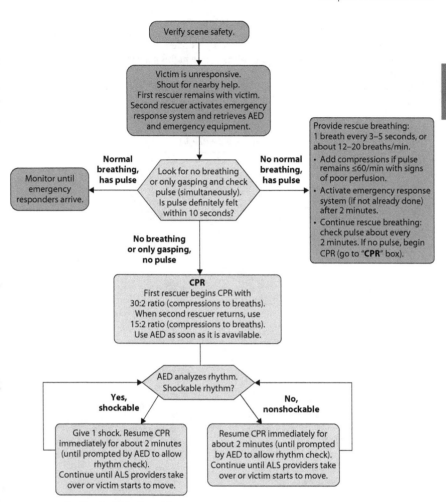

FIGURE 7-1 Pediatric BLS algorithm.
Reprinted with permission from Part 11: Pediatric Basic Life Support and Cardiopulmonary Resuscitation Quality. Atkins DL, et al. Circulation. 2015;132:S519-S525 ©2015 American Heart Association, Inc.

- Because the majority of pediatric cardiac arrests occur secondary to progressive asphyxia or ischemia, recognition and treatment of respiratory failure and shock states may prevent a number of arrest events from occurring.
- The Pediatric Advanced Life Support (PALS) course was designed to reduce the number of cardiac arrests by improving the early recognition of these conditions.
- Care during this phase should focus on:
  ○ Identifying and treating reversible conditions
  ○ Optimizing patient monitoring
  ○ Providing rapid emergency response for patients not already in a health care setting

NO FLOW (UNTREATED CARDIAC ARREST)

- During untreated cardiac arrest, circulation has stopped.
- Responders to cardiac arrest should minimize time in this state in order to optimize patient outcomes.
- Interventions should focus on the initiation of Basic and Advanced Life Support techniques.

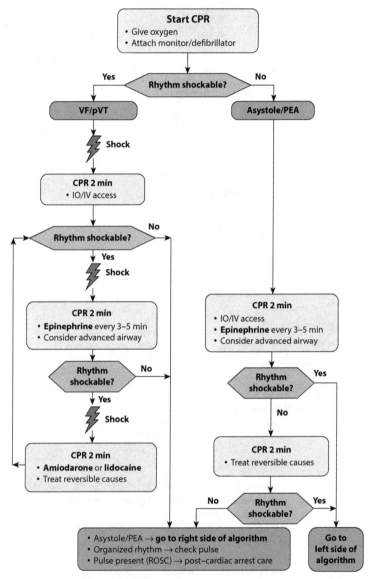

FIGURE 7-2 **Pediatric cardiac arrest algorithm.**
Used with permission from Part 14: Pediatric Advanced Life Support. Kleinman ME, et al. Circulation. 2010;122:S876-S908.

LOW FLOW (CPR)

- The low-flow phase begins with the initiation of resuscitation measures (chest compressions).
- Effective CPR improves coronary perfusion pressure and provides cardiac output to support organ viability.
- Even with optimal CPR, cardiac output is only 10% to 25% of normal. Basic Life Support (BLS) and PALS guidelines should be followed during the resuscitation phase.

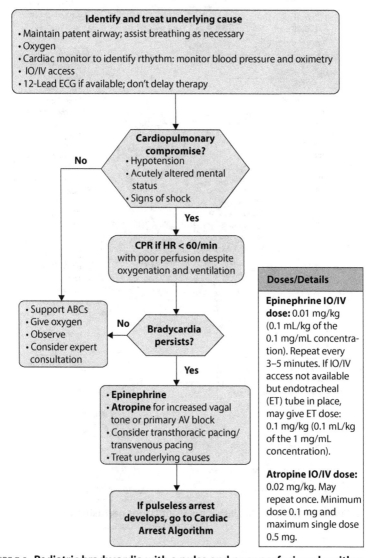

FIGURE 7-3 Pediatric bradycardia with a pulse and poor perfusion algorithm.
Used with permission from Part 14: Pediatric Advanced Life Support. Kleinman ME, et al. Circulation. 2010;122:S876-S908.

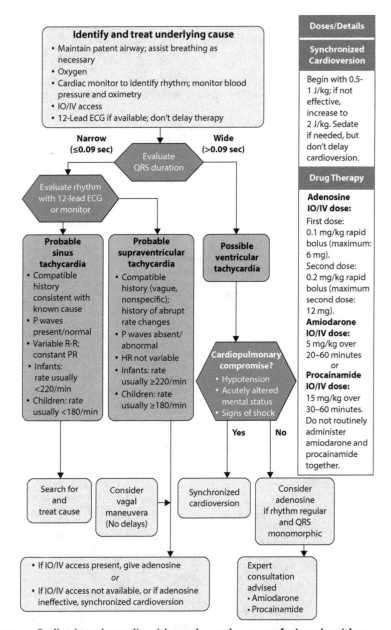

FIGURE 7-4 Pediatric tachycardia with a pulse and poor perfusion algorithm.
Used with permission from Part 14: Pediatric Advanced Life Support. Kleinman ME, et al. Circulation. 2010;122:S876-S908.

TABLE 7-1	Code Medications		
Drug	**Route**	**Dose**	**Special Considerations**
Epinephrine (1:10,000)	IV/IO	0.01 mg/kg/dose (max 1 mg/dose)	
Epinephrine (1:1,000)	ETT/Trach	0.1 mg/kg/dose (max: 2.5 mg/dose)	Dilute with 5 mL of NS; administer with 5 ventilations
Adenosine	IV/IO	0.1 mg/kg/dose (first dose, max 6 mg)	Must be given rapidly by IV push followed by NS flush
		0.2 mg/kg/dose (up to two additional doses, max dose 12 mg)	
Amiodarone	IV/IO	5 mg/kg/dose (max dose 300 mg; max daily dose 15 mg/kg)	
Atropine	IV/IO	0.02 mg/kg/dose (min dose 0.1 mg; max dose 0.5 mg for bradycardia, 1 mg for asystole/PEA)	
	ETT/Trach	0.04–0.06 mg/kg/dose	Dilute with 5 mL of NS, may repeat once
Calcium chloride	IV/IO	20 mg/kg/dose (max dose 2000 mg)	
Dextrose 10%	IV/IO	5 mL/kg/dose (max dose 25 g)	
Hydrocortisone	IV/IO/IM	1–2 mg/kg/dose or 50–100 mg/m^2/dose (max dose 100 mg)	
Lidocaine 1%	IV/IO	1 mg/kg/dose	
	ETT/Trach	2 mg/kg/dose (twice the IV dose)	Dilute with 5 mL of NS
Magnesium sulfate	IV/IO	25 mg/kg/dose (max dose 2000 mg)	
Sodium bicarbonate 8.4%	IV/IO	1 mEq/kg/dose (max dose 50 mEq)	
Procainamide	IV/IO	15 mg/kg/dose	Do not use routinely with amiodarone

- Responders should push hard and fast and should allow for complete chest recoil to maximize cardiac filling.
- Care should be taken to minimize interruptions to CPR and to avoid overventilation.
- Code medications should be administered according to PALS guidelines. See Table 7-1.
- Further research on goal-directed endpoints (end tidal CO_2, etc.) is necessary, but a sudden increase in end-tidal CO_2 suggests return of spontaneous circulation.

POSTRESUSCITATION

- The postresuscitation period involves the management of the physiologic derangements that occur after cardiac arrest.

- Cardiac issues:
  - During the initial period after cardiac arrest, patients are at high risk for ventricular arrhythmias and reperfusion injuries.

- Additionally, the myocardium may be stunned and require support with inotropes to maintain cardiac output.

- Neurologic issues:
  - The brain is at high risk of reperfusion injury, and care should be taken to minimize further neurologic injury during the recovery period.
  - Neuroprotection consists of maintaining:
    ○ Euglycemia
    ○ Normothermia
    ○ Normotension
    ○ Normocarbia
    ○ Normonatremia
    ○ Normoxia
  - Care should be taken to avoid hyperoxia to minimize the risk of further oxidative damage to the brain.
  - Standard guidelines do not exist regarding the length of optimal neuroprotection, but many centers maintain strict control of these parameters for 48 to 72 hours following cardiac arrest.
  - Electroencephalogram (EEG) monitoring may be used to monitor for subclinical seizures in comatose patients.
  - Seizures should be treated to minimize further neurologic injury.
  - Cerebral edema may develop in the 48 to 72 hours following a prolonged cardiac arrest.
  - Treatment should focus on maintaining cerebral perfusion pressure and may require the use of hyperosmolar therapy (e.g., mannitol or hypertonic saline).

OUTCOMES

- Improved likelihood of ROSC (Return of Spontaneous Circulation) is associated with:
  ○ Short time to initiation of adequate CPR
  ○ High-quality CPR
  ○ Shorter overall duration of resuscitation
  ○ Witnessed cardiac arrest
- Achievement of ROSC is not necessarily predictive of a favorable neurologic outcome.
- Further research is necessary to identify clinical data (biomarkers or radiographic data) that is predictive of patient outcome.

SUGGESTED READINGS

Atkins DL, Everson-Stewart S, Sears GK, et al. Epidemiology and outcomes from out-of-hospital cardiac arrest in children: the Resuscitation Outcomes Consortium Epistry—Cardiac Arrest. *Circulation.* 2009;119:1484-1491.

de Caen AR, Berg MD, Chameides L, et al. Part 12: pediatric advanced life support: 2015 American Heart Association Guidelines Update for Cardiopulmonary Resuscitation and Emergency Cardiovascular Care. *Circulation.* 2015;132:S526-S542.

Donoghue AJ, Nadkarni V, Berg RA, et al. Out-of-hospital pediatric cardiac arrest: an epidemiologic review and assessment of current knowledge. *Ann Emerg Med.* 2005;46:512-522.

Herlitz J, Bang A, Aune S, et al. Characteristics and outcome among patients suffering in-hospital cardiac arrest in monitored and non-monitored areas. *Resuscitation.* 2001;48:125-135.

Nadkarni VM, Larkin GL, Peberdy MA, et al. First documented rhythm and clinical outcome from in-hospital cardiac arrest among children and adults. *JAMA.* 2006;295:50-57.

Pitetti R, Glustein JZ, Bhende MS. Prehospital care and outcome of pediatric out-of-hospital cardiac arrest. *Prehosp Emerg Care*. 2002;6:283-290.

Richard J, Osmond MH, Nesbitt L, Stiell IG. Management and outcomes of pediatric patients transported by emergency medical services in a Canadian prehospital system. *CJEM*. 2006;8:6-12.

Slonim AD, Patel KM, Ruttimann U, Pollack MM. Cardiopulmonary resuscitation in pediatric intensive care units. *Crit Care Med*. 1997;25:1951-1955.

Young KD, Seidel JS. Pediatric cardiopulmonary resuscitation: a collective review. *Ann Emerg Med*. 1999;33:195-220.

Vascular Access

Although it is always best to utilize the least invasive access, central venous access is often required in the PICU. This chapter addresses central venous access and arterial access first and then addresses peripheral venous access and interosseus access. Ultrasound considerations are incorporated throughout the chapter.

CENTRAL VENOUS ACCESS

Central versus peripheral access: Peripheral access should be used whenever possible, unless specific indications for central venous access are present.

INDICATIONS

- Unable to achieve peripheral access
- Large volume resuscitation
- Need for vesicant, irritant, or hyperosmolar or highly concentrated solutions (including total parenteral nutrition [TPN], electrolyte replacement, greater than 12.5% dextrose, pH <5 or >9, or osmolarity >600 mOsm/L)
- Need for vasoactive support
- Need for hemodynamic monitoring, including central venous pressure, pulmonary artery pressure, or mixed venous saturation monitoring
- Frequent blood draws
- Need for prolonged access (chemotherapy, prolonged antibiotic course)

CONTRAINDICATIONS

- Increased bleeding risk secondary to thrombocytopenia or coagulopathy.
- Predisposition to sclerosis or thrombosis. Contraindicated in a vessel with a known thrombus.

RISKS/POTENTIAL COMPLICATIONS

- Bleeding: Assessment for thrombocytopenia and coagulopathy should occur prior to line placement
- Infection: Use sterile technique with full barrier to minimize infection
- Embolization of intravascular thrombus, guidewire, or air
- Vessel perforation

PREPARATION

- Materials
  - Sterile gloves, gown, drapes
  - Surgical hat, mask
  - Catheter (see Table 8-1 for size and length considerations)
  - Caps for each catheter lumen
  - Introducer needle
  - Syringe (non-Luer Lock) to attach to introducer needle and two to three additional 3-mL syringes
  - Guidewire (at least double the length of the catheter; verify that guidewire passes through needle prior to starting procedure)
  - Scalpel

TABLE 8-1.	Catheter Selection by Age	
Age	**Catheter Size (Fr)**	**Catheter Length (cm)**
< 28 weeks	UVC 3.5 — 5	
28 weeks to full term	UVC 5	
3 months	3	5–12
6 months to 1 year	3–4	5–12
5 years	4	5–15
10 years	4–5	8–20
12 – 16 years	5+	8–30

  ○ Tissue dilator
  ○ Suture
  ○ Kelly clamp
  ○ Additional syringes
• Medications
  ○ Lidocaine 1% for skin numbing (and appropriate needle for superficial injection)
  ○ Chlorhexidine (>2 months) or iodine (<2 months) for skin preparation
• Catheter selection

TECHNIQUE

• Preparation
  ○ Sterile procedure: Use cap/mask, gown, sterile gloves
  ○ Prepare the area with 2% chlorhexidine (>2 months) or 10% povidine-iodine (<2 months)
  ○ Catheter preparation
    ▪ Flush all ports and caps with normal saline or heparinized saline
    ▪ Clamp lumens after flushing
• Anesthesia
  ○ For use of systemic sedation or analgesia, ensure NPO status (6 hours for solids; 4 hours for clear liquids).
  ○ Inject local anesthetic (1% lidocaine) into the tissues at and below the venipuncture site. Withdraw prior to injection to avoid intravascular injection.
• Seldinger technique (Figure 8-1)
  ○ Puncture the skin using an introducer needle attached to non-Leur Lock syringe.
  ○ Advance until blood return is free-flowing, then remove syringe, keeping introducer needle in place. Place finger over open lumen on needle to avoid air entry.
  ○ Insert guidewire through introducer needle, keeping one hand on the guidewire at all times.
    ▪ Until the guidewire is removed, one hand should be kept on the guidewire for each subsequent step.
    ▪ Guide wire should enter without resistance and, if met with resistance, needle or guide-wire should be redirected prior to reattempting advancement.
  ○ When guidewire is in place, using a scalpel, make a small incision at the venipuncture site. Remove the introducer needle with the guidewire remaining in place.
  ○ Introduce the dilator over the guidewire. Use a twisting motion to advance through the skin as needed. Remove the dilator with the guidewire remaining in place.

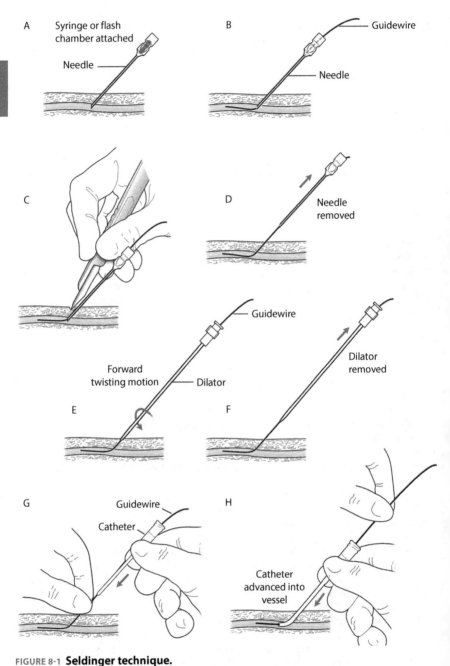

FIGURE 8-1 Seldinger technique.
Reproduced with permission from Michelson K. Chapter 10. Femoral Venous Catheterization. In: Goodman DM, et al., eds. *Current Procedures: Pediatrics* New York, NY: McGraw-Hill; 2007.

- Thread the catheter over the guidewire, retracting the guidewire through the catheter as needed until the guidewire is visible on the other side of the catheter.
- Once the catheter is in place, remove the guidewire.
- Aspirate blood through each port to ensure free flow. Flush each port. Take care to avoid introducing any air through the catheter.
- Suture the catheter in place.
- Attach caps to the catheter lumens.

CONFIRMATION OF PLACEMENT

- Blood gas
- Transduce pressure
- Imaging
  - Chest x-ray for internal jugular (IJ) or subclavian placement to verify positioning and evaluate for pneumothorax
  - Abdominal x-ray for femoral placement to verify positioning

REMOVAL OF CATHETER

- Remove as soon as the indication for a central venous line (CVL) is no longer present
- Remove sutures and retract catheter with pressure at the insertion site after removal

GENERAL PRINCIPLES FOR ULTRASOUND-GUIDED VASCULAR ACCESS

PREPARATION

- Materials
  - Ultrasound machine
  - High-frequency linear probe
  - Ultrasound gel

TECHNIQUE

- Preparation
  - Cover probe
  - Place gel over ultrasound probe
  - Vessel identification and confirmation
    - Veins compress more easily than arteries
    - Veins have thinner walls than arteries
    - Arteries have pulsatile flow; veins do not
  - Prescan along length of vessel to ensure its depth, course, and patency
  - Center vessel on screen
  - Confirm successful catheterization with catheter/wire visualized in vessel
- General technique
  - Position the ultrasound machine in the operator's direct line of site (usually on the opposite side of the patient's bed with the cord draped across the patient)
  - Orient the probe so that the left side of the probe corresponds to the left side of the ultrasound screen
  - Ultrasound probe held in operator's nondominant hand
  - Needle held in operator's dominant hand
- Short axis/transverse approach
  - Orient probe with its long axis perpendicular to the path of the vessel
  - Vessel will appear as black/anechoic circle with white/hyperechoic rim on screen

- o Brace fingers of hand holding probe on patient to ensure stability
- o Insert needle at skin at midpoint of probe of the long axis of the probe
- o Identify needle tip as bright white/hyperechoic dot on screen
- o Advance or slide ultrasound probe a few millimeters while advancing the probe
- o Adjust needle direction to ensure it is in line with the vessel
- o Ensure needle tip remains in view by tilting the probe back and forth
- o Poke needle through superficial wall into vessel
- o Shallow needle angle to allow passage of wire or catheter
- Long axis/longitudinal approach
  - o Orient probe with its long axis parallel to the path of the vessel
  - o Vessel will appear as black/anechoic tube with white/hyperechoic edges on screen
  - o Brace fingers of hand holding probe on patient to ensure stability
  - o Insert needle into the skin proximal to and at the midpoint of the short axis of the probe
  - o Identify needle tip and shaft as hyperechoic oblique line on screen
  - o Keep nondominant hand in place while vessel is in view
  - o Advance needle under direct ultrasound guidance
  - o Poke needle through superficial wall into vessel
  - o Shallow needle angle to allow passage of wire or catheter
- Short axis vs. long axis approach
  - o Short axis approach:
    - Allows simultaneous visualization of intended and neighboring vessels
    - Any point of the needle (tip and shaft) appears as a hyperechoic dot; if needle tip is not followed, one may poke inadvertently through the vessel
    - Some operators may find it difficult to manipulate the probe with their nondominant hand
  - o Long axis approach:
    - Allows visualization of the entire vessel and needle
    - The hand–eye coordination necessary to keep probe still while advancing the needle along its plane may be challenging
    - Limited space of a patient's short neck may preclude placing the probe in the long axis and a longitudinal approach

TYPES OF CENTRAL VENOUS ACCESS

FEMORAL CENTRAL VENOUS CATHETER

- Advantages
  - o Avoids device in neck or chest
  - o Able to control bleeding locally with pressure
- Drawbacks
  - o Unable to obtain a true mixed venous saturation, unless a long catheter is placed
  - o Central venous pressure (CVP) monitoring affected by intra-abdominal pressure; femoral CVLs should not be placed in the setting of acute intra-abdominal process or trauma
  - o Difficult when anatomic landmarks are distorted
  - o Excessive stooling increases infection risk
- Anatomy (Figure 8-2)
  - o Inguinal ligament runs from anterior superior iliac spine to the pubic symphysis
  - o Femoral artery and vein run in parallel and should be entered below the inguinal ligament
  - o "NAVEL" describes the structures from lateral to medial of importance: nerve, artery, vein, empty space, lymphatics

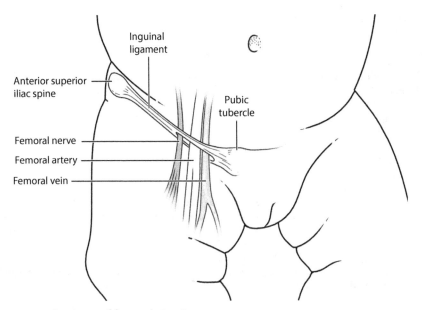

FIGURE 8-2 **Anatomy of femoral structures.**
Reproduced with permission from Noah Z. Chapter 11. Arterial Puncture. In: Goodman DM, et al., eds. *Current Procedures: Pediatrics* New York, NY: McGraw-Hill; 2007.

- Approach
  - Patient positioning
    - Supine position
    - Lift hips with leg on the side of the approach in slightly flexed, "frogleg" position
  - Palpate the femoral artery; the femoral vein will be just medial to the artery
  - With ultrasound:
    - Identify the femoral vein as the nonpulsatile, thinner-walled structure
    - Adjust leg position while visualizing the femoral vein and artery so as to minimize femoral vein overlap of the femoral artery and reduce risk of inadvertent femoral artery puncture
  - Enter the skin 1 to 2 cm inferior to the inguinal ligament at a 30- to 45-degree angle aimed toward the umbilicus
  - Place the line using the Seldinger technique
- Specific complications
  - Impaired lower extremity venous return with lower extremity swelling
  - Thrombus
  - Misplacement of the catheter; placement into the lumbar venous plexus can result in mortality

INTERNAL JUGULAR (IJ) CENTRAL VENOUS CATHETER

- Advantages
  - Avoids femoral access
  - Allows for more reliable hemodynamic monitoring (CVP, mixed venous saturation)
  - Better control of bleeding than subclavian
  - Potential access point for pacing wire

- Drawbacks
  - Difficult with tracheostomy stoma and ties
  - May impair cerebral venous drainage in the setting of increased intracranial pressure
- Anatomy (Figure 8-3)
  - Triangle formed by clavicle and two bellies of the sternocleidomastoid
- Approach
  - Patient positioning
    - Supine and head slightly down (Trendelenburg) 15 to 30 degrees
    - Roll under shoulders
    - Head turned contralateral to puncture site
  - Right IJ preferred to avoid injury to thoracic duct, left brachiocephalic vein, or superior vena cava (SVC)
  - With ultrasound:
    - Identify the internal jugular vein as the nonpulsatile, thinner-walled structure
    - Adjust neck position while visualizing the internal jugular vein and carotid artery so as to minimize overlap of the internal jugular vein and carotid artery and reduce the risk of inadvertent arterial puncture
  - Three approaches (the middle is the most common)
    - Anterior – introduce the needle along the anterior margin of the sternocleidomastoid between the mastoid process and sternum; aim for the ipsilateral nipple
    - Middle
      - Enter apex of triangle formed by two muscle bellies and clavicle
      - Enter at 30-degree angle
      - Aim for ipsilateral nipple
    - Posterior
      - Introduce the needle along the posterior border of the sternocleidomastoid cephalad to the division into anterior and sternal heads
      - Aim toward the suprasternal notch
- Complications
  - Pneumothorax or hemothorax
  - Arrhythmia
  - Pericardial tamponade
  - Left-sided approach can lead to thoracic duct injury or injury to the SVC or left brachiocephalic vein

SUBCLAVIAN CENTRAL VENOUS CATHETER

- Advantages
  - Avoids femoral access or neck access
  - Better hemodynamic monitoring than femoral
- Drawbacks
  - Coagulopathy – more difficult to control bleeding because cannot apply direct pressure to the artery or vein
- Anatomy (Figure 8-3)
  - Entry point is at the junction of the middle and medial thirds of the clavicle
- Approach
  - Patient positioning
    - Head down (Trendelenburg) 30 degrees
    - Neck may be extended with neck roll, neutral, or slightly flexed with head turned to direction of needle entry

A

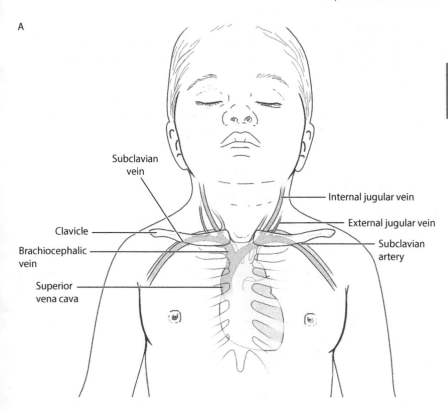

B

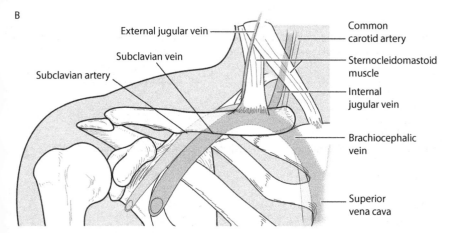

FIGURE 8-3 **A: Vessel location for percutaneous placement of central venous catheters. B: Landmarks used to guide central venous catheter placement.**
Reproduced with permission from Michelson K. Chapter 57. Internal Jugular and Subclavian Catheterization. In: Goodman DM, et al., eds. *Current Procedures: Pediatrics*. New York, NY: McGraw-Hill; 2007.

- Shoulders neutral with arms beside patient
  - Introduce needle at the inferior aspect of the clavicle at the junction of the middle and medial thirds of the clavicle and advanced while applying negative pressure to attached syringe
  - With ultrasound:
    - Supraclavicular and infraclavicular approaches are options
    - Adjust neck position while scanning to maximize visualization of subclavian vein
    - Identify pleura just deep to the subclavian vein
  - Insert needle parallel to patient and direct medially and slightly cephalad toward finger placed in the sternal notch
  - Introduce guidewire during inspiration on ventilator and on expiration in spontaneously breathing patient to avoid air embolus
  - Complete placement using Seldinger technique
- Complications
  - Pneumothorax – risk is reduced by using expiratory hold or hemothorax
  - Arrhythmia
  - Pericardial tamponade

ARTERIAL ACCESS

INDICATIONS

- Continuous blood pressure monitoring when noninvasive blood pressure monitoring is inaccurate (morbidly obese, very thin, burns)
- Frequent blood laboratory sampling
- Frequent arterial blood gas sampling

CONTRAINDICATIONS

- Absent pulse
- Full-thickness burn
- Inadequate circulation, including Raynaud's
- Relative: anticoagulation, partial-thickness burn, inadequate collateral flow, local infection at insertion site, vascular graft, surgical site at insertion site

PREPARATION

- For Seldinger technique
  - Arterial catheter
  - Finder needle
  - Guidewire
- For non-Seldinger technique use an IV catheter or arterial catheter with a catheter over the needle technique
- Chlorhexidine solution
- Gauze
- Sterile towels/drape
- Sterile gloves, gown, hat

PROCEDURE

- Identify site for cannulation
  - Radial artery most common (Figure 8-4). Allen test (Figure 8-5) should be performed to evaluate for dual perfusion to the hand. The patient opens and closes the hand multiple times and then squeezes tightly. The examiner then compresses over both the radial and

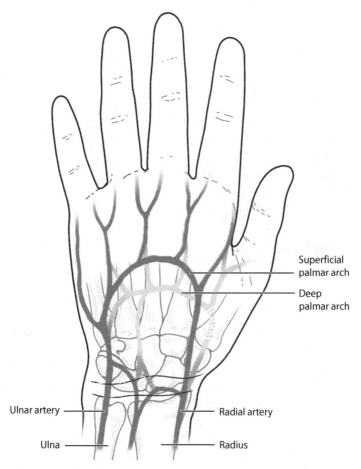

FIGURE 8-4 Anatomy of radial artery.
Reproduced with permission from Noah Z. Chapter 11. Arterial Puncture. In: Goodman DM, et al., eds. *Current Procedures: Pediatrics* New York, NY: McGraw-Hill; 2007.

ulnar arteries and then releases the ulnar artery. The hand should reperfuse when the artery is released. This should be repeated with the radial released to ensure dual hand perfusion and can be compared to the contralateral side.

- Other sites include ulnar, posterior tibialis, dorsalis pedis, axillary, and femoral (for central arterial cannulation). Brachial is not recommended due to absence of collateral circulation.
- Prepare and drape the area as described earlier for central venous cannulation.
- Feel arterial pulsation prior to inserting catheter.
- For Seldinger technique.
  - Insert finder needle until blood return is obtained. Alternatively, the needle can be advanced fully through the vessel until flow stops (to transfix the vessel) and then the needle pulled back until flow starts again.

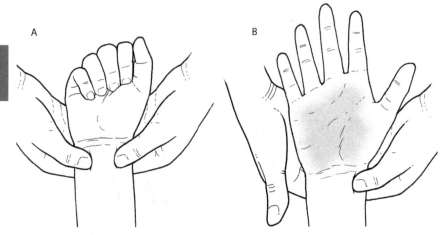

FIGURE 8-5 Modified Allen test.
Reproduced with permission from Noah Z. Chapter 11. Arterial Puncture. In: Goodman DM, et al., eds. *Current Procedures: Pediatrics.* New York, NY: McGraw-Hill; 2007.

- Advance the wire through the needle. Rotate the needle 90 to 180 degrees if difficulty with passing wire to avoid blockage from an intimal flap.
- Once wire is in place, advance catheter over wire. No dilation of the vessel is generally required (unless central cannulation is performed).
- For the catheter over needle technique, once the needle is introduced with blood return, advance the catheter over the needle.
- Attach catheter to arterial line pressure monitoring system and secure with sterile dressing (procedure similar to dressing of peripheral IV lines for peripheral arterial lines and central venous lines for central arterial line).

Complications (most are rare with proper technique)
- Hematoma/bleeding
- Local site infection
- Sepsis
- Ischemic damage (may be permanent)
- Thrombosis
- Air embolism
- Compartment syndrome
- Nerve injury
- For femoral cannulation, femoral artery dissection, pseudoaneurysm

Ultrasound considerations (see General Principles for Ultrasound-Guided Vascular Access for complete description of technique)

- Indications
  - Ultrasound-guided placement improves success rate and reduces complications
  - Inability to palpate artery secondary to obesity, edema, or multiple prior attempts
- Preparation, materials, and technique
  - Cover ultrasound probe with sterile sheath
  - Use sterile gel outside the sheath
  - Scan at site of insertion to ensure artery is free of clots

o Either short axis/transverse approach or long axis/longitudinal approach may be used (see General Principles for Ultrasound-Guided Vascular Access for details)
o Insert needle at appropriate angle to ensure sufficient catheter length

PERIPHERAL VENOUS ACCESS

INDICATIONS

- IV fluid or medication administration
- Blood sampling
- Peripheral IV nutrition
- Blood product administration
- Contrast administration for imaging
- There are no absolute contraindications, but should avoid placement in an injured, infected, or burned extremity

PROCEDURE

- Preparation
  o Choose a catheter size appropriate for the indication. Smaller catheters will risk less damage to vessels. Larger catheters are preferred for high volume or resuscitation.
  o Venous engorgement will aid cannulation and can be accomplished by placing the target vein in a dependent position, tourniquets, and "pumping" the muscle to create contractions around the vessel.
  o Transillumination with a *cold* light source (usually fiber-optic) in a dark room can help to illuminate veins in neonates and infants.
- Materials
  o Chlorhexidine or alcohol to decontaminate the skin
  o IV cannula
  o Sterile syringe with normal saline
  o Three-way connector or T-connector
  o Sterile dressing (e.g., Tegaderm)
  o Tape
  o Gauze
  o Board to secure/immobilize extremity following placement
  o Blood tubes if needed to send blood
  o Gloves
- Technique (Figure 8-6)
  o Stabilize extremity at joints above and below entry site if necessary
  o Apply tourniquet if needed with care not to compress arterial flow
  o Decontaminate using chlorhexidine or alcohol; do not touch site after decontamination
  o Insert needle at a 10- to 15-degree angle, advancing the needle 1 to 2mm after entering the vessel
  o Advance the catheter over the needle into the vessel
  o Secure the hub of the needle at the skin entry point
  o Attach saline-filled three-way connector and flush IV
  o Consider placing a small piece of gauze under the hub of the needle to avoid pressure on the skin
  o Attach using tape crossed over the cannula and at the hub with the skin entry point remaining visible
  o Place a clear dressing over the catheter
  o Secure extremity to board or place immobilizer around extremity as needed

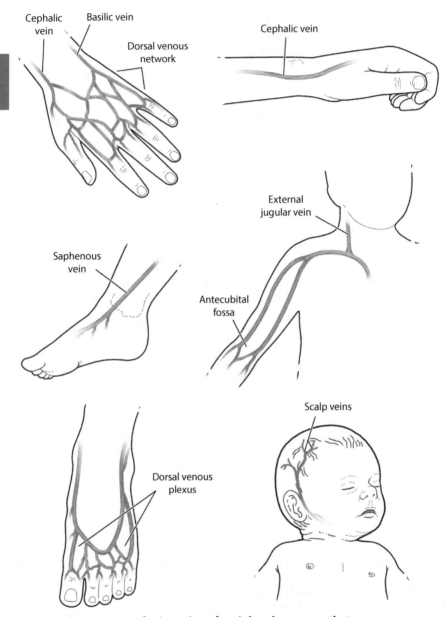

FIGURE 8-6 Common sites for insertion of peripheral venous catheter.
Reproduced with permission from Noah Z. Chapter 8. Peripheral IV Insertion. In: Goodman DM, et al., eds. *Current Procedures: Pediatrics.* New York, NY: McGraw-Hill; 2007.

Ultrasound Considerations (see General Principles for Ultrasound-Guided Vascular Access for complete description of technique)

- Indications
  - Difficult access secondary to edema, obesity, multiple prior vascular attempts, or inability to visualize veins
  - Desire to avoid/limit central access
- Preparation and materials
  - Cover ultrasound probe with adhesive dressing or sterile sheath
  - Superficial vessels are preferred, as they are associated with a higher success rate of cannulation
  - Choose longer (>2 inches) catheters, as they have less risk of premature failure secondary to dislodgement as compared to shorter catheters
- Technique
  - Scan at site of insertion to ensure vein is free of clots and valves
  - Either short axis/transverse approach or long axis/longitudinal approach may be used (see General Principles for Ultrasound-Guided Vascular Access for details)
  - Insert needle at appropriate angle to ensure sufficient catheter length

INTRAOSSEOUS ACCESS

- General considerations
  - An intraosseous (IO) line may be used for venous access whenever a peripheral IV is needed and cannot be accomplished.
  - IO lines should be removed within hours of placement or earlier as soon as peripheral or central access is achieved.
  - Special IO needles with stylets should be used.
- Procedure (Figure 8-7)
  - Identify site for placement
    - Infants: Distal femur, proximal tibia
    - Children/adolescents: Distal femur, proximal tibia, distal tibia
    - Other sites: Anterior superior iliac spine, calcaneus, humerus, radius, sternum (adults)
  - Stabilize the extremity without placing hand behind the area where the IO line will be inserted.
  - For proximal tibia, insertion should be on the flat anteromedial surface, 1 to 2 centimeters distal to the tibial tuberosity.
  - For distal femur, insertion should be 3 cm above the lateral condyle in the midline.
  - For distal tibia in older children, insertion should be on the medial surface 2 cm above the medial malleolus.
  - The needle is held firmly in the palm of the hand not being used to stabilize the extremity and inserted using moderate pressure and a rotary motion aimed away from the direction of the joint, stopping when a "pop" marks penetration of the cortex. Semi-automatic (spring- or battery-powered) devices may be used to aid insertion.
  - The needle should be stabilized once the cortex has been penetrated and the needle is in the medullary cavity to avoid crossing the cortex on the other side of the bone.
  - Once the cavity is entered, the stylet is removed and the IO can be used.
- Complications
  - Advancing the needle too far can result in exiting the opposite cortex and soft tissue infusion of IV products
  - Osteomyelitis
  - Bleeding
  - Compartment syndrome

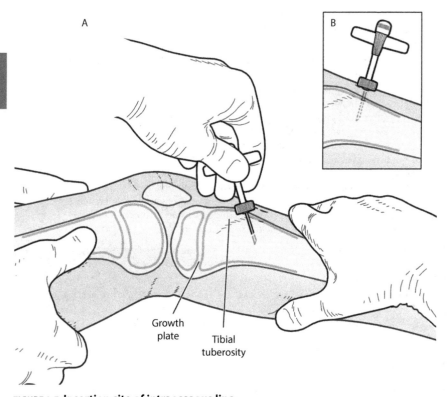

FIGURE 8-7 Insertion site of intraosseous line.
Reproduced with permissio from Noah Z. Chapter 9. Intraosseous Line Insertion. In: Goodman DM, et al., eds. *Current Procedures: Pediatrics.* New York, NY: McGraw-Hill; 2007.

Ultrasound Considerations (see General Principles for Ultrasound-Guided Vascular Access for complete description of technique)

○ Confirmation of placement
○ Place high-frequency linear probe proximal or distal to IO needle in transverse or longitudinal orientation (with respect to bone)
○ The accessed bone will appear as a hyperechoic line
○ Use color Doppler or power Doppler for placement confirmation
○ Appropriate placement will reveal flow within the IO channel (visualized deep to the bony cortex)
○ Placement failure will be seen as flow superficial or lateral to bone

SUGGESTED READINGS

Aouad-Maroun M, Raphael CK, Sayyid SK, Farah F, Akl EA. Ultrasound-guided arterial cannulation for paediatrics. *Cochrane Database Syst Rev.* 2016;9:CD011364. doi:10.1002/14651858.CD011364.pub2.

Feldman R. Venipuncture and peripheral intravenous access. In: E. Reichman & R. Simon, eds. *Emergency Medicine Procedures.* New York: McGraw Hill; 2004:297-313.

Franco R, Soni NJ. Central Venous Access. In: Soni NJ, Arntfield R, Kory P, eds. *Point-of-Care Ultrasound*. Philadelphia, PA: Elsevier Saunders, Inc.; 2015:225-232.

Keim S, ed. Procedures. In: Gomella LG, Series Ed. *Emergency Medicine on Call*. New York: The McGraw-Hill Companies, Inc.; 2004:417-478.

Kohn LT, Corrigan JM, Donaldson MS, eds. *To Err Is Human: Building a Safer Health System (2000)*. Institute of Medicine; Committee on Quality of Health Care in America. Washington, DC: National Academy Press; 2000.

Michelson K. Femoral venous catheterization. In: Goodman DM, Green TP, Unti SM, Powell EC, eds. *Lange Current Procedures: Pediatrics*. New York: The McGraw-Hill Companies, Inc.; 2007:48-53.

Michelson K. Internal jugular and subclavian catheterization. In: Goodman DM, Green TP, Unti SM, Powell EC, eds. *Lange Current Procedures: Pediatrics*. New York: The McGraw-Hill Companies, Inc.; 2007:244-248.

Milzma D, Janchar T. Arterial puncture and cannulation. In: Roberts JR, Hedges JR, eds. *Clinical Procedures in Emergency Medicine*. 4th ed. Philidelphia: W.B. Saunders; 2004:384-400.

Nichols DG, Stephen M. Schexnayder, Praveen Khilnani, Naoki Shimizu, Arno Zaritsky. Invasive procedures. In: *Rogers' Textbook of Pediatric Intensive Care*. Philadelphia: Lippincott Williams & Wilkins; 2008:355-371.

Noah Z. Arterial puncture. In: Goodman DM, Green TP, Unti SM, Powell EC, eds. *Lange Current Procedures: Pediatrics*. New York: The McGraw-Hill Companies, Inc.; 2007:54-57.

Noah Z. Intraosseous line insertion. In: Goodman DM, Green TP, Unti SM, Powell EC, eds. *Lange Current Procedures: Pediatrics*. New York: The McGraw-Hill Companies, Inc.; 2007:44-47.

Noah Z. Peripheral IV insertion. In: Goodman DM, Green TP, Unti SM, Powell EC, eds. *Lange Current Procedures: Pediatrics*. New York: The McGraw-Hill Companies, Inc.; 2007:38-43.

Patient Monitoring

INTRODUCTION

The aim of this chapter is to introduce the reader to commonly deployed patient monitoring devices in critical care medicine. It is necessary to have a basic understanding of how these devices work to have an ability to recognize potential pitfalls in interpretation of the data they generate.

HEMODYNAMIC MONITORING

Invasive hemodynamic monitoring remains the accepted reference standard for blood pressure monitoring of hemodynamically unstable patients.

- **Transducers:** Integral to monitoring of all pressure waveforms is the transducer. Transducers contain a fluid-filled interface that detects changes in pressure. The transducer contains a diaphragm that interfaces with a column of fluid extending from the cannula inserted into the blood vessel, through the pressure tubing, to the transducer.
- **How it works:** Changes in intravascular pressure result in pulsations in the column of saline in the tubing between the cannula in the blood vessel and the transducer. The pulsations displace the diaphragm on the transducer, which transmits the waveform to the monitor and converts this waveform into an electrical signal displaying the pressure.
- **Zeroing/positioning:** All transducers must be zeroed and placed in the appropriate location relative to the patient.
  - Zeroing negates the influence of external pressures (like atmospheric pressure) and occurs when the stopcock connecting the cannula to the noncompressible pressure tubing is opened to ambient atmospheric pressure. Consequently, all pressures displayed account for the external pressures like atmospheric pressure.
  - Transducer position is often aligned either with the blood vessel or cavity against which the pressure will be measured or at the level of cannula insertion. For example, the central venous pressure (CVp) transducer should be aligned with the upper fluid level of the right atrium (typically 5 cm posterior to the right sternal border at the fourth intercostal space). If the transducer changes position, then the blood pressure will be incorrect secondary to the effects of hydrostatic pressure from the tubing. For example, if the transducer is too low, the fluid in the tubing above the transducer will exert a greater pressure on the transducer than at the location at which it was zeroed, resulting in a falsely high blood pressure.

INVASIVE ARTERIAL PRESSURE MONITORING (SEE FIG. 9-1)

- Indications include the following: Blood pressure monitoring in the hemodynamically unstable patient, frequent sampling of arterial blood gases or other laboratory tests.
- Potential complications of arterial cannulation: Infection, pain, bleeding, embolus, impaired arterial circulation in the extremity cannulated. Retroperitoneal hematoma may occur in femoral arterial line placement.
- Locations for arterial cannulation: Radial, dorsalis pedis, and posterior tibial arteries are most commonly the first sites accessed. If unable to cannulate these areas, alternative areas to consider include ulnar (smaller, more challenging, and less desirable if the radial artery is in the same side previously cannulated, as this would compromise blood flow to that hand), femoral, or axillary arteries. Brachial arterial lines are often avoided, as compromise to this artery may result in impaired blood flow to the distal part of that limb and possible limb loss in extreme cases.

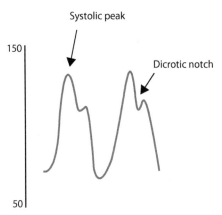

FIGURE 9-1 **The normal arterial waveform.** This waveform demonstrates the systolic peak and dicrotic notch.

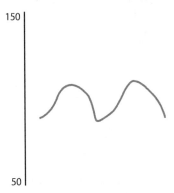

FIGURE 9-2 **Arterial line "fling" (underdamping).** This artifact tends to result in overestimation of systolic blood pressure and underestimation of diastolic blood pressure.

- Waveform artifacts due to technical errors include damping (overdamping vs. underdamping), fling (whip). See normal arterial waveform in Figure 9-1.
  - Damping is when the waveform amplitude is reduced. Some amount of damping is desired in order to reduce the inherent resonant frequency of the monitoring system or to eliminate the contributions of the physical forces of the system and only measure the patient's pressure waveform. If the system is overdamped (See Fig. 9-2) (by an air bubble, partially closed stopcock, or soft tubing that absorbs the pressure waves), then the pressure will be underestimated with a low-amplitude waveform. An underdamped system occurs when there is too high a frequency response in the system, causing a large-amplitude waveform and an overestimation of the systolic blood pressure.
  - Arterial catheter fling (whip) (See Fig. 9-3) occurs when the peak pressure "overshoots," resulting in a falsely high systolic blood pressure. This can result from significant catheter tip movement or overfilling of the transducer.

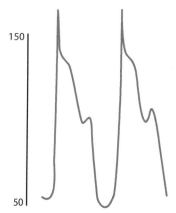

FIGURE 9-3 Overdampened arterial pressure. This tends to underestimate systolic blood pressure and overestimate diastolic blood pressure.

- o Resonance: The arterial waveform is composed of multiple sine waves with each wave having a specific frequency. If any of these frequencies are the same as the resonant frequency inherent in the transduction system, distortion of the signal will occur, leading to erroneous measurements. The equipment used is specifically designed to maintain a natural frequency above the frequencies of the arterial waveforms to eliminate this problem.

CENTRAL VENOUS PRESSURE (CVp) MONITORING (SEE FIG. 9-4)

- Indications: In patients with hemodynamic instability, CVp monitoring provides an assessment of intravascular volume as well as an assessment of right ventricular end diastolic pressure (RVEDp) in patients without tricuspid stenosis. Central lines also offer stable vascular access for infusion of vesicants, inotropes, and parenteral nutritional support, as well as a means of obtaining blood samples for laboratory testing.
- Potential complications: Infection, pain, bleeding, vascular injury, pulmonary embolus, air embolus, hemothorax, and pneumothorax.
- Sites: Femoral, internal jugular, subclavian. Note: Due to line characteristics that lead to inaccuracy (i.e., length and distensibility), peripherally inserted central catheter (PICC) lines are generally undesirable for CVp monitoring.
- Waveforms:

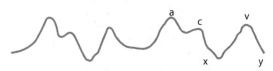

FIGURE 9-4 The normal CVp tracing. The waveform consists of a, c, and v waves, as well as a systolic x descent and diastolic y descent.

a wave = atrial contraction
c wave = ventricular contraction
v wave = atrial filling driven by systemic venous return
x descent = atrial relaxation
y descent = rapid emptying of atrium following opening of tricuspid valve

An understanding of the components of the CVp is crucial, as the waveform undergoes characteristic changes in certain pathologic states:

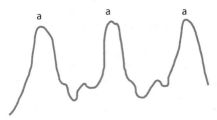

FIGURE 9-5 **The figure shows cannon a-waves associated with atrial systole against a closed atrioventricular valve.** This is usually diagnostic of a loss of atrioventricular synchrony.

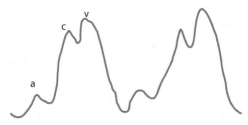

FIGURE 9-6 **The figure shows a regurgitant cv-wave and is associated with clinically important tricuspid regurgitation.**

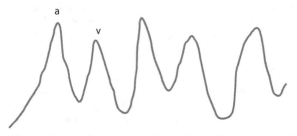

FIGURE 9-7 **The figure shows the accentuation of a and v waves as well as steep systolic (x) and diastolic (y) descents associated with pericardial constriction/myocardial restriction.** The other characteristic of the CVp in these situations is an elevated actual value.

Central venous vessels are very sensitive to changes in intrathoracic pressure during the respiratory cycle. This respiratory variation in the CVp tracing is accentuated in conditions that promote an excessively negative intrathoracic pressure (like upper airway obstruction) and in patients experiencing positive pressure ventilation.

NONINVASIVE BLOOD PRESSURE (BP) MEASUREMENT

• Methods include auscultation, palpation, and oscillometry.
• Auscultation: Auscultation over the brachial artery while a cuff is inflated. Systolic pressure is identified when Korotkoff sounds occur. Diastolic blood pressure is identified by the loss

of all sounds. This methodology is often inaccurate and often user dependent. Diastolic values are less accurate than systolic values.

- Palpation: A cuff is inflated to above systolic pressure, preventing arterial pulsations from occurring. The cuff is then deflated to the point where pulsations are palpated. This is the systolic blood pressure. No diastolic blood pressure is obtained. This methodology is easy to perform, though often inaccurate. Shown to underestimate systolic blood pressure.
- Oscillometer: This is an automatic measurement using a self-inflating cuff. The cuff inflates above systolic pressure, eliminating arterial pulsations, then deflates either continuously or in steps until pulsations reappear. The electronic transducer detects this and notes the pressure at which the oscillations (pulsations) occurring within the artery are greatest, and this is systolic pressure. The cuff continues to deflate, and when the oscillations are the smallest, this is noted as diastolic pressure. Mean arterial pressure and systolic pressure are the most accurate in this method. These values are compared to standard BP calculation equations included in the system by the manufacturer where:
  - Mean BP $= [\text{Systolic BP} + (2 \times \text{Diastolic BP})] / 3$

CARBON DIOXIDE AND OXYGEN MONITORING

- **Transcutaneous carbon dioxide (CO_2) monitoring:**
  - Measures the skin-surface partial pressure of CO_2 as an estimate of the partial pressure of arterial CO_2 ($PaCO_2$).
  - Mechanism: The monitor is placed on an adhesive ring containing saline or glue and causes the capillaries to dilate by increasing the temperature of the skin at the site where it is applied using a heating electrode. This allows the skin to become more permeable to gases. Using a temperature correction factor, it calculates the CO_2 value electrochemically by detecting a change in the pH of the solution present between the skin and the electrode.
  - Limitations: Device must be calibrated and allowed several minutes to begin reading accurately. Can cause damage to skin due to local increases in skin temperature. Trapped air bubbles in the solution between the skin and monitor will result in inaccurate readings. Vasoconstriction due to hypothermia, shock states, etc., will reduce system accuracy.
- **Near-Infrared Spectroscopy (NIRS)**
  - NIRS is a spectroscopic method that relies on the relative transparency of the skin to the near-infrared region of the electromagnetic spectrum (700–2500 nm) to determine tissue oxygenation. By monitoring absorption at wavelengths where oxyhemoglobin, deoxyhemoglobin, and cytochrome aa3 differ, it is possible to calculate local hemoglobin–O_2 saturation.
  - Although both pulse oximetry and NIRS monitors use near-infrared light to determine O_2 saturation, due to differences in how the strong pulsatile (the focus of pulse oximetry) and weaker nonpulsatile (the focus of NIRS) signals of the waveform are processed, NIRS monitors are less susceptible to errors from poor perfusion.
  - The designation of the regional saturation being measured depends on where the probe is placed. If measuring a specific tissue saturation (e.g., limb), the value is designated StO_2 (tissue); if cerebral venous saturation is being measured, the value is recorded as ScO_2 (cerebral), and rSO_2 (regional) if used to estimate splanchnic perfusion by placement on the patient's flank.
  - Somanetics devices in clinical practice are not very accurate when compared to a weighted average of absolute tissue oxygenation (10%–15% error), but are more accurate in measuring a change in saturation ($+/- 5\%$) and are therefore best interpreted as a trend rather than an absolute value.

- **Pulse Oximetry**
  - Transmissive pulse oximetry involves the placement of a sensor that has small light-emitting diodes (LEDs) facing a photodetector and a processor. Two wavelengths (660 nm and 940 nm) of light that are differentially absorbed by oxyhemoglobin and deoxyhemoglobin are passed through the tissue, and changing absorbance at each wavelength allows determination of absorbances due to arterial pulsation with correction for tissue absorbance. The ratio of red to infrared measurement is calculated by the processer and converted to the SpO_2 by reference to tables of empiric observation.

$$SpO_2 = HbO_2 / total\ Hb$$

  - Limitations: Accurate readings are very dependent on perfusion and movement. Pulse oximetry is not a measure of circulatory sufficiency; significant anemia with tissue hypoxia can exist in spite of high measured oxygen saturations. Because oximetry is only measuring the percentage of bound hemoglobin, false readings occur when hemoglobin binds something other than oxygen.
    - Falsely high values occur with carbon monoxide poisoning and cyanide exposure
    - Falsely low readings occur with methemoglobinemia (classically 80%–85%)
- **End Tidal Capnography ($EtCO_2$)** (See Fig. 9-8)
  $EtCO_2$ refers to the graphical measurement of the partial pressure of CO_2 (mmHg) during exhalation.
  - Indications: Monitoring of adequacy of ventilation, verifying correct placement of an endotracheal tube, measuring efficacy of CPR, assessing for return of spontaneous circulation, and assessment of pulmonary pathology (obstruction, shunt thrombosis, pulmonary embolus).
  - Measurement: Measurement can involve either mainstream (in line with the endotracheal tube) or sidestream techniques (which are more appropriate for extubated patients).
  - Interpretation: An elevated end tidal CO_2 could indicate inadequate ventilation (i.e., a generous $paCO_2$) or an increase in deadspace ventilation. An abrupt decrease in the measured partial pressure of CO_2 by capnography could indicate a sudden decrease in pulmonary blood flow, as would occur with pulmonary embolism or shunt thrombosis. A gradual decrease in $EtCO_2$ likely indicates overgenerous minute ventilation. It is necessary to also note the morphology of the $EtCO_2$ waveform, as this provides additional information about pathologic processes as indicated by Figures 9-8 and 9-9.

INTRACRANIAL PRESSURE MONITORING

- Indications: Continuous measurement of intracranial pressure (ICP) in the critically ill patient with brain injury (for example, patients with closed head injury).
- ICP waveforms: The ICP wave is a combination of two pulsatile waves. The first is secondary to arterial pulsations from vessels within the brain. This results in an ICP waveform similar to the arterial waveform. The second waveform is a result of respirations altering the central venous pressure waveform. This represents intrathoracic pressure. The two patterns are superimposed and result in an overall ICP wave form.
- Methodology: Two common forms of continuous ICP measurement are used currently: an intraventricular drain (commonly referred to as an external ventricular drain [EVD]) and the catheter-tip transducer (bolt).
  - Intraventricular drain, commonly referred to as the external ventricular drain (EVD): This is considered to be the gold standard of ICP measurement. The drain is connected to an external pressure transducer (see Transducers earlier) with the reference point at the foramen of Monro or at the midway point between the two external auditory canals.

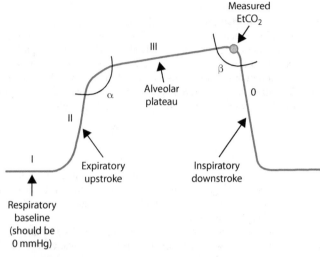

FIGURE 9-8 **Phases of the capnogram.**
Phase I – Indicates deadspace
Phase II – Transition from deadspace to alveolar gas flow
Phase III – Peak expiratory flow
Phase 0 – Inspiratory point

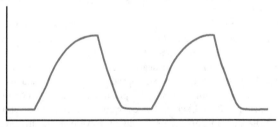

FIGURE 9-9 **Typical capnogram pattern associated with lower airway obstruction.**
Due to difficulty generating expiratory flow in conditions like asthma and chronic obstructive pulmonary disease (COPD), there is a gradual upslope of phase II and little or no plateau (phase III).

- Benefits include the ability to drain cerebrospinal fluid (CSF) while transducing ICP and calculating cerebral perfusion pressure (CPP), as well as the ability to rezero the system (has an external transducer).
- Limitations include injury of nearby regions of brain, increased risk of infection, overdrainage of CSF, bleeding with placement, and difficulty with insertion if small ventricle size (i.e., in setting of significant cerebral edema).
- $CPP = MAP - ICP$
  - Catheter-tip transducer (bolt): There are three kinds: parenchymal (inserted into brain parenchyma; reduced risk of hemorrhage and infection), subdural (inserted into subdural space; may not reflect pressure changes within brain), and ventricular (inserted into ventricle; can drain CSF and measure ICP).

- Limitations include inability to rezero after insertion due to internal transducer (vs. external transducer with EVD), leading to possibly false estimates of ICP (drift). Drift is loss of measurement accuracy usually after approximately 5 days. Also ICP may not be uniform throughout the brain; thus measurements from one location may not reflect ICP elsewhere.

INDIRECT CALORIMETRY

- Indications: Accurate assessment of resting energy expenditure (REE) in patients to determine precise fluid and nutritional needs.
- Methodology: Calorimetry classically measures heat transfer as a means of registering changes in state. In living organisms, metabolic processes generate heat. Due to the challenges associated with the direct measurement of heat production, indirect measurement of metabolic activity by consumption of oxygen or elimination of carbon dioxide and nitrogen waste have become the gold standard. Respiratory indirect calorimetry (IC) has an error rate of <1% and is a highly reproducible method that measures oxygen consumed (VO_2) and carbon dioxide produced (VCO_2). Measured values are then entered in the modified Weir equation to calculate REE.

$$\text{Resting energy expenditure (REE)} = [(3.94 \times VO_2) + (1.1 \times VCO_2)] \times 1440 \text{ min/day}$$

- This technique also allows for calculation of the respiratory quotient: $RQ = VCO_2/VO_2$. Normal values of the RQ range from ~0.7 for pure fat oxidation, to 0.8 for pure protein oxidation, to 1.0 for pure carbohydrate oxidation in states of metabolic balance.
- Considerations:
  ○ REE usually accounts for 75% to 90% of total energy expenditure, but does not accommodate activity.
  ○ Brain, heart, liver, and kidney metabolism account for 60% to 70% of REE.
  ○ REE increases up to 13% per degree (C) of fever.
  ○ Illness affects REE, but not always predictably (~60% of critically ill patients are hypermetabolic with the other ~40% being evenly divided between normometabolic and hypometabolic).
  ○ REE should not be performed in patients on high FiO_2 (>0.6), patients on high positive end-expiratory pressure (PEEP) (>14), or in patients with known circuit leaks or chest tubes due to pneumothorax, as these conditions lead to inaccuracy in measurement.

SUGGESTED READINGS

Burns DA, Ciurczak EW. *Handbook of Near-Infrared Analysis*. 3rd ed. Practical Spectroscopy, CRC Press; 349–369.

Czosnyka M, Pickard JD. Monitoring and interpretation of intracranial pressure. *J Neurol Neurosurg Psychiatry*. 2004;75(6):813-821.

Esper SA, Pinsky MR. Arterial waveform analysis. *Best Pract Res Clin Anaesthesiol*. 2014;28(4):363-380.

Ferrannini E. The theoretical bases of indirect calorimetry: a review. *Metabolism*. 1988;37(3):287-301.

Gilbert M. Principles of pressure, transducers, resonance, damping, and frequency response. *Anaesth Intensive Care Med*. 2011;13(1):1-6.

Jones A, Pratt O. Physical principles of intra-arterial blood pressure measurement. *Anesthesia Tutorial of the Week*. 2009;137:1-8.

Krogh A, Lindhard J. The relative value of fat and carbohydrate as sources of muscular energy: with appendices on the correlation between standard metabolism and the respiratory quotient during rest and work. *Biochem J.* 1920;14(3-4):290-363.

Long CL, Schaffel N, Geiger JW, Schiller WR, Blakemore WS, et al. Metabolic response to injury and illness: estimation of energy and protein needs from indirect calorimetry and nitrogen balance. *J Parenter Enteral Nutr.* 1979;3(6):452-456.

Millikan GA. The oximeter: an instrument for measuring continuously oxygen saturation of arterial blood in man. *Rev Sci Instrum.* 1942;13(10):434-444.

Raemer DB, Calalang I. Accuracy of end-tidal carbon dioxide tension analyzers. *J Clin Monit.* 1991;7(2):195-208.

Restrepo RD, Hirst KR, Wittnebel L, Wettstein R. AARC clinical practice guideline: transcutaneous monitoring of carbon dioxide and oxygen: 2012. *Respir Care.* 2012;57(11):1955-1962.

Ward M, Langton JA. Blood pressure measurement. *Continuing Education in Anaesthesia, Critical Care & Pain.* 2007;7(4):122-126.

Wolf M, Ferrari M, Quaresima V. Progress of near-infrared spectroscopy and topography for brain and muscle clinical applications. *J Biomed Opt.* 2007;12(6):062104.

10 Other Critical Care Procedures

NEEDLE CRICOTHYROTOMY

This procedure involves the creation of a communication between airway and skin via the cricothyroid membrane. An over-the-needle catheter is then passed through the membrane. This procedure provides a temporary secure airway to oxygenate and ventilate a patient in severe respiratory distress when less invasive measures have failed or are unlikely to be successful.

A high pressure gas source such as Jet Ventilation or percutaneous transtracheal ventilation (PTV) is then used to deliver oxygen to the lungs through the catheter. The gas source attaches to the inserted catheter through an improvised device. One can attach the catheter to a 3-mL syringe with the plunger removed and then attach the syringe to the proximal connection piece of a 7.5-mm internal diameter endotracheal tube (Figure 10-1). Alternatively, one can insert an endotracheal tube into the barrel of the 3-mL syringe and inflate the cuff.

Needle cricothyrotomy is considered preferable in children less than 12 years of age because of the membrane's small size and close proximity of vascular structures

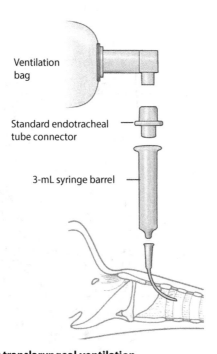

Ventilation bag

Standard endotracheal tube connector

3-mL syringe barrel

FIGURE 10-1 **Setup for translaryngeal ventilation.**
Reproduced with permission from Michelson K. Chapter 5. Cricothyrotomy. In: Goodman DM, et al., eds. *Current Procedures: Pediatrics* New York, NY: McGraw Hill; 2007.

Advantages over tracheostomy:
  Simplicity
  Speed
  Bloodless field
  Minimal training required
  Avoidance of hyperextension of neck

Indications:
  Inability to intubate
  Inability to ventilate
  Rescue laryngeal mask airway cannot be inserted/passed

Contraindications:
  Injury to larynx with damage to cricoid cartilage
  Laryngeal fracture
  Tracheal rupture
  Relative contraindications include anterior neck swelling that distorts anatomic landmarks, anatomic anomalies that distort the larynx or trachea, and bleeding disorders.
  In most cases, the need for securing an airway will outweigh the risks involved in this procedure.

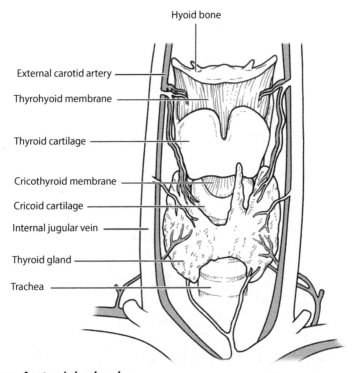

FIGURE 10-2 **Anatomic landmarks.**
Reproduced with permission from Michelson K. Chapter 5. Cricothyrotomy. In: Goodman DM, et al., eds. *Current Procedures: Pediatrics* New York, NY: McGraw Hill; 2007.

TECHNIQUE

1. Position patient supine with neck extended, if possible
2. Identify surface landmarks: thyroid cartilage, cricoid cartilage, and cricothyroid membrane (Figure 10-2)
3. Clean and sterile drape (universal precautions)
4. If time, inject 1% lidocaine into the skin, through the cricothyroid membrane and into airway, to anesthetize the airway and suppress the cough reflex
5. Palpate landmarks; fix thyroid cartilage with the first and third fingers of the nondominant hand, leaving the second finger to locate/palpate the cricothyroid membrane
6. With the dominant hand, pass a 12- or 14-gauge intravenous cannula attached to a syringe filled with sterile saline through the membrane, angling the needle caudally or inferiorly at 45-degree angle (Figure 10-3)
7. Apply negative pressure to the syringe; if in the trachea, escaping air should create air bubbles in the syringe
8. Advance the cannula and remove the needle
9. Secure catheter
10. Attach Jet ventilator and ventilate at 15 L/min
11. Monitor adequacy of ventilation by chest wall movement and breath sound auscultation. Can also interpose $ETCO_2$ in the circuit to monitor exhalation

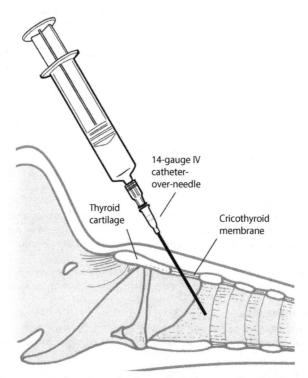

14-gauge IV catheter-over-needle

Thyroid cartilage

Cricothyroid membrane

FIGURE 10-3 **Percutaneous transtracheal ventilation or needle cricothyrotomy.**
Reproduced with permission from Michelson K. Chapter 5. Cricothyrotomy. In: Goodman DM, et al., eds. *Current Procedures: Pediatrics* New York, NY: McGraw Hill; 2007.

Complications:
Pneumothorax
Subcutaneous and mediastinal emphysema
Bleeding
Esophageal puncture
Respiratory acidosis secondary to hypoventilation

Caveats:
Cricothyroidotomy is typically performed as an emergency procedure that is temporizing only:
Ventilation via needle cricothyrotomy is only effective for approximately 45 minutes secondary to inadequate ventilation and CO_2 accumulation. This can be particularly injurious to head injury patients, as hypoventilation will lead to intracranial pressure (ICP) increase.
The patient should be intubated (if possible) or formal tracheostomy performed within 24 hours to avoid glottic or subglottic stenosis.
Complete upper airway obstruction proximal to the cricothyrotomy is a contraindication because of the risk of devastating barotrauma to the lungs.

PERICARDIOCENTESIS

Pericardiocentesis is the aspiration of fluid from the pericardial space that surrounds the heart. It is typically performed in patients experiencing cardiac tamponade and may be lifesaving.
Echocardiography is now the most facile way to identify pericardial effusions, characterize their size and location, and assess dynamic findings associated with tamponade. Hemodynamic effects can be assessed by determining abnormal septal motion, right atrial or right ventricular inversion, and decreased respiratory variation of the inferior vena cava (IVC) diameter.

INDICATIONS

Emergent pericardiocentesis:
The presence of life-threatening hemodynamic alterations in a patient with suspected cardiac tamponade.
Nonemergent pericardiocentesis:
The aspiration of pericardial fluid in hemodynamically stable patients may be used for diagnostic, palliative, or prophylactic reasons. This procedure should be performed under ultrasonography, fluoroscopic visualization, or computerized tomography.
Contraindications:
No absolute contraindications exist in the hemodynamically unstable patient. Even the aspiration of small amounts of fluid may improve the patient's status and prevent arrest.
Relative contraindications:
Uncorrected bleeding disorders and traumatic cardiac tamponade. Some experts believe that tamponade caused by trauma should be treated via emergency thoracotomy.
Materials:
Antiseptic solution
Sterile drapes, gown, mask

1% lidocaine
Small and large syringes
Needles
Pericardiocentesis kit

EMERGENT NEEDLE PERICARDIOCENTESIS POSITIONING AND TECHNIQUE

The patient can be positioned either supine or in a semirecumbent position at a 30- to 45-degree angle. This brings the heart closer to the anterior chest wall.

The patient should have at *least* one intravenous line, should be receiving supplemental oxygen, and should be connected to a cardiac monitor and continuous pulse oximetry. If time permits, placement of a nasogastric tube is advised to decompress the stomach and decrease the chance of gastric perforation.

Identify the anatomic landmarks, including the xiphoid process and the fifth and sixth ribs, and select a site for needle insertion. The subxiphoid approach is most commonly used, followed by the left sternocostal margin. See Figure 10-4.

Sterilely clean and drape the subxiphoid area using universal precautions (if time allows).

Create a skin wheal with local anesthetic solution, and use that wheal to infiltrate and anesthetize subcutaneous and deeper tissue and sternocostal margins.

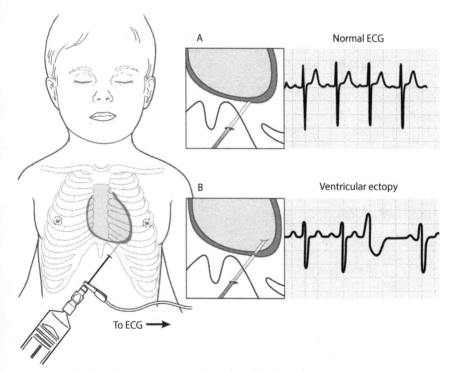

A

Normal ECG

B

Ventricular ectopy

To ECG ➡

FIGURE 10-4 **Pericardiocentesis may trigger ventricular ectopy.**
Reproduced with permission from Pophal S. Chapter 22. Pericardiocentesis. In: Goodman DM, et al., eds. *Current Procedures: Pediatrics* New York, NY: McGraw Hill; 2007.

Connect a large syringe (20 or 60 mL) to the spinal needle, and aspirate 5 mL of normal saline into the syringe. Occasional injection of small amounts of saline can help keep your needle patent and free of clots or debris. If time allows, connect an alligator clip to the base of the spinal needle and connect it to the V1 lead of an electrocardiogram (ECG) machine (see Figure 10-4).

Insert the spinal needle at the subxiphoid area at a 45-degree angle to the abdominal wall and direct toward the left shoulder at 45 degrees off the midline sagittal plane. If time permits, needle insertion should be done under ultrasonographic guidance.

While applying negative pressure on the syringe, slowly advance the needle until there is return of fluid, cardiac pulsations are felt, or there is a change in ECG waveform. If the ECG waveform is consistent with myocardial injury (ST segment elevation), this may mean the needle is in direct contact with the myocardium; slowly withdraw the needle until the tracing returns to normal.

Withdraw as much fluid as possible. One may want to configure a setup using a three-way stopcock in order to limit movement of the needle and syringe if there is a need to remove a large volume/effusion.

Remove the needle once fluid can no longer be aspirated.

CONFIRMATION TESTS TO DETERMINE IF FLUID IS PERICARDIAL VS. INTRACARDIAC

Pericardial aspirate should not form a clot, whereas intracardiac blood will clot.

Pericardial aspirate should have a **lower** hemoglobin concentration than peripheral blood.

Fluorescein test: Intracardiac injection of fluorescein should cause a fluorescent flush when examining a patient's conjunctiva.

CHEST TUBE INSERTION

Chest tubes are used to remove air (pneumothorax), fluid (pleural effusion, blood), or pus (empyema) in the thoracic space. To accomplish this task, either a needle thoracentesis or percutaneous thoracostomy can be performed.

INDICATIONS

Pneumothorax (spontaneous, iatrogenic, tension)
Hemothorax
Parapneumonic effusion (if complex)
Empyema
Recurrent malignant effusion
Chylothorax
Penetrating chest trauma
Bronchopleural fistula

NEEDLE THORACENTESIS

Equipment
• Needle size (dependent on patient size)
• Infant: #23 to 25 gauge butterfly needle or #22 to 24 gauge IV catheter
• Child: #18 gauge needle or #18 gauge angiocath
• Young adult: #14 gauge needle (2″ catheter-over-needle)
• Approved cleansing solution (chlorhexidine, povidone-iodine)
• Sterile gown, gloves, mask, and cap/sterile drapes

- Three-way stopcock, "T" connector/extension tubing
- 20 mL syringe
- 1% lidocaine
- Sterile 2″ × 2″ gauze pads
- Paper tape

Patient preparation

1. Place the patient in the supine position (ensure thermoregulation is maintained in infants).
2. Augment oxygen concentration and delivery and/or ventilation as needed.
3. Monitor heart rate, color, and oxygen saturation.

TECHNIQUE

(Needle decompression in emergent situations)

1. Locate landmarks on the chest to find the second intercostal space (Figure 10-5).
2. Cleanse the insertion site with cleansing solution. Work from the identified site of insertion and clean in a concentric pattern outward. Allow ~1 minute to dry. Drape with sterile field/towels.
3. Using 1% lidocaine, initially anesthetize the insertion site subcutaneously (above the rib to avoid the neurovascular bundle) and then advance to anesthetize the costal margins and deeper to the muscle and parietal pleura.

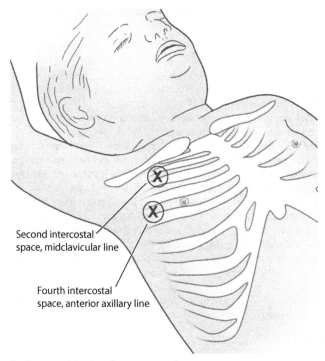

Second intercostal space, midclavicular line

Fourth intercostal space, anterior axillary line

FIGURE 10-5 **Patient positioning for pneumothorax.**
Reproduced with permission from Prestridge A. Chapter 20. Thoracentesis. In: Goodman DM, et al., eds. *Current Procedures: Pediatrics* New York, NY: McGraw Hill; 2007.

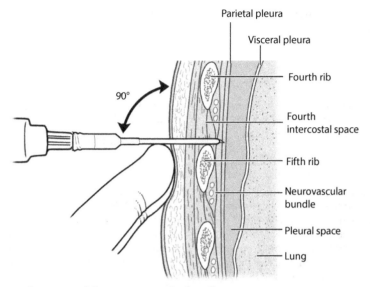

FIGURE 10-6 Anatomy of the neurovascular bundle.
Reproduced with permission from Prestridge A. Chapter 20. Thoracentesis. In: Goodman DM, et al., eds.
Current Procedures: Pediatrics New York, NY: McGraw Hill; 2007.

4. Insert the needle firmly into the second intercostal space, midclavicular line, just above the top of the third rib (again, inserting the needle at the superior edge of the rib avoids the neurovascular bundle) (Figure 10-6).
5. The operator can connect the needle/angiocath to extension tubing and a three-way stopcock set up with a 20-mL syringe attached to facilitate safe drainage.
6. As the needle is being advanced into the pleural cavity, a small amount of negative pressure should be exerted on the syringe plunger. Advance the needle until a "pop" is felt, signifying pleural entry. Air or fluid may rapidly flow into the syringe. Once the pleural space has been entered, the needle should be held steady and advanced no farther. If aspiration is not successful, then imaging (typically ultrasound) should be obtained.
7. For a tension pneumothorax, the inserted thoracentesis needle hub should be connected to extension tubing that is attached to a water seal/Pleur-evac. This will prevent air from being entrained and entering the pleural cavity and allows any trapped air to escape.
8. Needle thoracentesis is typically a temporary measure (unless being performed for diagnostics). A chest tube should be placed for more definitive treatment when the patient is stable.
9. Once the withdrawal of air or fluid is complete, withdraw the needle. Monitor the patient vigilantly for any signs of reaccumulation.

PERCUTANEOUS THORACOSTOMY

Equipment
- Sterile gloves, gown, mask, and cap
- Sterile surgical drapes

- Chest tube tray that contains (at minimum):
  - Scalpel and blade
  - Two straight hemostats
  - Suture scissors
  - Needle driver
  - Two curved Kelly hemostats
- 3.0 silk suture
- Chest tubes of age-appropriate size
- Antiseptic skin preparation
- 1% lidocaine
- 3 mL sterile syringe
- Occlusive dressing
- Sterile gauze pads (4 × 4)
- Chest drainage device (e.g., Heimlich one-way flutter valve, Pleur-evac)

CHEST NEEDLE AND CHEST TUBE INSERTION

Preparation

1. Administer sedation as required.
2. Place the patient in a supine position. The patient's arm can be raised/taped above the head on the insertion side to facilitate exposure.
3. Augment oxygen concentration and delivery and/or ventilation as needed. Monitor heart rate, color, and oxygen saturation.
4. For chest tubes placed along the anterior axillary line, the head of the bed can be elevated 30 to 60 degrees, lowering the diaphragm and decreasing the risk of injury to the diaphragm, liver, or spleen.

Technique

1. Apply mask, perform sterile scrub, and don sterile gown and gloves.
2. Estimate insertion distance. Using the chest tube, measure the distance from the insertion site to the lung apex and make a note of this.
3. Identify appropriate landmarks on the chest
   - The nipple is an anatomic landmark for the fourth intercostal space. Avoid the pectoralis muscle and the axillary artery.
   - Choose the appropriate insertion site at the fourth or fifth intercostal space at the midaxillary line.
4. Prepare the catheter for insertion. Close the hemostat or forceps around the insertion end of the chest tube. Clamp the end of the chest tube that will be connected to the Pleur-evac so that air cannot enter the pleural cavity once the chest tube is inserted.
5. Cleanse the identified insertion site with chlorhexidine 2%, cleaning from the insertion site outward in concentric circles. Allow to dry for 1 to 2 minutes.
6. Drape the desired anatomic region with a sterile drape or towels to create a surgical field. Make sure you can still view the patient's head and neck.
7. Using 1% lidocaine, anesthetize the insertion site. Some operators create a wheal. Infiltrate subcutaneous tissue first and then proceed to muscle, periosteum, and pleura. Infiltrating the pleura is vital to minimize discomfort in the awake patient.
8. Create a 2-cm superficial skin incision immediately above the rib, parallel to the rib and intercostal space. This will avoid injury to the neurovascular bundle if your incision extends more deeply than intended.
9. Insert a forceps or Kelly clamp into the incision to perform blunt dissection down to the intercostal space. This process may require several scissoring and separating maneuvers.

Once the operator has dissected down to the pleura, gently advance the forceps in the closed position until the pleura is penetrated. Once pleural penetration is achieved, open the forceps to spread and dissect, creating a subcutaneous tunnel in the parietal pleura and intercostal muscles (Figure 10-7).

10. After penetrating the pleura with the instrument, a rush of air/fluid is often audible.

11. Grasp the curved hemostat that is holding the catheter and direct the catheter through the incision into the pleural cavity. Once this is achieved, stabilize the catheter with the opposite hand and release it from the hemostat. Slowly remove the hemostat from the chest and advance the catheter to the desired position. Condensation in the lumen of the tube indicates that it has entered the pleural space. Its entry site should be palpated to ensure that it is not in the subcutaneous tissue.

12. In most cases, the catheter will need to be directed anteriorly and superiorly. Advance the chest tube after releasing the hemostat. Ensure that the eyes/holes of the catheter are within the pleural space. Moisture that is present within the tube usually confirms its proper placement within the pleural space.

13. A purse string suture may be placed around the tube and the chest tube secured by wrapping and then tying the skin suture around the tube.

14. Cover the insertion site with an occlusive dressing. The use of Tegaderm over the insertion site permits visualization of the field.

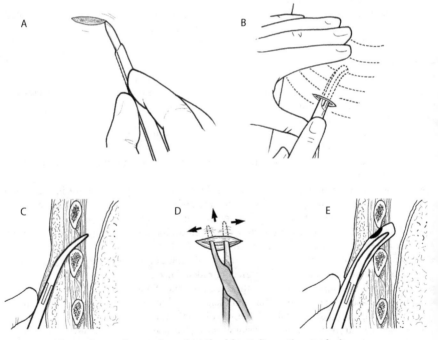

FIGURE 10-7 **Inserting a chest tube using the blunt dissection technique.**
Reproduced with permission from Prestridge A. Chapter 21. Chest Tube Insertion. In: Goodman DM, et al., eds. *Current Procedures: Pediatrics* New York, NY: McGraw Hill; 2007.

15. After securing the chest tube, connect the chest tube to a Pleur-evac or similar device. If the chest tube is draining fluid, the operator may want to control the volume of drainage with intermittent clamping to avoid rapid fluid shifts and re-expansion pulmonary edema, especially in smaller children.

Do not unclamp the chest tube until the drainage system is attached. This will prevent the inspiration of air into the pleural space.

PARACENTESIS

Abdominal paracentesis is a bedside procedure in which a needle is inserted into the peritoneal cavity and ascitic fluid is obtained. Diagnostic paracentesis involves the removal of a small amount of fluid for testing. Diagnostic peritoneal lavage is usually performed by a surgeon to rule out internal bleeding after a trauma and will not be explained here in detail. Therapeutic paracentesis typically involves the removal of a large volume of ascitic fluid to reduce intra-abdominal pressure and its associated symptoms (abdominal pain, dyspnea, feeding intolerance).

Indications:
Evaluation of new-onset ascites
Diagnostic sampling of ascitic fluid (rule out bleeding, chyle leak, malignancy, or infection)
Therapeutic removal of ascitic fluid

CONTRAINDICATIONS

Absolute
Patient instability (unstable airway or hemodynamics)
Intestinal perforation

Relative
Potential sites on abdomen infected or compromised
Coagulopathy or bleeding diathesis
Recent intestinal tract surgery (<1 month)

Equipment
Sterile gloves, gown, mask, and cap
Sterile surgical drapes
Antiseptic skin preparation
Local anesthetic (1% lidocaine)
21 or 23 gauge needles
Angiocatheters with syringes
Large-bore needle with plastic catheter
Sterile gauze pads (4 × 4)
Sterile containers for fluid collection
Culture tubes for samples

Risks
Perforation of bowel or solid organs
Bleeding
Infection
Pneumoperitoneum
Ascites leak

TECHNIQUE

Place the patient in a supine or side position.

Cleanse the insertion site with cleansing solution. Work from the identified site of insertion and clean in a concentric pattern outward. Allow ~1 minute to dry. Drape with sterile field/towels.

Ultrasound guidance is recommended (if available) to locate the optimal pocket of fluid.

Using 1% lidocaine, initially anesthetize the insertion site; injecting the skin first and then deeper into the subcutaneous layer.

The anterosuperior iliac spine should be located and a site chosen that is ~3 cm medial and ~ 3 cm cephalad to this landmark (Figure 10-8). The inferior epigastric arteries run from a point just lateral to the pubic tubercle cephalad within the rectus sheath and should be avoided due to the risk of bleeding. Insert the tap needle into the anesthetized area. In most children, depending on size and body habitus, fluid can be obtained by inserting the needle 1 to 2 inches into the abdomen. To prevent ascites leak after the procedure, the Z-track technique can be utilized, which creates a nonlinear track to prevent direct connection between the ascitic fluid in the peritoneal cavity and the skin (Figure 10-9).

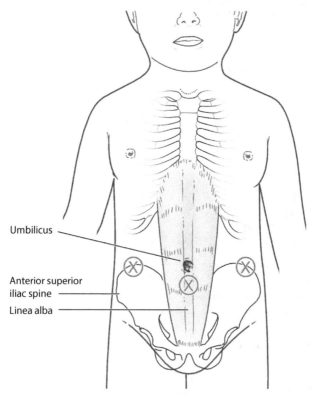

FIGURE 10-8 Anatomic landmarks and sites of entry.
Reproduced with permission from Sudel B, Li BK. Chapter 28. Paracentesis/Peritoneal Lavage. In: Goodman DM, et al., eds. *Current Procedures: Pediatrics* New York, NY: McGraw Hill; 2007.

If a large volume of paracentesis is required, connecting the insertion needle to a three-way stopcock may facilitate removal so that the operator does not need to disconnect the syringe from the needle and risk migration of the needle/catheter setup.

Obtain as much fluid as desired for laboratory sampling or therapeutic relief.

Remove the needle and place a pressure dressing at the insertion site.

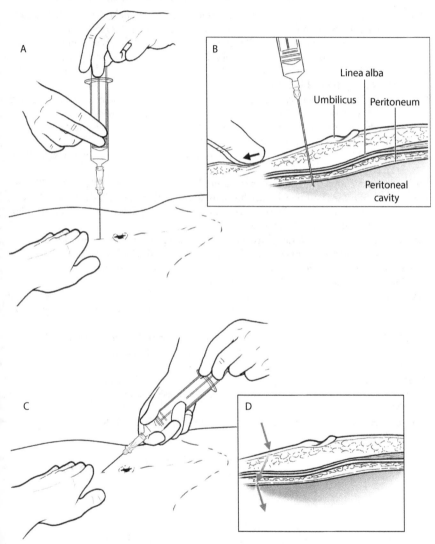

FIGURE 10-9 **The Z-track. A:** Needle is inserted perpendicular to the skin while the skin is pulled taut. **B:** Sagittal view. **C:** Alternatively, the needle can be inserted at 45 degrees to the skin and aimed caudally. **D:** Resultant Z-track (arrows).

Reproduced with permission from Sudel B, Li BK. Chapter 28. Paracentesis/Peritoneal Lavage. In: Goodman DM, et al., eds. *Current Procedures: Pediatrics* New York, NY: McGraw Hill; 2007.

Colloid replacement is controversial and likely unnecessary unless removing more than 5 liters of fluid in larger children. Some studies suggest the use of colloid replacement when draining >200 mL/kg (dry weight) in children to prevent circulatory changes and potential renal compromise.

SUGGESTED READINGS

Dev S, Nascimiento B, Simone C, et al. Chest tube insertion. *N Engl J Med*. 2007;357:e15.

Fagan J. Cricothyroidotomy and needle cricothyrotomy. In: *Open Access Atlas of Otolaryngology, Head and Neck Operative Surgery*. 2017. http://www.entdev.uct.ac.za/guides/open-access-atlas-of-otolaryngology-head-neck-operative-surgery/.

Goodman DM, Green TP, Unti SM, Powell EC, eds. *Current Procedures: Pediatrics*. New York, NY: McGraw-Hill; 2007.

Havelock T, Teoh R, Laws D, et al. Pleural procedures and thoracic ultrasound: British Thoracic Society Pleural Disease Guideline 2010. *Thorax*. 2010;65:ii61-ii76.

Light RW, MacGregor MI, Luchsinger PC, et al. Pleural effusions: the diagnostic separation of transudates and exudates. *Ann Intern Med*. 1972;77:507-513.

McElnay PJ, Lim E. Modern techniques to insert chest drains. *Thorac Surg Clin*. 2017;27(1):29-34.

Runyon B. Paracentesis of ascitic fluid: a safe procedure. *Arch Intern Med*. 1986;146:2259-2261.

Runyon MS, Marx JA. Peritoneal procedures. In: Roberts JR, Hedges JR, Custalow CB, et al., eds. *Roberts and Hedges' Clinical Procedures in Emergency Medicine*. 6th ed. Philadephia, PA: Elsevier Saunders; 2014:852-872.

Sabato SC, Long E. An institutional approach to the management of the 'Can't Intubate, Can't Oxygenate' emergency in children. *Paediatr Anaesth*. 2016;26(8):784-793.

Scrase I, Woollard M. Needle vs. surgical cricothyroidotomy: a short cut to effective ventilation. *Anaesthesia*. 2006;61(10):962-974.

Sen Sarma M, Yachha SK, Bhatia V, et al. Safety, complications and outcome of large volume paracentesis with or without albumin therapy in children with severe ascites due to liver disease. *J Hepatol*. 2015;63(5):1126-1132.

Van Heeckeren DW, Moss MM. Pericardiocentesis and pericardial tube insertion. In Blumer JL, ed. *A Practical Guide to Pediatric Intensive Care*. St. Louis, MO: Mosby-Year Book; 1990.

Wong C, Holroyd-Leduc J, Thorpe K, et al. Does this patient have bacterial peritonitis or portal hypertension? How do I perform a paracentesis and analyze the results? *JAMA*. 2008;299:1166-1178.

Zahn EM, Houde C, Benson L, et al. Percutaneous pericardial catheter drainage in childhood. *Am J Cardiol*. 1992;70:678-680.

Surgical Critical Care

Postoperative Monitoring

LINES, DRAINS, AND TUBES

NASOGASTRIC AND OROGASTRIC TUBES

1. Indications:
   a. Management of bowel obstruction
   b. Symptom relief in patients with nausea and/or emesis (e.g., acute pancreatitis).
2. Types of tubes:
   a. Salem sump – standard double-lumen gastric tube. The larger lumen allows for evacuation of air and fluid. The smaller-vent lumen allows for air to be drawn into the stomach to equalize pressures. Available in multiple sizes from 6 to 18 Fr.
   b. Andersen – very soft, comfortable double-lumen tube made from vinyl.
   c. Replogle – used most commonly for evacuating proximal esophageal pouch in unre- paired esophageal atresia.
3. Management: Can be placed to gravity drainage or to low intermittent wall suction. Suction provides better decompression but risks gastric irritation. Ventilation port must remain unoccluded for proper function. If occluded, the drainage port should be flushed with water and the ventilation port with air.
4. Removal: Generally removed when gastric output is nonbilious and output volume is decreased. Some surgeons opt to continue nasogastric/orogastric (NG/OG) decompres- sion until return of bowel function.
5. EBM Pearl: Routine nasogastric drainage after abdominal surgery is not indicated. A Cochrane review demonstrated that NG tubes are associated with delayed return of bowel function, with no difference in anastomotic leak, wound infection, or other complications.[1]

SURGICAL DRAINS

1. Indications:
   a. Prevention of seroma or hematoma under flaps
   b. Monitoring and control of biliary or pancreatic leak following biliary or pancreatic anastomosis, liver resection, or pancreatic resection
   c. Monitoring and control of chyle leak following extensive retroperitoneal dissection
   d. Monitoring and control of urine leak following partial nephrectomy, bladder augmen- tation, and other urologic procedures
   e. Drainage of abscess cavity
   f. Monitoring and drainage following esophageal or duodenal perforation +/− repair
   g. Drainage of neonatal perforation in extremely low-birth-weight (ELBW) infants (<1 kg) with Penrose drain
2. Types of drains:
   a. Jackson-Pratt – closed suction drain with suction provided by compressed bulb. Often used intra-abdominally or under skin flaps.
   b. Hemovac – closed suction drain with suction provided by spring-loaded accordion- type container.
   c. TLS – small-caliber closed suction drain with suction provided by Vacutainer. Often used in head and neck surgery or other times when output is expected to be low.
   d. Penrose – open drain. Tube provides passive route of egress for fluid and air.

3. Management:
   a. Stripping and flushing – closed suction drains may require stripping and/or flushing to maintain patency, especially when drainage is thicker (blood or abscess). Flushing must be performed using sterile technique. Drains are flushed with saline to maintain patency. Tissue plasminogen activator (tPA) can also be used if the drain is clotted or if trying to break up loculations in an abscess cavity.
   b. Drains should be emptied and output volume recorded at least every shift and more frequently if needed.
4. Removal:
   a. Timing – dependent on indication. Drains placed to monitor for bile, pancreatic, or chyle leak should remain until patient is on a general diet. If monitoring for a leak following a biliary, pancreatic, or urologic procedure, it is sometimes helpful to check a drain bilirubin, amylase, or creatinine, respectively, prior to removal. Abdominal drains are removed, even with moderately high volume of output, if character is sero-sanguinous. Drains in subcutaneous flaps require lower volume (approximately 10–20 mL/day) for removal.
   b. Technique – drains should be taken off suction for removal. Drains can be removed outright or slowly backed out in cases where the clinician is trying to establish a fistula tract (e.g., bile leak).
5. EBM Pearl: Routine abdominal drainage is not indicated for preventing postoperative abscess, nor should they be used routinely around surgical anastomoses. A Cochrane review found that routine drain placement following complicated appendectomy increased length of stay without reducing the risk of intraperitoneal abscess or wound infection.[2]

URETHRAL CATHETERS AND OTHER UROLOGIC TUBES

1. Indications: The Centers for Disease Control and Prevention (CDC) provides guidelines for the prevention of catheter-associated urinary tract infections, which include guidelines for appropriate indications for urethral catheterization.[3]
   a. Urinary retention
   b. Need for accurate urine output measurement in critically ill patients
   c. Selected perioperative indications
      i. Urologic surgery or other surgery on genitourinary (GU) structures
      ii. Prolonged duration of surgery (remove ASAP postoperatively)
      iii. Patients receiving large fluid volume or diuretics in surgery
      iv. Need for intraoperative monitoring of urine output
   d. To assist healing of perineal or sacral wounds in incontinent patients
   e. Patient requiring prolonged immobilization
   f. To improve comfort in end-of-life care
2. Types of catheters:
   a. Foley urethral catheter – standard urethral catheter comes in a variety of sizes
   b. Coude – curved tip useful when placement is difficult, especially in males with enlarged prostrate
3. Management: maintain a closed drainage system. Keep the drainage tubing unkinked and the urine collection bag below the level of the bladder.
4. Bladder irrigation: irrigation only indicated when obstruction is anticipated, such as with bleeding or mucus production after bladder surgery. In general, urethral catheters should be maintained as a closed drainage system. However, after urologic surgery, irrigation (manual or continuous) is often also necessary to remove clots or mucus within the bladder.
5. Removal: remove as soon as possible when the previous indications no longer apply.

6. Other urologic tubes:
   a. Suprapubic tubes – placed percutaneously or during open bladder surgery. Catheter goes directly into the bladder in patients for whom urethral catheterization is contraindicated or not possible, or as an extra drainage tube after major urologic reconstruction. Maintenance similar to uretheral tubes. Cannot be exchanged for several weeks until a tract has formed.
   b. Percutaneous nephrostomy tubes – tube placed through renal parenchyma and into the collecting system to treat hydronephrosis when transurethral drainage is contraindicated or not possible. Also occasionally placed during a definitive urologic procedure as a postoperative drainage modality. Can be flushed with sterile saline to maintain patency.
   c. Vaginostomy tubes – tube placed percutaneously into the vagina, most commonly in girls with a cloaca in whom urine refluxes back into the vagina, creating a massive hydrocolpos, which compresses the bladder and urethra. Maintenance similar to suprapubic tube.
7. EBM Pearl: Although data is still limited, there is mounting evidence that urethral catheters can be removed in patients with thoracic epidurals with a low incidence of urinary retention.[4]

CENTRAL VENOUS CATHETERS AND CENTRAL VENOUS PRESSURE

1. Indications: central venous catheters are often placed at the time of surgery. These lines serve three main purposes in the perioperative patient:
   a. Access for medication and volume infusion
   b. Repeated blood draws
   c. Monitoring of central venous pressure
2. Types of catheters:
   a. Nontunneled central lines – nontunneled lines (e.g., Cook or Arrow) can be placed in the internal jugular, subclavian, or femoral veins at the time of surgery. They are indicated for short-term access.
   b. PICC – peripherally inserted central venous catheters work well for infusion and aspiration, but are less reliable for central venous pressure measurement.
   c. Tunneled central lines – tunneled lines (e.g., Broviac, Hickman, etc.) are typically placed in neonates or in children with malignancy or short gut syndrome who require frequent (often daily) access.
   d. Implantable venous port – placed in children who require ongoing, but intermittent, access. Can be utilized in the perioperative period.
3. Management:
   a. A sterile dressing should be maintained. Sterile dressing changes are performed according to each hospital's policy.
   b. Central venous pressure (CVP) is measured at the level of the heart with the patient lying flat. CVP is utilized to guide fluid resuscitation and/or diuresis, as well as to monitor for acute perioperative complications such as acute pulmonary hypertensive crisis. Fluid resuscitation beyond a CVP of around 15 mm Hg is unlikely to be beneficial.
4. Removal: temporary lines placed for perioperative use can be removed when no longer needed for volume or medication infusion (including total parenteral nutrition [TPN]), repeated blood draws, or CVP monitoring. Lines should be removed as soon as peripheral access will suffice to reduce the risk of central line–associated bloodstream infection (CLABSI). To reduce the risk of air embolus, lines are removed with the patient lying flat and creating positive intrathoracic pressure (e.g., by humming). Pressure is held over the venipuncture site and a sterile dressing is applied.

5. EBM Pearl: The implementation of central line insertion and maintenance bundles has been shown to reduce the risk of CLABSI, from 6.4 per 1,000 catheter days to 2.5 per 1,000 catheter days in one meta-analysis of adult, pediatric, and neonatal patients.[5]

CHEST TUBES

1. Indications:
   a. To evacuate fluid or air following chest surgery
   b. To monitor for air leak following lung surgery
   c. To monitor for and manage leaks following esophageal surgery
   d. To drain a pulmonary abscess or empyema
   e. Management of spontaneous pneumothorax
2. Types of catheters:
   a. Standard chest tubes – can be placed using a standard open technique or via the Seldinger technique using progressive dilators over a wire (e.g., QuickThal kits). Available in sizes from 12 Fr to 40 Fr. Larger-caliber tubes used for draining empyemas and hemothorax.
   b. Pigtail catheters – placed percutaneously using the Seldinger technique. Indicated for draining air and/or thin fluid.
   c. Blake drains – silicone drain with four grooved channels around a solid core center. Can be placed to Pleur-evac for drainage or to bulb suction.
3. Management:
   a. Chest tubes are generally connected to a Pleur-evac to allow evacuation of fluid and air without allowing air to be entrained into the chest. These devices combine three separate components (fluid collection, water seal, and suction control) into one box. A closed system should be maintained. If the Pleur-evac needs to be exchanged, it should be done using sterile technique.
   b. Routine radiographs – although many surgeons elect to obtain a chest x-ray daily in patients with a chest tube, this is not always necessary. An x-ray should be obtained immediately following surgery, following a change in management such as a decrease in the level of suction, and as indicated for signs and symptoms.
   c. Checking for air leak – modern Pleur-evacs contain an air leak detection chamber. This chamber should be observed at baseline and with the patient creating positive intrathoracic pressure (e.g., coughing) to check for bubbles. Many systems contain graduated air leak monitors, which allow you to quantify the number of chambers, for example, ranging from 1 (low) to 5 (high).
   d. Level of suction – suction is used as needed to optimize drainage of fluid from the chest or to keep the lung fully expanded. A suction level of −10 mm Hg in neonates and −20 mm Hg in children and adults is generally utilized, but can be increased up to −40 mm Hg as needed. Patients can be disconnected from suction (i.e. placed to water seal), even in the immediate postoperative period and/or in the presence of a small air leak, so long as the lung remains expanded and the chest adequately evacuated.
   e. Heimlich valve – these small one-way flutter valves are generally used to replace the Pleur-evac in children with minimal volume output but persistent small air leaks. In rare cases this can allow for discharge home with a chest tube remaining in place.
4. Removal: a chest tube can be removed when the indication for placement is no longer present (e.g., no evidence of air leak, low volume output, no evidence of esophageal leak, etc.). The tube is disconnected from suction for removal and is removed quickly with the patient maintaining positive intrathoracic pressure (e.g., by humming). If a "U" stitch was placed around the tube at the time of placement, this can be quickly tied by one person while another pulls the tube. An occlusive sterile dressing is placed over the chest tube site.

5. EBM Pearls:
   a. Although many surgeons leave a chest tube after most or all thoracic operations, there is some evidence that no chest tube is needed following operations with a very low risk of air leak such as lung biopsy, resection of an extralobar sequestration, Nuss procedure, resection of esophageal masses/duplications, and thymectomy.[6]
   b. Post-pull chest radiograph – although most surgeons obtain a "post-pull" chest radiograph, retrospective evidence suggests this is unnecessary. Small atmospheric post-pull pneumothoraces are relatively common, but only those with symptoms require a change in management. An exception may be patients going home immediately after tube removal.[7]

NEGATIVE PRESSURE WOUND THERAPY (NPWT OR "WOUND VAC")

1. Indications:
   a. Management of wounds (acute, chronic, traumatic, dehisced)
   b. Open abdomen management
   c. Skin grafts – as an alternative to a standard bolster dressing
2. Products:
   a. Control unit – a multitude of products are available from various companies. These units provide carefully regulated continuous or intermittent negative pressure, as well as sensors to detect leak from nonocclusive dressings.
   b. Sponges – various sponges from a multitude of companies are available. All are cut to fit within the surgical wound. They are designed to promote formation of granulation tissue, to help evenly distribute the negative pressure, and to allow for evacuation of exudative fluid. KCI makes a WhiteFoam dressing, which is premoistened and less adherent to underlying tissue and may be preferable for skin grafts or open abdomens. A WhiteFoam sponge can also be safely applied over exposed critical structures (nerves, blood vessels) to temporize contaminated wounds until they are ready for definitive soft tissue reconstruction.
   c. Open abdomen systems – these commercial systems include a fenestrated drape which lies below the abdominal wall but above the viscera to protect the abdominal organs yet allow efflux of peritoneal fluid. A foam dressing is applied above this drape to deliver uniform negative pressure, and then a clear adhesive barrier is applied over the foam to achieve a seal.
3. Management
   a. Settings – the clinician must select a pressure, an intensity, and a mode (continuous or intermittent). An intensity of -125 mm Hg is typically used for soft tissue wounds in older children and adults. Less negative pressures may be required for younger children, for open abdomens, or whenever there is concern for adverse effects of excessive negative pressure. The intensity regulates the speed with which the set pressure is achieved.
   b. Leaks – most NPWT systems will alert when a leak is detected. When this occurs, the clinician should ensure that all connections are secure and then assess for areas where the dressing has become nonocclusive. Dressings can be reinforced as needed to achieve a seal.
   c. Blockage – most NPWT systems will alert if a blockage is detected. The clinician should check to make sure the tubing is not clamped or kinked. The tubing can be "stripped" to attempt to clear visible clots. If these maneuvers fail to resolve the blockage, the tubing and/or vac dressing may need to be replaced.
   d. Dressing changes – dressing changes are typically performed every 3 to 5 days. Most dressing changes can be performed using aseptic technique at the bedside with appropriate pain control or sedation. The existing dressing and sponge are removed. A new

sponge is cut to the desired size, placed in the wound, and covered with the provided adhesive dressing. A small hole is cut in the adhesive dressing, over which the circular dressing attached to the tubing is applied.

4. EBM Pearl: A Cochrane review found insufficient evidence to permit any conclusions regarding the potential benefits of NPWT for partial-thickness burns.[8]

OTHER POSTOPERATIVE MONITORING

MICROVASCULAR SURGERY MONITORING

Free tissue transfers ("free flaps") rely on surgically created microanastomoses of arteries and veins for the transplanted tissue to survive. There are several methods of monitoring these flaps to alert the clinician to a microvascular problem before it might be clinically detectable. Any concern for thrombosis or change in Doppler tones is an indication for evaluation by the plastic surgery service at the least, and is often an indication for emergent surgical re-exploration. Because thrombotic events are most likely to occur in the first 24 hours following surgery, these patients are typically kept NPO the night of surgery.

1. Flap appearance – the gold standard of evaluation, with a healthy flap appearing warm, pink, and with capillary refill of <2 seconds. A flap with arterial thrombosis will have insufficient blood flow to the transplanted tissue and will appear pale and cool. Furthermore, a needle can be used to poke the flap to detect any bleeding from the tissues. An absence of bright red blood following needle stick is also suggestive of arterial insufficiency, most often caused by thrombosis. On the contrary, a flap that appears dark with overly brisk capillary refill is likely too engorged with blood and may be the result of venous thrombosis, where inflow is maintained, but outflow is obstructed. In this setting, needle stick will result in brisk bleeding of dark, deoxygenated venous blood.

2. Doppler assessment – of the many available tools for monitoring flaps, Doppler assessment is most commonly utilized. Branches of the main flap artery arborize to reach the surface component of the flap and can be detected using a handheld "pencil" Doppler. These sites are typically marked by the surgeons in the operating room with a staple, stitch, or marker, and the Doppler tones are checked every 30 minutes to 1 hour for the first 24 hours following surgery. Due to the potential for false-positive readings with this method, some surgeons choose not to rely on pencil Dopplers and instead use them as a backup or not at all. Venous Dopplers can be implanted using a small silastic cuff that surrounds the recipient vein of the microanastomosis and provides a continuous assessment of venous flow out of the transplanted tissue. Due to their small size and delicate nature, these devices may require some troubleshooting from time to time, but are considered more reliable than monitoring arterial tones.

3. Transcutaneous tissue oximetry - several devices are available that utilize transcutaneous tissue oximetry within a flap. While the early results of head-to-head comparisons with more traditional monitoring techniques have demonstrated earlier detection of thrombotic events and increased rates of flap salvage, these remain less commonly utilized at present. One limitation to these technologies is that they require the flap to have a skin component for placement of the probe.

DOPPLER TONES

Doppler tone assessment may be indicated following a variety of procedures other than microvascular surgery, including orthopedic, vascular, or transplant operations, to monitor arterial or venous flow.

1. Distal perfusion – arterial Doppler tones are often checked in the upper or lower extremities following a trauma or operation with the potential to compromise distal perfusion. This could include a vascular reconstruction or bypass, a fracture reduction, or an injury with concern for compartment syndrome. This can be assessed by simple evaluation of the strength and character of the tones or by measurement of an ankle-brachial index (ABI) or brachial-brachial index (BBI). In those cases, the systolic pressure in the involved limb is compared to that in an uninvolved arm using a blood pressure cuff while listening distally to the Doppler tones.

2. Liver transplant – hepatic artery thrombosis is a serious complication following liver transplant, which can lead to ischemic cholangiopathy. Some surgeons utilize an implantable Doppler probe on the hepatic artery to allow for continuous monitoring and early intervention.

INTRA-ABDOMINAL PRESSURE (BLADDER PRESSURE) MONITORING

Measurement of intra-abdominal pressure (IAP) should be performed in children with concern for abdominal hypertension or abdominal compartment syndrome.[9] This can include children with significant abdominal or pelvic trauma, bowel distention, postoperative intra-abdominal bleeding, etc. IAP is measured at end expiration in the supine position. Abdominal muscle contractions must be absent. Pressure is measured via the Foley catheter with 25 mL of sterile saline instilled in the bladder. Intra-abdominal hypertension is defined as IAP >12 mm Hg. Abdominal compartment syndrome (ACS) is defined as IAP >20 mm Hg in conjunction with organ dysfunction. ACS requires urgent surgical evaluation for decompressive laparotomy.

REFERENCES

1. Nelson R, Edwards S, Tse B. Prophylactic nasogastric decompression after abdominal surgery. *Cochrane Database Syst Rev.* 2005(1):CD004929.

2. Cheng Y, Zhou S, Zhou R, et al. Abdominal drainage to prevent intra-peritoneal abscess after open appendectomy for complicated appendicitis. *Cochrane Database Syst Rev.* 2015(2):CD010168.

3. CDC. Catheter-associated Urinary Tract Infections (CAUTI) | HAI | CDC https://www.cdc.gov/hai/ca_uti/uti.html accessed 12/19/17.

4. Zaouter C, Ouattara A. How long is a transurethral catheter necessary in patients undergoing thoracotomy and receiving thoracic epidural analgesia? Literature review. *J Cardiothorac Vasc Anesth.* 2015;29(2):496-501.

5. Ista E, van der Hoven B, Kornelisse RF, et al. Effectiveness of insertion and maintenance bundles to prevent central-line-associated bloodstream infections in critically ill patients of all ages: a systematic review and meta-analysis. *Lancet Infect Dis.* 2016;16(6):724-734.

6. Ponsky TA, Rothenberg SS, Tsao K, Ostlie DJ, St Peter SD, Holcomb GW 3rd. Thoracoscopy in children: is a chest tube necessary? *J Laparoendosc Adv Surg Tech A.* 2009;19(Suppl 1):S23-S25.

7. Cunningham JP, Knott EM, Gasior AC, et al. Is routine chest radiograph necessary after chest tube removal? *J Pediatr Surg.* 2014;49(10):1493-1495.

8. Dumville JC, Munson C, Christie J. Negative pressure wound therapy for partial-thickness burns. *Cochrane Database Syst Rev.* 2014(12):CD006215.

9. WSACS. WSACS consensus guidelines summary. https://www.wsacs.org/education/definitions-recommendations/summary.html. Accessed June 11, 2016.

Pediatric Trauma

EPIDEMIOLOGY

- Approximately 17,000 children and adolescents die from injuries, intentional and unintentional, each year.[1]
- Injury is the leading cause of death and disability in children.

EVALUATION AND ASSESSMENT

ADVANCED TRAUMA LIFE SUPPORT (ATLS)

- ATLS Sequence:[2-3] Outlines a standard approach to trauma patients that reduces mortality and morbidity. The evaluation and assessment are critical for appropriate triage, diagnosis, and treatment of the trauma patient.
- Primary survey and resuscitation: Serves to identify life-threatening conditions and should take only a few minutes.
  - *Assess for a pulse*: if no pulse is present, initiate cardiopulmonary resuscitation (CPR).
  - *Assess the airway*: determine if blood, stomach contents, edema, foreign bodies, or facial trauma is present; the presence of a closed head injury may lead to airway instability and be signified by the presence of stridor or inability to maintain a patent airway.
  - *Assess breathing*: breathing may be impaired by neurologic process, airway obstruction, chest wall, or respiratory pathology.
  - *Major hemorrhage*: all efforts should be made to control bleeding.
  - *Assess disability and exposure*: by evaluating neurologic status using the Glasgow Coma Scale (GCS) (Table 12-1)
    - Assess pupil size and reactivity to help ascertain underlying neurologic injury
    - Patient's clothes should be fully removed to facilitate a full exam
    - Remove any hazardous material
    - Reduce risk of hypothermia from saturated clothing; avoid hyperthermia
  - *Inline stabilization*: should be used to avoid worsening of potential cervical cord injury; cervical spine injury should be assumed; even though the incidence is rare, the consequences are devastating.
- Secondary survey: goal is to identify any other injury
  - More thorough history and examination; the practitioner can determine which laboratory and diagnostic tests are indicated to rule out underlying injury
  - "Pan-scanning" of pediatric trauma patients is not recommended, but further imaging is recommended when history and physical examination indicate suspicion for injury

IMAGING STUDIES (SEE TABLE 12-2)

- Guided by the primary and secondary surveys
- Undertaken with a direct indication in mind in order to reduce radiation exposure and guided by the primary and secondary surveys

TABLE 12-1	Glasgow Coma Scale[8]	
Behavior	**Response**	**Score**
Eye Opening Response	Spontaneously	4
	To speech	3
	To pain	2
	No response	1
Verbal Response	Oriented to time, place, and person	5
	Confused	4
	Inappropriate words	3
	Incomprehensible sounds	2
	No response	1
Best Motor Response	Obeys commands	6
	Moves to localized pain	5
	Flexion withdrawal from pain	4
	Abnormal flexion (decorticate)	3
	Abnormal extension (decerebrate)	2
	No response	1

TABLE 12-2	Imaging modalities in pediatric trauma with indications for use	
Modality	**Anatomic Location**	**Timing**
Plain X-Rays	C-spine	If clinical clearance of C-spine is unable to be determined, films can be done when patient is hemodynamically stable
	Chest, pelvic, extremity	External signs of injury over the areas concerned or physiologic signs of injury on exam
CT	Head	Based on risk assessment determined by mechanism of injury and age* or
		GCS <15 or
		Symptoms concerning for neurologic process
		Presence of altered mental status or
		Palpable skull fracture
	Abdomen	ALT >125 or AST >200
		Gross hematuria or microhematuria (>5 RBC/HPF)
		Clinical signs/symptoms of abdominal injury
	C-spine	If clinical clearance or neck films not able to be obtained
	CTA	Blunt cerebrovascular injury suspected

*Patients under 2 years of age are considered at higher risk of head injury without obvious signs and should warrant a lower threshold for imaging.

UNIQUE CONSIDERATIONS FOR THE PEDIATRIC PATIENT

Multisystem injury[4]:
- In general, children have less fat and more elastic tissues, which make them prone to multisystem injury.
- The chest walls of children are more compliant and can absorb and distribute forces more evenly then adults, leading to fewer rib fractures; however, this can also mask serious underlying injury.
- The relative large size of solid organs in relationship to total body combined with minimal subcutaneous fat and thinner muscular structure make pediatric patients more prone to abdominal injury.

Hypothermia and fluid losses:
- Higher risk of hypothermia due to the larger body surface area to body mass index
- Greater insensible fluid losses

Shock:
- Children can compensate with normal blood pressures even when they lose up to 30 percent of their blood volume from hemorrhage.

NONACCIDENTAL TRAUMA (NAT):

- Epidemiology: leading cause of childhood injury and death[5-6]
  - 2 to 3.5/100,000 die each year from abuse and neglect
  - Greatest risk is from ages 0 to 3
  - 4,500 hospitalized per year for physical abuse
- Risk factors:
  - Child risk factors: younger age (<2); history of prematurity or medical conditions; history of perinatal condition; no consensus on gender or race, although black children have higher mortality
  - Perpetrators: history of abuse as a child, young parent, female (although male perpetrators more likely to be responsible in lethal child abuse)
  - Family/situational risk factors: abuse is higher during economic recession and in high poverty counties, 66 percent of families live in inner cities, 76 percent received public assistance, parents with lack of community support, decreased self-esteem, mental health or substance abuse issues, parent in foster care, unwanted pregnancy, engagement in criminal activity, less prenatal care, history of problems with adults, shorter birth intervals between children, history of separation from child in the first year of life, familial history of corporal punishment
- Clinical presentations:
  - Bruising: look for bruising not on bony prominences such as cheeks, ears, neck, genitals, buttocks, and back (and consider further imaging if you suspect fracture underlying); consider patterned bruising such as from fingers, kitchen utensils, cords, shoes; exclude Mongolian spots and hemangiomas on your exam
  - Burns: up to 35 percent of burns are due to abuse, so have a high index of suspicion; hands, legs, feet, and buttocks more likely to be involved in abuse; scald burns due to hot liquids are often characterized by forced immersion patterns like sharp demarcations of the burn edge with sparing of flexed areas rather than splatter burns; thermal injuries can be seen due to forced contact with a hot object like an iron, cigarette, utensils
  - Fractures: ribs common with forced squeezing; long bones with spiral or oblique fractures from twisting, metaphyseal chip fractures more likely accidental, any femur fracture in nonambulating child, rarely spine injury (most are younger than 2 and have multilevel trauma)

- Abusive head trauma (AHT): nonspecific presentation of vomiting, poor feedings, irritability or lethargy, seizures may lead to AHT being missed; primary injuries may include skull fractures, hemorrhage, cortical contusion, diffuse axonal injury; secondary injuries include cerebral edema, infarction, infection, herniation
- Ocular manifestations: periorbital hematomas, lacerations, subconjunctival hemorrhage, subluxed lens, glaucoma, papilledema; retinal hemorrhage often occurs in multiple layers and occurs in 60 to 85 percent of nonaccidental head injuries (sensitivity is 75 percent and 93 percent specific for child abuse when severe retinal hemorrhages present, 100% specific for NAT)
- Evaluation for NAT[7]:
  - History of bleeding disorders in patient or family
  - Labs: prothrombin time (PT), activated partial thromboplastin time (aPTT), factor VIII level, factor IX level, complete blood count (CBC), D-dimer, fibrinogen; urine and stool screens for blood, trauma labs as indicated, may require further testing for coagulopathy or osteogenesis imperfecta or causes of bone fragility such as calcium and vitamin D
  - Skeletal survey for any child <2 years of age with any evidence of abuse, and any child <5 or unable to communicate with suspicious fracture; may consider bone scan and repeat skeletal survey in 7 to 10 days if initial survey is negative but index of suspicion is high
  - Intracranial imaging – computerized tomography (CT), magnetic resonance imaging (MRI), or both
  - Abdominal imaging
  - Ophthalmologic exam – dilated fundoscopic exam when clinical status allows, may also see retinal hemorrhages on MRI with an orbit Susceptibility weighted imaging (SWI) protocol
  - Early electroencephalogram (EEG) in AHT – risk for subclinical seizures
- Treatment – treatment of found injuries, victims of AHT more likely to need neurosurgical intervention than accidental head injuries, consider antiepileptic treatment
- Outcome – high morbidity in children <2 years who suffered head injury for neurologic deficit (50 percent) and mortality (15 to 38 percent), reduced rates of regaining independent ambulation and expressive language in child of abuse rather than accidental injury, high rates of seizures early after AHT; this remains an issue for patients with more severe AHT who survive

ORGAN-SPECIFIC INJURIES

INTRATHORACIC INJURIES

- Clinical: include pulmonary contusions, pneumothorax, tracheal disruption, flail chest or rib fractures; cardiac injury is rarer. Should be suspected in any patient with signs of external bruising on the chest wall, irregular breathing patterns, unequal breath sounds, hypoxemia and/or hemodynamic instability. Additional workup for intrathoracic injury should include a 12-lead electrocardiogram (ECG) and chest x-ray.[4]
- Epidemiology: relatively rare in pediatrics; often in the setting of blunt force trauma either in motor vehicles or bicycle injuries; risk of mortality is higher (between 15 and 26 percent)[1] in part due to the association with other injuries.
- Flail chest: occurs when a segment of one or more ribs fractures at two distinct points, creating paradoxical movement with respiration.
  - Caused by high-energy injuries

- Rare in children due to the increased elasticity of their chest wall
- When it is present, it is often associated with pulmonary contusions, which contribute to hypoxemia and VQ mismatch.
- Pulmonary contusion: direct mechanical injury to the lung parenchyma, which results in hematoma within lung tissue itself
  - It is not always present initially on chest x-ray and may not become evident until hours after the initial trauma and resuscitation.
  - Treatment is conservative management with support of oxygenation.
- Pneumothorax/hemothorax: occurs when air or blood, respectively, accumulates in the pleural space.
  - *Hemothorax*: the cause is often related to the rupture of intercostal vessels or a broken rib; if not controlled, hemothorax can lead to hemorrhagic shock.
  - *Pneumothorax*: typically a tension pneumothorax from alveolar or tracheobronchial rupture.
  - Treatment is chest tube placement and supportive care with blood transfusion as needed. Emergent decompression when tamponade physiology is present may be indicated prior to thoracostomy tube placement if the patient is quickly deteriorating.
- Diaphragmatic rupture: occurs with blunt abdominal trauma; high pressure in the abdominal compartment results in herniation of abdominal contents into the chest; can lead to shock by impeding blood return to the heart and requires emergent surgical intervention.
- Tracheal or bronchial disruption: rare injuries occur when there are tears, most commonly close to the carina and posteriorly directed.
  - They should be suspected in the presence of dyspnea and subcutaneous emphysema.
  - They are also often associated with pneumothorax or pneumomediastinum.
  - Treatment includes preventing infection with antibiotic therapy, bronchoscopy, and ultimately surgical repair if conservative supportive medical management is not successful.
  - These injuries increase the risk of bronchopleural fistula formation.
- Cardiac injury: cardiac injuries are uncommon but life-threatening conditions.
  - *Commotio cordis* is a specific type of injury described after sudden impact to the anterior chest wall that may cause the heart to stop or induce arrhythmia; frequently described with projectile injury rather than with blunt trauma.
  - *Cardiac tamponade*: sudden decompensation can also indicate cardiac tamponade.
    - Blood quickly accumulates in the pericardial space and restricts filling of the myocardium, reducing cardiac output, which is exaggerated by shifting of the intraventricular septum into the left ventricular outflow tract and further impeding cardiac output.
    - Signs and symptoms of cardiac tamponade include tachycardia, narrow pulse pressure, jugular venous distention, and pulsus paradoxus. Breath sounds are normal which can help distinguish from a tension pneumothorax.
    - The definitive treatment is pericardiocentesis.
  - *Cardiac contusion*: the heart is also susceptible to wall contusions if the mechanism of injury is a high-energy accident creating chest wall compression.
    - Manifests as arrhythmias or lack of response to volume resuscitation.
    - Diagnosis can be made by echocardiography which will show dyskinetic wall motions.
    - Vasoactive medications should be used cautiously, as they increase myocardial oxygen demand but may have little contractility of the contused muscle.
  - *Cardiac rupture*: extremely rare and highly fatal; occurs in the setting of high-energy motor vehicle accidents or extremely high falls, and mortality occurs within seconds to minutes.

INTRA-ABDOMINAL INJURIES

- **Clinical:** most common trauma-related injury to go unrecognized, likely due to diversion by other external or more obvious injuries; liver and spleen are the most commonly injured structures in the abdomen. Due to their highly vascular nature, these injuries can lead to hemorrhagic shock.
  - *Signs:* include abrasions or bruising over the abdomen or back. In motor vehicle accidents, a "seat belt" sign may be present, which indicates bruising at the site of restraint and warrants further workup for internal injuries.
  - *Initial management:* nasogastric tube placement for decompression and Foley placement for assessment of the genitourinary (GU) tract, monitoring of fluid balance, and decompression of enlarged bladder.
  - *Imaging:* The Focused Assessment with Sonography in Trauma (FAST) exam can be used as a quick screening test for intra-abdominal injuries, but the presence or absence of solid organ injury is usually evaluated by CT scan.
- **Epidemiology:** third leading cause of traumatic death behind head and thoracic injury. Nearly one third of children with major trauma will have significant intraperitoneal injuries.
- **Splenic injury:** in addition to external signs of injury on the abdomen with tenderness, splenic injuries should be considered in patients who have blunt mechanisms directly to the abdomen, left shoulder pain (which is referred pain from diaphragmatic irritation), and shock.
  - These injuries are also diagnosed and graded based on CT imaging findings.
  - *Treatment:*
    - The higher-grade injuries require close monitoring and likely surgical intervention.
    - For lower-grade injuries with no hemodynamic compromise, conservative management with fluids and transfusions as needed with close monitoring is recommended.
    - Nonoperative management is successful in as many as 97 percent of cases of splenic injury.[4]
- **Liver injury:** similar to splenic injuries, liver injury can cause referred pain to the right shoulder.
  - These also may be detected by elevations in alanine aminotransferase (ALT) or aspartate aminotransferase (AST).
  - Liver injury is often seen with other associated injuries and can be diagnosed by CT scan.
  - *Treatment:*
    - Degree of injury is again graded on radiographic findings, with a higher degree indicative of the need for operative repair.
    - Conservative management is recommended in the absence of hemodynamic instability.
    - Close monitoring, fluid, and blood transfusions as needed are the mainstay of interventions.
- **Bowel injury:** less common then splenic and liver injury; require a higher index of suspicion for diagnosis.
  - Diagnostic studies, including CT scans, can be falsely reassuring; therefore, serial abdominal exams are the gold standard for diagnosis.
  - Suspicion should be high if there was a restraining seatbelt, handlebar, or nonaccidental injury involved in the trauma.
  - *Treatment:* surgery is often indicated to remove limited segments of affected area and to avoid ischemic strictures.

- Renal injury: should be suspected if there is penetrating right upper quadrant or left upper quadrant flank injury or a hematoma, pain, or tenderness in those areas, gross hematuria or micro-hematuria as evidenced by >5 RBCs/HPF on urine analysis.
  - Diagnose by abdominal imaging with a CT; graded based on radiologic findings on a scale of I to V.
  - *Treatment:*
    - If abdominal CT confirms injury, urology should be consulted.
    - Management can be conservative for low-grade injury, but patient should remain NPO until an observation period confirms stability.
    - For higher-grade injury (grades III to V), intensive care admission is required for closer monitoring, and surgical intervention would be recommended if there is hemodynamic instability.
    - Foley placement should await urologic evaluation if there are signs of blood at the meatus of the urethra; otherwise close monitoring of fluid balance is recommended.

*For intracranial and spinal injuries, please see Chapters 39 and 41.

NEAR DROWNING

- Epidemiology: approximately 15,000 to 70,000 near drownings occur in the United States each year.[1,4] Mortality is more likely with acute respiratory distress syndrome (ARDS) patients and often occurs directly from respiratory failure or indirectly from sepsis, multi-organ failure, or air leak syndrome.

  Depending on age, the location of near drownings varies:
  - Infants less than 1 year of age are most likely to drown in bathtubs.
  - Older children between the ages of 1 year and 4 years of age are likely to experience near drowning in pools.
  - Young adolescents are more likely to have near drowning experiences in fresh water.
- Prognosis is poor if:
  - Submersion was longer than 25 minutes
  - Delay in CPR
  - Severe acidosis on presentation
  - Arrival to an emergency department still pulseless
  - Elevated blood sugar on arrival
  - Dilated and fixed pupils on arrival
  - Abnormal initial CT
  - Initial GCS <5
- Pathophysiology:
  - Near drownings result in injury due to hypoxemia, which results after an apneic period.
  - Laryngospasm and pulmonary aspiration may contribute to the injury.
  - These insults then lead to acute lung injury, which may progress into ARDS. ARDS may occur after initial recovery.
  - Profound cardiovascular instability is often seen after an episode of severe near drowning.
  - Life-threatening arrhythmias such as ventricular tachycardia or fibrillation and asystole are most often a result of hypoxemia.
  - Cardiogenic shock may result from hypoxic damage to the myocardium.
  - Hypoxia, sufficiently prolonged, causes profound disturbances of central nervous system (CNS) function.
  - The severity of brain injury depends on the magnitude and duration of hypoxia.

- Treatment:
  - Supportive management focuses on respiratory support through mechanical ventilation. Patients often require high FIO_2 and high positive end-expiratory pressure (PEEP).
  - There is no evidence for the initial use of steroids or antibiotics unless superinfection is suspected.
  - Monitor for hypothermia, as it can lead to arrhythmias, acidosis, and coagulopathy. Treatment includes increasing ambient temperature, removal of wet clothing, heating blankets, and warm fluids.
  - Close monitoring is recommended for all near drowning admissions.
  - Arterial and central venous pressure (CVP) monitoring is often required.
  - Extracorporeal membrane oxygenation (ECMO) may be considered in patients with severe lung injury or severe hypothermia.

REFERENCES

1. Kenefake ME, Swarm M, Walthall J. Nuances in pediatric trauma. *Emerg Med Clin North Am*. 2013;31(3):627-652.
2. van Olden GDJ, Dik Meeuwis J, Bolhuis HW, Boxma H, Goris RJA. Clinical impact of advanced trauma life support. *Am J Emerg Med*. 2004;22(7):522-525.
3. Bell RM, Krantz BE, Weigelt JA. ATLS: a foundation for trauma training. *Ann Emerg Med*. 1999;34(2):233-237.
4. Zamakhshary M, Wales PW. *Hospital for Sick Children Manual of Pediatric Trauma*. Lippincott: Philadelphia, PA; 2008:145-160.
5. Paul AR, Adamo MA. Non-accidental trauma in pediatric patietns: a review of epidemiology, pathophysiology, doagnosis, and treatment. *Transl Pediatri*. 2014;3(3):195-207.
6. Farrell CA, Fleegler EW, Monuteaux MC, Wilson CR, Christian CW, Lee LK. Community poverty and child abuse fatalities in the United States. *Pediatrics*. 2017;139(5):1-9.
7. Campbell KA, Olson LM, Keenan HT. Critical elements in the medical evaluation of suspected child physical abuse. *Pediatrics*. 2015;136(1):35-43.
8. Teasdale G, Jennett B. Assessment of coma and impaired consciousness. A practical scale. *Lancet*. 1974;304(7872):81-84.

Pharmacology

In addition to medications in this formulary chapter, the following categories of medications can be found in the identified chapters:

Intubation Medications - see chapter 6
Code Medications - see chapter 7
Cardiovascular Medications - see chapter 14
Sedation/Analgesia/Neuromuscular Blockade - see chapter 15
Anti-infective Medications - see chapter 16

Respiratory			
Medication	**Dose**	**Mechanism**	**Comment**
Albuterol	Intermittent 2.5 mg nebulization or Continuous nebulization from 5–20 mg/hr	ß2-agonist: bronchodilation via airway smooth muscle relaxation	Frequent re-evaluation needed, especially if tachycardic Side effects: tremor, tachycardia, agitation, hypokalemia
Acetylcysteine	Infants: 1–2 mL of 20% solution or 2–4 mL of 10% solution (undiluted); three to four times daily Children and adolescents: 3–5 mL of 20% solution or 6–10 mL of 10% solution (undiluted); administer three to four times daily	Exerts mucolytic action through its free sulfhydryl group, which opens up the disulfide bonds in the mucoproteins, thus lowering mucous viscosity	
Ipratropium	125–500 mcg nebulization q6–8 hr	Inhaled anticholinergic (inhibit cGMP) bronchodilator	Systemic SEs rare due to poor absorption from lung
Saline nebulization 0.9%, 3%, 7%	3% solution: 4 mL inhaled every 2 hr ≥6 years and adolescents: inhalation: 7% solution: 4 mL inhaled twice daily		Pretreatment with a bronchodilator is recommended to prevent potential bronchospasm
Terbutaline	Load: 2–10 mcg/kg IV Infusion: 0.08–1 mcg/kg/min	Systemic ß2-agonist	SEs same as albuterol Stop infusion and obtain ECG for chest pain or ST changes

SE: Side Effects

Neurologic			
Medication	**Route**	**Dose**	**Mechanism**
Midazolam	IV bolus	Loading dose: 0.15–0.2 mg/kg	Enhances GABA activity
	IV infusion	0.06–0.5 mg/kg/hr	
	Intramuscular	0.2 mg/kg/dose, may repeat every 10–15 min, maximum dose: 6 mg	
	Buccal	0.2–0.5 mg/kg once; maximum dose: 10 mg	
	Intranasal	0.2 mg/kg once; maximum dose: 10 mg	
Lorazepam	IV bolus	0.1 mg/kg maximum: 4 mg, slow IV over 2–5 min; may repeat in 5–15 min	
Diazepam	IV bolus	0.1–0.3 mg/kg/dose given over 3–5 min, every 5–10 min; maximum dose: 10 mg/dose	
	Rectal	2–5 years: 0.5 mg/kg	
		6–11 years: 0.3 mg/kg	
		≥12 years and adolescents: 0.2 mg/kg	
Fosphenytoin	IV bolus	15–20 mg PE/kg; maximum dose: 1500 mg PE	Stabilizes voltage-gated sodium channels
		Administer at 1–3 mg PE/kg/min up to a maximum of 150 mg PE/min	
Levetiracetam	IV bolus	20–60 mg/kg; dose should not exceed adult initial range: 1000–3000 mg	Thought to have multiple sites of action, including calcium channels, glutamate receptors, and GABA modulation
Pentobarbital	IV bolus	Loading dose: 5 mg/kg	Enhances GABA activity
	IV infusion	Initial: 0.5–1 mg/kg/hr	
Phenobarbital	IV bolus	15–20 mg/kg; maximum dose: 1000 mg	

PE: Phenytoin equivalent; GABA: gamma-aminobutyric acid.

Miscellaneous			
Medication	**Dose**	**Mechanism**	**Comment**
Albumin	0.5–1 g/kg/dose IV Use 5% in hypovolemic or intravascularly depleted patients Use 25% in fluid/Na restricted patients	Provides increase in intravascular oncotic pressure	Administration rate: 5% = 2–4 mL/min 25% = 1 mL/min (after initial volume replacement)
Diphenhydramine	0.5 mg/kg/dose IV/PO Maximum dose: 50 mg	Antihistamine	
Haloperidol	Limited data available ≥3 months, children, and adolescents: IV (lactate, immediate release): loading dose: 0.15–0.25 mg/dose infused slowly over 30–45 min	Nonselectively blocks postsynaptic dopaminergic receptors in the brain	Use has been associated with adverse effects, including cardiac effects, circulatory and respiratory insufficiency, extrapyramidal symptoms, and neuroleptic malignant syndrome
Mannitol	IV bolus 0.25–1 g/kg/dose infused over 20–30 min	Osmotic diuresis, decrease in ICP through osmosis and reduction in blood viscosity	
Metoclopramide	0.1 mg/kg/dose IV/PO	Enhances motility and accelerates gastric emptying	
Naloxone	Full reversal: 0.1 mg/kg/dose IV (2 mg max) For respiratory depression: 0.001–0.005 mg/kg/dose	Opioid antagonist	
Octreotide	Load: 1–2 mcg/kg bolus IV over 2–5 min Maintenance: IV: 1–10 mcg/kg/hr continuous infusion	Mimics natural somatostatin	Consider tapering dose for discontinuation
Ondansetron	0.1 mg/kg/dose IV/PO	Selective 5-HT_3-receptor antagonist	

ICP: Intracranial pressure.

Systemic Steroids

Medication	Dose	Mechanism	Comment
Prednisolone (PO)	Load: 2 mg/kg Max: usually 60 mg Maintenance: 0.5–1 mg/kg q6 hr Max: usually 60 mg/dose	Decrease inflammation, mucus production, and mediator release	Stress dosing may be needed for patients on long-term steroids Max effect 6–12 hr No Δ PO/IV dose
Methylprednisolone (IV)	Load: 2 mg/kg Max: usually 60 mg Maintenance: 0.5–1mg/kg q6 hr max: usually 60 mg/dose		
Hydrocortisone	Shock: IV 50–100 mg/m²/day divided every 6 hr Physiologic replacement: IV/PO 8–10 mg/m²/day divided every 8 hr	Decreases inflammation and reverses increased capillary permeability	No Δ PO/IV dose
Dexamethasone	Croup: 0.6 mg/kg/dose IV/PO once	Decreases inflammation and mediator release	No Δ PO/IV dose

Glucorticoid Equivalency Table

Glucocorticoid	Equivalent Dose (mg)	Routes	Relative Anti-inflammatory Potency	Relative Mineralo-corticoid Potency	Elimination Half-Life (hr)
Cortisone	25	PO, IM	0.8	0.8	~0.5
Hydrocortisone	20	IM, IV	1	1	~2
MethylPREDNISolone	4	PO, IM, IV	5	0	1–2
PrednisoLONE	5	PO	4	0.8	2–4
PredniSONE	5	PO	4	0.8	2–3
Dexamethasone	0.75	PO, IM, IV	25–30	0	~4
Fludrocortisone	—	PO	10	125	~3.5

Electrolytes

Medication	Dose	Max Dose	Max Rate
3% Sodium chloride	Increased intracranial pressure: 2–5 mL/kg/dose Na def = [desired sodium (mEq/L) − actual sodium (mEq/L)] × [0.6 × wt (kg)] 3% has 513 mEq Na/L		1 mEq/kg/hr 10 mEq/kg/hour when treating acute, life-threatening ICP elevation
Arginine chloride	To correct hypochloremia: (mEq) = 0.2 × kg × [103 − Cl⁻] give ¹/₂ to ²/₃ of calculated dose and reevaluate	Supplements chloride ions Potassium chloride and sodium chloride supplementation should be considered	
Calcium chloride	10–20 mg/kg/dose IV/IO; slow IV push Calcium chloride is three times more potent than calcium gluconate	1 gm/dose [2 gm/dose: CV arrest]	IVP = 50–100 mg/min Infusion = 45–90 mg/kg over 1hr
Calcium gluconate	100 mg/kg/dose IV/IO over 15–20 min 1 gm Ca gluc = 90 mg elemental Ca = 4.5 mEq Ca	2–3 gm/dose	IVP = 50–100 mg/min Infusion = 200 mg/min
Magnesium sulfate	25–50 mg/kg/dose IV/IO/IM	2 gm	Pediatric: 125 mg/kg/hr Adult: 2 gm/hr; can give over 15–20 min in emergent situations
Potassium chloride	0.5–1 mEq/kg/dose IV over 2–3 hr	40 mEq	Infuse at 0.5 mEq/kg/hour or 10 mEq/hour (whichever is slower)
Potassium phosphate	0.16–0.36 mmol/kg/dose IV over 6 hr 3 mmol phos + 4.4 mEq potassium per mL	Dose limit: 27 mmol Phos = 40 mEq K	0.06 mmol/kg/hr
Sodium bicarbonate 4.2% (0.5 mEq/ml) (for <2 yr old)	1 mEq/kg/dose IV/IO; do not administer through UAC	50 mEq	IVP: 10 mEq/min Infusion: 0.33 mEq/kg/hr
Sodium bicarbonate 8.4% (1 mEq/ml) (For >2 yr old)	1 mEq/kg/dose IV/IO; do not administer through UAC	50 mEq	IVP: 10 mEq/min Infusion: 0.33 mEq/kg/hr
Sodium phosphate	0.16–0.36 mmol/kg/dose IV over 6 hr 3 mmol phos + 4 mEq Na/ml		0.06 mmol/kg/hr

Diuretics				
Loop Diuretic	**Dose**	**Bioavailability (PO/IV dose ratio)**	**Equivalent Dosing**	**Max Daily Dose**
Diuretic that inhibits reabsorption of sodium and chloride in the ascending loop of Henle and proximal renal tubule				
Furosemide IV	1–2 mg/kg/dose every 6–12 hr	100%	1 mg/kg	8 mg/kg/day Up to 8 gm/day in adults
Furosemide PO	1–2 mg/kg/dose every 6–12 hr	~50% (2:1)	2 mg/kg	8 mg/kg/day Up to 8 gm/day in adults
Bumetanide IV	0.015–0.1 mg/kg/dose every 6–24 hr (max dose: 10 mg/day)	100%	0.025 mg/kg	0.2 mg/kg/day
Bumetanide PO	0.015–0.1 mg/kg/dose every 6–24 hr	80%–90% (1:1)	0.025 mg/kg	0.2 mg/kg/day (max dose: 10 mg/day)
Torsemide (Demadex) PO	Adult: 20 mg once daily	80%–100% (1:1)	0.5 mg/kg	4 mg/kg/day Max adult: 200 mg/day

Thiazide-Like Diuretics	**Dose**	**Biovailability (PO/IV dose ratio)**	**Equivalent Dosing**	**Max Daily Dose**
Diuretic that inhibits sodium reabsorption in the distal tubules				
Chlorothiazide (Diuril) IV	IV: 5–10 mg/kg/day in two divided doses	100%	1 mg/kg	40 mg/kg/day Or Adult max: 2000 mg/day
Chlorothiazide (Diuril) PO	20–40 mg/kg/day in two divided doses	65%–75% (~1:0.7)	1 mg/kg	40 mg/kg/day Or Adult max: 2000 mg/day
Hydrochlorothiazide (HydroDIURIL) PO	1–2 mg/kg/day in one to two divided doses	65%–75% (NA)	0.1 mg/kg	4 mg/kg/day Or Adult max: 200 mg/day
Metolazone (Zaroxolyn) PO	0.2–0.4 mg/kg/day divided every 12–24 hr	40%–65% (NA)	0.01 mg/kg	0.4 mg/kg/day Or Adult max: 20 mg/day

Other Diuretics	Dosing	Bioavailability	Equivalent Dosing	Max Daily Dose
Diuretic working in the distal renal tubules, increasing sodium chloride and water excretion while conserving potassium				
Spironolactone (Aldactone) PO	1–3.3 mg/kg/day	50%–80% (NA)	NA	3.5 mg/kg/day Or Adult max: 400 mg/day
Carbonic anhydrase inhibitors; reduced HCO_3 reabsorption in the renal proximal tubule				
Acetazolamide	Acetazolamide (5 mg/kg q24–q8)	Dose dependent	NA	

FREQUENTLY USED PARENTERAL FLUIDS (MEQ PER LITER)

Liquid	Na	Cl−	K+	Ca+	Lactate (~HCO_3)	mOsm/L
D5W	–	–			–	252
0.9% NS	154	154			–	308
3% NS	513	513			–	1027
Lactated Ringer's (LR)	130	109	4	2.7	28	273

SUGGESTED READINGS

Abend N, Dlugos D. Treatment of refractory status epilepticus: literature review and a proposed protocol. *Pediatr Neurol.* 2008;38:377-390.

Acetylcysteine [package insert]. Shirley, NY: American Regent, Inc.; 2011.

Asare K. Diagnosis and treatment of adrenal insufficiency in the critically ill patient. *Pharmacotherapy.* 2007;27(11):1512-1528.

Ashrafi MR, Khosroshahi N, Karimi P, et al. Efficacy and usability of buccal midazolam in controlling acute prolonged convulsive seizures in children. *Eur J Paediatr Neurol.* 2010;14:434-438.

Auron M, Raissouni N. Adrenal insufficiency. *Pediatr Rev.* 2015;36(3):92-102.

Ausejo M, Saenz A, Pham B, et al. The effectiveness of glucocorticoids in treating croup: meta-analysis. *BMJ.* 1999;319:595-600.

Bailie MD. Diuretic treatment agents. *Adv Pediatr.* 1993;40:273-285.

Baliga R, Lewy JE. Pathogenesis and treatment of edema. *Ped Clin North Am.* 1987;34(3):693-648.

Bogie AL, Towne D, Luckett PM, Abramo TJ, Wiebe RA. Comparison of intravenous terbutaline versus normal saline in pediatric patients on continuous high-dose nebulized albuterol for status asthmaticus. *Pediatr Emerg Care.* 2007;23(6):355-361.

Brenkert TE, Estrada CM, McMorrow SP, Abramo TJ. Intravenous hypertonic saline use in the pediatric emergency department. *Pediatr Emerg Care.* 2013;29(1):71-73.

Brophy GM, Bell R, Claassen J, et al. Guidelines for the evaluation and management of status epilepticus. *Neurocrit Care.* 2012;17:3-23.

Chemtob S, Kaplan BS, Sherbotie JR, et al. Pharmacology of diuretics in the newborn. *Ped Clin North Am*. 1989;36(5):1231-1250.

Dellon EP, Donaldson SH, Johnson R, et al. Safety and tolerability of inhaled hypertonic saline in young children with cystic fibrosis. *Pediatr Pulmonol*. 2008;43(11):1100-1106.

Diastat [package insert] Bridgewater, NJ. Valeant Pharmaceuticals; 2016.

Felker GM, Lee KL, Bull DA, et al. Diuretic strategies in patients with acute decompensated heart failure. *N Engl J Med*. 2011;364(9):797-805.

Frey BM, Frey FJ. Clinical pharmacokinetics of prednisone and prednisolone. *Clin Pharmacokinet*. 1990;19(2):126-146.

Holsti M, Dudley N, Schunk J, et al. Intranasal midazolam vs rectal diazepam for the home treatment of acute seizures in pediatric patients with epilepsy. *Arch Pediatr Adolesc Med*. 2010;164(8):747-753.

Hunt SA, Abraham WT, Chin MH, et al. ACC/AHA 2005 guideline update for the diagnosis and management of chronic heart failure in the adult-summary article: a report of the American College of Cardiology/American Heart Association Task Force on Practice Guidelines (Writing Committee to Update the 2001 Guidelines for the Evaluation and Management of Heart Failure). *J Am Coll Cardiol*. 2005;46(6):1116-1143.

Kohr LM, O'Brien P. Current management of congestive heart failure in infants and children. *Nur Clin North Am*. 1995;30(2):261-290.

Kuzik BA, Al-Qadhi SA, Kent S, et al. Nebulized hypertonic saline in the treatment of viral bronchiolitis in infants. *J Pediatr*. 2007;151(3):266-270, 270.e1.

Lactated Ringer's [package insert]. Deerfield, IL. Baxter Healthcare Corp.; 2013.

National Asthma Education and Prevention Program (NAEPP). Expert Panel Report 3 (EPR-3): Guidelines for the Diagnosis and Management of Asthma, Clinical Practice Guidelines. National Institutes of Health, National Heart, Lung, and Blood Institute, NIH Publication No. 08-4051, prepublication 2007, Bethesda, MD; available at http://www.nhlbi.nih.gov/guidelines/asthma/asthgdln.htm.

Phelps S, Hageman T, Lee K, Thompson A, eds. *Pediatric Injectable Drugs: The Teddy Bear Book*. American Society of Health Systems Pharmacists, Bethesda, MD; 2013.

Roehr CC, Jung A, Proquitté H, et al. Somatostatin or octreotide as treatment options for chylothorax in young children: a systematic review. *Intensive Care Med*. 2006;32(5):650-657.

van der Vorst MM, Kist JE, van der Heijden AJ, et al. Diuretics in pediatrics: current knowledge and future prospects. *Paediatr Drugs*. 2006;8(4):245-264.

Wells TG. The pharmacology and therapeutics of diuretics in the pediatric patient. *Ped Clin North Am*. 1990;37(2):463-504.

Witte MK, Stork JE, Blumer JL. Diuretic therapeutics in the pediatric patient. *Am J Card*. 1986;57:44a-53a.

Antiarrhythmic Medications	Class	Dose	Mechanism
Procainamide	Ia	IV: Loading dose: 10–15 mg/kg over 30–60 min; in adults, maximum dose range: 1000–1500 mg	Decreases atrial and ventricular automaticity, vagolytic effect
		Maintenance: Continuous IV infusion: 20–80 mcg/kg/minute; maximum daily dose: 2000 mg/24 hr	
Lidocaine	Ib	IV: Loading dose: 1 mg/kg/dose; follow with continuous IV infusion; may administer second bolus if delay between initial bolus and start of infusion is >15 min	Affects ventricular tissue
		Continuous IV infusion: 20–50 mcg/kg/min	
Mexiletine		PO: 1.4–5 mg/kg/dose (mean: 3.3 mg/kg/dose) given every 8 hr	
Phenytoin		IV/PO: Loading dose: 15–20 mg/kg	
		Maintenance therapy: Initial: 5 mg/kg/day in divided doses	
Flecainide	Ic	PO: Initial: 1–3 mg/kg/day or 50–100 mg/m^2/day in three divided doses	Slows conduction velocities throughout the myocardium
Propafenone		PO: Initial 200–300 mg/m^2/24 hr divided in three or four equal doses or 8–10 mg/kg/24 hr in three or four equal doses	
Esmolol	II	Initial IV bolus: 100–500 mcg/kg over 1 min	Lowers heart rate, decreases automaticity, slows AV nodal conduction
		Continuous IV infusion: Initial rate: 25–100 mcg/kg/min	
Propranolol		PO: Initial: 0.5–1 mg/kg/day in divided doses every 6–8 hr; max 16 mg/kg/day	
Metoprolol		PO: Initial: 0.5–1 mg/kg/dose (maximum initial dose: 25 mg/dose) twice daily	
Ibutilide	III	<60 kg: 0.01 mg/kg over 10 min	Prolongs repolarization and refractoriness of atrial, nodal, and ventricular tissue
		≥60 kg: 1 mg over 10 min	

(continued)

Antiarrhythmic Medications	Class	Dose	Mechanism
Sotalol		Initial: Infants, children, and adolescents: 2 mg/kg/day divided every 8 hr	
Amiodarone		IV: Loading dose: 5 mg/kg (maximum: 300 mg/dose) given over 60 min	
		Continuous IV infusion (if needed): Initial: 5 mcg/kg/min; increase incrementally as clinically needed	
Verapamil	IV	IV:	Slows conduction in sinus and AV nodes
		0.1–0.3 mg/kg/dose (usual dose: 2–5 mg/dose); maximum dose: 5 mg/dose; may repeat dose in 15–30 min if response inadequate	
Diltiazem		Adults:	
		Initial bolus dose: 0.25 mg/kg actual body weight over 2 min	
Digoxin	Misc	Please consult pharmacy for patient-specific dosing	Directly suppresses AV node conduction
Adenosine	Misc	Rapid IV, IO: Initial: 0.1 mg/kg (maximum initial dose: 6 mg/dose)	
Magnesium	Misc	IV, IO: 25–50 mg/kg/dose	
Atropine	Misc	IV, IO: 0.02 mg/kg/dose; minimum dose recommended by pediatric advanced life support (PALS): 0.1 mg; is not recommended in patients <5 kg	
Isoproterenol	Misc	Continuous IV infusion:	
		0.05–2 mcg/kg/min; titrate to effect	

Continuous Infusion Medications	Dose Range (route = IV)	Mechanism
Alprostadil	0.01–0.4 mcg/kg/min	Vasodilation by means of direct effect on vascular and ductus arteriosus smooth muscle
Amiodarone	Load 5 mg/kg over 60 min Drip 3–15 mcg/kg/min	Class III antiarrhythmic; alpha- and beta-blocking properties; affects sodium, potassium, and calcium channels; prolongs the action potential and refractory period in myocardial tissue; decreases AV conduction and sinus node function

Continuous Infusion Medications	Dose Range (route = IV)	Mechanism
Bumex (bumetanide)	0.008–1 mg/hr	Diuretic that inhibits reabsorption of sodium and chloride in the ascending loop of Henle and proximal renal tubule
Dobutamine	2–20 mcg/kg/min	Beta-adrenergic receptors and some alpha-receptor agonism, resulting in increased contractility and heart rate, also stimulates beta- and alpha-receptors in the vasculature
Dopamine	2–20 mcg/kg/min	Direct and indirect action via release of norepinephrine
Epinephrine	0.02–1 mcg/kg/min	Endogenous catecholamine with potent alpha and beta effects
Esmolol	Load: 500 mcg/kg over 1 min Maintenance: 50–500 mcg/kg/min	Blocks response to beta-adrenergic stimulation
Furosemide	0.05–10 mg/hr	Diuretic that inhibits reabsorption of sodium and chloride in the ascending loop of Henle and proximal renal tubule
Heparin	Load: 75 units/kg 10–35 units/kg/hr	Inhibits thrombin-activated conversion of fibrinogen to fibrin
Isoproterenol	0.02–2 mcg/kg/min	Stimulates beta-receptors, resulting in increased heart rate and contractility
Lidocaine	Load: 1 mg/kg, repeat 10–15 min for two doses Maintenance: 20–50 mcg/kg/min	Blocks fast sodium channels with rapid association dissociation
Milrinone	0.1–0.75 mcg/kg/min	Phosphodiesterase inhibitor in cardiac and vascular tissue, resulting in vasodilation and inotropic effects
Nicardipine	0.5–5 mcg/kg/min	Inhibits calcium ion uptake, resulting in a relaxation of coronary vascular smooth muscle and coronary vasodilation
Nitroglycerin	0.25–20 mcg/kg/min	Vasodilating agent that dilates peripheral veins and arteries
Nitroprusside	0.3–10 mcg/kg/min	Direct-acting vasodilator

(continued)

Continuous Infusion Medications	Dose Range (route = IV)	Mechanism
Norepinephrine	0.01–2 mcg/kg/min	Stimulates beta-adrenergic receptors and alpha-adrenergic receptors, causing increased contractility and heart rate, as well as vasoconstriction
Phenylephrine	0.05–0.5 mcg/kg/min	Direct-acting alpha-adrenergic agonist
Procainamide	Load: 3-6 mg/kg/dose over 5 min (Max dose: 100 mg/dose) Maintenance: 20–80 mcg/kg/min Max: 2 g/day	Blocks fast sodium channels with intermediate association/dissociation
Vasopressin (bleeding)	2–10 milliunits/kg/min	Acts on smooth muscle receptors (V_2) in the capillaries and small arterioles, causing them to vasoconstrict
Vasopressin (shock)	0.17–8 milliunits/kg/min Usual range: 0.3–2 milliunits/kg/min	

Antihypertensive Medications	Mechanism of Action	Dose	Route	Side Effects/ Precautions
Enalapril	Angiotensin-converting enzyme (ACE) inhibitor	Enalapril: 0.1–0.5 mg/kg/day divided q12 hr	Enalapril: oral	May exacerbate renovascular hypertension Can cause hyperkalemia
Enalaprilat		Enalaprilat: 5–10 µg/kg/dose, repeated every 6–24 hr as needed	Enalaprilat: intravenous bolus	Can cause cough from bradykinin accumulation
Captopril	ACE inhibitor	Infants: 0.1–0.5 mg/kg/dose every 6–12 hr Children: 0.3–0.5 mg/kg/dose every 6–12 hr	Oral	Same as for enalapril
Clonidine	Central alpha-agonist	3–10 µg/kg/day every 6–8 hr up to 25 µg/kg/day	Oral (also available in patch for chronic usage)	Can cause sedation Useful adjunct for pain or drug withdrawal

Antihypertensive Medications	Mechanism of Action	Dose	Route	Side Effects/ Precautions
Hydralazine	Direct vasodilator	0.1–0.2 mg/kg/ dose as starting dose, can escalate to 20 mg total dose. Can be dosed every 4–6 hr. Max of 3.5 mg/kg/day	Intravenous bolus Intramuscular	Can cause reflex tachycardia, fluid retention
Labetalol	Alpha and beta receptor blocker (beta >> alpha)	0.2–1 mg/kg bolus, up to 40 mg total dose. Can repeat every 10 min. Infusion dose: 0.25–3 mg/ kg/hr	Intravenous bolus Intravenous infusion	Relative contraindication in reactive airway diseases and decompensated heart failure
Nifedipine	Calcium channel blocker	0.1–0.25 mg/kg/ dose every 4–6 hr	Oral	
Phentolamine	Alpha receptor blocker	0.05–0.1 mg/kg bolus dose Maximum of 5 mg	IV bolus	Indicated for pheochromocytoma, generally 1–2 hr prior to surgery

Diuretics: For diuretic medications other than bumetanide and furosemide continuous infusion described earlier, please see Chapter 13.

SUGGESTED READINGS

Barrington KJ. The myth of a minimum dose for atropine. *Pediatrics.* 2011;127(4):783-784.

Chang PM, Silka MJ, Moromisato DY, et al. Amiodarone versus procainamide for the acute treatment of recurrent supraventricular tachycardia in pediatric patients. *Circ Arrhythm Electrophysiol.* 2010;3(2):134-140.

Cuneo BF, Zales VR, Blahunka PC, et al. Pharmacodynamics and pharmacokinetics of esmolol, a short-acting beta-blocking agent in children. *Pediatr Cardiol.* 1994;15(6):296-301.

de Caen AR, Berg MD, Chameides L, et al. Part 12: pediatric advanced life support: 2015 American Heart Association guidelines update for cardiopulmonary resuscitation and emergency cardiovascular care. *Circulation.* 2015;132(18 Suppl 2):S526-S542.

Figa FH, Gow RM, Hamilton RM, et al. Clinical efficacy and safety of intravenous amiodarone in infants and children. *Am J Cardiol.* 1994;74(6):573-577.

Garson A, Kugler JD, Gillette PC, et al. Control of late postoperative ventricular arrhythmias with phenytoin in young patients. *Am J Cardiol.* 1980;46:290.

Guyatt GH, Akl EA, Crowther M, et al. Executive summary: antithrombotic therapy and prevention of thrombosis, 9th ed: American College of Chest Physicians Evidence-Based Clinical Practice Guidelines. *Chest.* 2012;141(2 Suppl):7-47.

Ibutilide [package insert]. Rockford, IL: Mylan Institutional LLC. 2012.

Kavey RE, Daniels SR, Flynn JT. Management of high blood pressure in children and adolescents. *Cardiol Clin.* 2010;28(4):597-607.

Kleinman ME, Chameides L, Schexnayder SM, et al. Part 14: Pediatric advanced life support: 2010 American Heart Association Guidelines for Cardiopulmonary Resuscitation and Emergency Cardiovascular Care. *Circulation.* 2010;122(18 Suppl 3):876-908.

Läer S, Elshoff JP, Meibohm B, et al. Development of a safe and effective pediatric dosing regimen for sotalol based on population pharmacokinetics and pharmacodynamics in children with supraventricular tachycardia. *J Am Coll Cardiol.* 2005;46(7):1322-1330.

Moak JP, Smith RT, Garson AJr. Mexiletine: an effective antiarrhythmic drug for treatment of ventricular arrhythmias in congenital heart disease. *J Am Coll Cardiol.* 1987;10(4):824-829.

National Institutes of Health, National Heart, Lung, and Blood Institute. Expert panel on integrated guidelines for cardiovascular health and risk reduction in children and adolescents. Clinical Practice Guidelines, 2011. http://www.nhlbi.nih.gov/guidelines/cvd_ped/peds_guidelines_full.pdf. Accessed May 2, 2017.

Neumar RW, Otto CW, Link MS, et al. Part 8: adult advanced cardiovascular life support: 2010 American Heart Association guidelines for cardiopulmonary resuscitation and emergency cardiovascular care. *Circulation.* 2010;122(18 Suppl 3):729-767.

Phelps SJ, Hagemann, TM, Lee KR, et al. *Pediatric Injectable Drugs (The Teddy Bear Book)* (10th ed.); American Society of Health Systems Pharmacists; Bethesda, Maryland. 2013.

Sullivan JE, Witte MK, Yamashita TS, et al. Dose-ranging evaluation of bumetanide pharmacodynamics in critically ill infants. *Clin Pharmacol Ther.* 1996;60(4):424-434.

The fourth report on the diagnosis, evaluation, and treatment of high blood pressure in children and adolescents. *Pediatrics.* 2004;114:555-576.

Weesner KM. Hemodynamic effects of prostaglandin E1 in patients with congenital heart disease and pulmonary hypertension. *Cathet Cardiovasc Diagn.* 1991;24(1):10-15. [PubMed 1913785]

Yancy CW, Jessup M, Bozkurt B, et al. American College of Cardiology Foundation/American Heart Association Task Force on Practice Guidelines. 2013 ACCF/AHA guideline for the management of heart failure: a report of the American College of Cardiology Foundation/American Heart Association Task Force on practice guidelines. *Circulation.* 2013;128(18):e240-e327.

15 Sedation, Analgesia, Neuromuscular Blockade and Withdrawal

I. **Nonpharmacologic strategies should be used prior to any pharmacologic intervention to reduce pain and anxiety. Sample strategies include, but are not limited, to the following:**
   a. Positioning
   b. Massage
   c. Distraction
      i. Music (live or from device)
      ii. Technology devices (e.g., video gaming, television, videos, etc.)
   d. Environmental changes
      i. Room temperature
      ii. Lighting
   e. Inclusion of family to promote comfort
      i. Story telling
      ii. Singing
      iii. Soothing touch
   f. Miscellaneous
      i. Bundling (age appropriate)
      ii. Non-nutritive suck (age appropriate)
      iii. Application/removal of blankets
      iv. Application/removal of warm/cool packs
      v. Active and passive range of motion
II. **Topical analgesia**
   a. Indications
      i. Minor procedures
         1. Intravenous catheter placement (peripheral or central)
         2. Arterial line catheter placement
         3. Lumbar puncture
         4. Phlebotomy
   b. Types available
      i. Lidocaine and prilocaine
         1. Apply to intact skin with occlusive dressing
         2. Remains on skin 20 to 60 min prior to procedure depending on formulation
      ii. Buffered lidocaine
         1. Needle-free pressurized delivery system into the subcutaneous tissue
         2. Allow 2 minutes for maximum anesthesia
         3. 1 mL bicarbonate/9 mL 1% lidocaine
      iii. Intradermal lidocaine
         1. Needle injection
         2. Maximum dose of lidocaine
            a. 4.5 mg/kg without epinephrine
            b. 7 mg/kg with epinephrine
III. **Nonopioid analgesia**
   a. Indications
      i. Reduce pain
      ii. Minor procedures
      iii. Facilitate medical therapies

IV. **Sedation and analgesia**
    a. Indications
        i. Reduce anxiety and pain
        ii. Procedures
        iii. Facilitate medical therapies
        iv. Airway control
        v. Decrease the work of breathing
        vi. Decrease oxygen demand

V. **Neuromuscular blocking agents (NMBAs)**
    a. Important notes
        i. ALWAYS ensure ability to bag-mask ventilate the patient prior to administration of NMBA
        ii. ALWAYS be prepared to manage the airway of a patient receiving NMBA
        iii. NEVER administer NMBA to a patient without assuring adequate sedation/analgesia beforehand
        iv. Ensure routine monitoring of depth of muscle blockade to reduce subsequent weakness and use minimum effective dose
    b. Indications
        i. Facilitate procedures
            1. Surgical relaxation
            2. Endotracheal intubation
            3. Vascular access
        ii. Facilitate medical therapies
            1. Decrease O_2 consumption
            2. Prevent shivering (hypothermia)
            3. Reduce metabolic expenditure
            4. Limit mechanical ventilator dyssynchrony
            5. Unconventional modes of ventilation
            6. Transport of patient

VI. **Medications** (See Tables 15-1–15-6)

TABLE 15-1	Nonopioid Pain Control	
Medication	**Dose**	**Mechanism**
Acetaminophen	IV: Infants to <2 yr: 7.5 mg/kg/dose IV q6 hr; max of 60 mg/kg/day Adolescents 2–12 yr <50 kg: 15 mg/kg/dose IV q6 hr; max of 75 mg/kg/day (max 3750 mg/day) ≥50 kg 1000 mg IV q6 hr PO: 10–15 mg/kg/dose every 4–6 hr as needed; do not exceed 5 doses in 24 hr; maximum: 75 mg/kg/day	Inhibits the synthesis of prostaglandins in the central nervous system and works peripherally to block pain impulse generation; produces antipyresis from inhibition of hypothalamic heat-regulating center

TABLE 15-1	(continued)	
Medication	**Dose**	**Mechanism**
	Rectal:	
	Infants and children <12 yr: 10–20 mg/kg/dose every 4–6 hr	
Ibuprofen	PO:	Reversibly inhibits cyclooxygenase-1 and 2 (COX-1 and 2) enzymes, which results in decreased formation of prostaglandin precursors; has antipyretic, analgesic, and anti-inflammatory properties
	Infants and children <50 kg: limited data available	
	Infants <6 mo: 4–10 mg/kg/dose every 6–8 hr; max daily dose: 40 mg/kg/day	
	≥12 yr and adolescents: 200 mg every 4–6 hr as needed; if pain does not respond, may increase to 400 mg; maximum daily dose: 1200 mg/day	
Ketoralac	IV:	
	<2 yr: limited data available	
	Multiple-dose treatment: IV: 0.5 mg/kg every 6–8 hr, not to exceed 48–72 hr	
	2–16 years or adolescents >16 yr <50 kg: 0.5 mg/kg every 6 hr; maximum dose: 30 mg/dose, usual reported duration: 48–72 hr; not to exceed 5 days of treatment	
Naproxen	PO:	
	<60 kg: 5–6 mg/kg/dose every 12 hr;	
	≥60 kg: 250–375 mg twice daily; maximum daily dose: 1000 mg/day	
Lidocaine	Local injectable dose varies with procedure, degree of anesthesia needed, vascularity of tissue, duration of anesthesia required, and physical condition of patient. Maximum dose: 5 mg/kg/dose	Blocks both the initiation and conduction of nerve impulses by decreasing the neuronal membrane's permeability to sodium ions.
Lidocaine and epinephrine	Local infiltration dosage varies with the anesthetic procedure, but should not exceed 7 mg/kg/dose	Lidocaine: Blocks both the initiation and conduction of nerve impulses by decreasing the neuronal membrane's permeability to sodium ions. Epinephrine: Increases the duration of action of lidocaine by causing vasoconstriction, slowing the vascular absorption of lidocaine.

TABLE 15-2	Analgesic Agents for Pain Management or Sedation Adjunct		
Medication	**Dosing**	**Onset and Duration**	**Comments**
Fentanyl	IV: 1–2 mcg/kg/dose Infusion: 1–2 mcg/kg/hr	Onset: 2–3 min Duration: 30–60 min	• More expensive than morphine but less histamine release • Reverse with naloxone • Reduce dose when combined with benzodiazepines
Hydromorphone	<u>Infants</u> >6 mo, >10 kg IV: 0.01 mg/kg/dose Infusion: 0.003–0.005 mg/kg/hr <u>Children</u> <50 kg IV: 0.015 mg/kg/dose Infusion: 0.003–0.005 mg/kg/hr <u>Children</u> >=50 kg IV: 0.2–0.6 mg/dose	Onset: 5 min Duration: 3–4 hr	• Contraindicated in acute or severe asthma • Reverse with naloxone • Reduce dose when combined with benzodiazepines
Ketamine	IV: 0.5–2 mg/kg IM: 2–5 mg/kg	IV: Onset: 1 min Duration: 5–10 min IM: Onset: 3–4 min Duration: 15–30 min	• Hallucinations may be blunted with benzodiazepine use • Hypersalivation (decreased by use with atropine 0.02 mg/kg) • Relatively contraindicated in conditions associated with elevated intracranial pressure (ICP) • Cautious use in hypertension
Morphine	IV: 0.05–0.2 mg/kg Infusion: 0.01–0.04 mg/kg/hr	Onset: 5 min Duration: 3–5 hr	• Life-threatening respiratory depression • Histamine release may result in hypotension

TABLE 15-2 (continued)			
Medication	**Dosing**	**Onset and Duration**	**Comments**
			• Contraindicated in acute/severe asthma if lack monitoring and resuscitation equipment, gastrointestinal (GI) obstruction
			• Reverse with naloxone
			• Reduce dose when combined with benzodiazepines

mg, milligrams; mcg, micrograms; kg, kilograms; IV, intravenous; hr, hour; min, minutes; PO, oral.

TABLE 15-3	Patient-Controlled Analgesia/Nurse-Controlled Analgesia Dosing Guidelines			
Medication	**PCA Bolus Dose**	**PCA Basal Infusion**		
Morphine	0.01–0.03 mg/kg	0.01–0.03 mg/kg/hr		
Hydromorphone	2–4 mcg/kg	2–4 mcg/kg/hr		
Fentanyl	0.5–1 mcg/kg	0.2–0.5 mcg/kg/hr		
PCA/NCA SIDE EFFECT MANAGEMENT				
Nausea and vomiting	Naloxone	0.05–1.5 mcg/kg/hr	IV infusion	First-line
	Ondansetron+	0.1–0.15 mg/kg/dose	IV/PO every 6 hr	
Pruritus	Naloxone	0.05–1.5 mcg/kg/hr	IV infusion	First-line
	Diphenhydramine	0.5 mg/kg/dose	IV/PO every 6 hr	
Sedation	Tolerance typically develops			
Respiratory depression	Hold medication and administer naloxone 0.001–0.003 mg/kg/dose for significant bradypnea			
Constipation	Tolerance does not develop. Routine prophylaxis with bowel regimen, including stool softeners and laxatives.			
	May also use enteral naloxone			

mg, milligrams; mcg, micrograms; kg, kilograms; IV, intravenous; hr, hour; min, minutes; PO, oral
+Although ondansetron has been used in clinical practice and clinical research protocols evaluating efficacy of *other agents* (i.e., naloxone) for PCA-associated nausea and vomiting, no current research exists specifically demonstrating the efficacy of ondansetron.

TABLE 15-4 Sedative and Hypnotic Agents

Medication	Indications	Dosing	Onset and Duration	Comments
Clonidine	Sedation, withdrawal control	PO: 1–5 mcg/kg/dose every 6–8 hr	Onset: 30–60 min Duration: 6–10 hr	• May cause hypotension and bradycardia • May convert to transdermal dosing • May also be used as analgesic
Dexmedetomidine	Sedation	IV bolus dose: 0.5–1 mcg/kg Infusion: 0.2–1 mcg/kg/hr	Onset: 5–10 min Duration: 1–2 hr	• Loading dose optional if using for intensive care unit (ICU) sedation • Bradycardia, hypotension
Etomidate	Procedural sedation	IV: 0.1–0.3 mg/kg	Onset: 30–60 sec Duration (dose dependent): 3–5 min, up to 10 min	• Given risk of adrenal suppression, dose with stress-dose steroids • May exacerbate underlying myocardial dysfunction
Lorazepam	Sedation, motion control, anxiolysis	IV/PO: 0.05–0.1 mg/kg	Onset: IV 5–20 min PO within 60 min Duration: 6–8 hr	• Hypotension • Respiratory depression when combined with opioid administration • Reduce dose when combined with opioids • Reversible with flumazenil • Cautious use in children with hepatic and/or kidney dysfunction

TABLE 15-4	(continued)			
Medication	**Indications**	**Dosing**	**Onset and Duration**	**Comments**
Midazolam	Sedation, motion control, anxiolysis	IV: 0.05–0.1 mg/kg PO: 0.25–0.5 mg/kg Infusion: 0.06–0.12 mg/kg/hr	Onset: IV: 3–5 min PO: 10–20 min Duration: IV: less than 2 hr	• Respiratory depression and respiratory arrest • Use only in setting with continuous monitoring • Hypotension • Cautious use in children with hepatic and/or kidney dysfunction • Reduce dose when combined with opioids • Reversible with flumazenil
Pentobarbital (fail standard therapy)	Sedation, motion control, anxiolysis	IV load: 1 mg/kg Infusion: 1–6 mg/kg/hr	Onset: Near immediate Duration: 15–45 min	• Hypotension • Respiratory depression secondary to narrow toxic window
Propofol	Procedural sedation	IV: Initial dose: 1–2 mg/kg Follow initial dose with 0.5 mg/kg every 3–5 min as needed Infusion: 9 mg/kg/hr (150 mcg/kg/min) titrated as required	Onset: 30 sec Duration: Dose and duration dependent, but 3–10 min	Propofol-related infusion syndrome (PRIS) is associated with higher doses and prolonged use Propofol injection contains ~0.1 g of fat/mL (1.1 kcal/mL)

mg, milligrams; mcg, micrograms; kg, kilograms; IV, intravenous; hr, hour; min, minutes; PO, oral

TABLE 15-5	Reversal Agents			
Medication	**Type**	**Dosing**	**Onset and Duration**	**Comments**
Flumazenil	Benzodiazepine antidote	IV: 0.01 to maximum 0.2 mg/kg one-time dosing	Onset: 1–2 min Duration: ~ 1 hr, depending on dose given and plasma levels of benzodiazepine	• May be repeated every 1 min up to four times for max cumulative dose of 1 mg or 0.05 mg/kg (whichever is lower) • Resedation may occur ~1 hr after administration • May result in seizures, especially in those receiving benzodiazepines long term • May cause vomiting
Naloxone	Narcotic antidote, opioid antagonist	***Opioid overdose*** *PALS guidelines* Children <5 yr or <20 kg (off label) <u>IV/IO/subQ/IM: 0.1 mg/kg/dose</u> Children >5 yr or >20 kg <u>IV/IO/subQ/IM: 2 mg</u> *Manufacturer's labeling (all ages)* IV: 0.01 mg/kg/dose if no response; subsequent dose is 0.1 mg/kg IM/subQ: 0.01 mg/kg/dose; if no response repeat at 0.1 mg/kg dosing Intranasal: 4 mg as single dose divided by half in each nare if using injectable solution ***Respiratory depression associated with therapeutic opioid dosing*** *PALS guidelines* IV: 0.001–0.005 mg/kg/dose, titrate to effect *Manufacturer's labeling* 0.005–0.01 mg/kg/dose, repeat every 2–3 min as needed	Onset: IV → 2 min ET/IM/subQ → 2–5 min Intranasal onset is delayed compared to other routes	• IO and ET dosing are off-label routes • May use IM/ET or SubQ route, but onset of action may be delayed • Optimal ET dose is unknown; two to three times the IV dose is recommended • SubQ and IM doses should be divided injections • May induce acute withdrawal symptoms in children who routinely take opioids • May result in cardiac arrest or seizures secondary to acute opioid withdrawal

mg, milligrams; kg, kilograms; IV, intravenous; IM, intramuscular; IO, intraosseous; ET, endotracheally; subQ, subcutaneously; hr, hour; min, minutes

TABLE 15-6	Neuromuscular Blocking Agents (NMBAs)			
Medication	**Type**	**Dosing**	**Onset and Duration**	**Comments**
Cisatracurium	Nondepolarizing agent	IV: 0.1–0.15 mg/kg of ideal body weight Infusion: 1–4 mcg/kg/min	Onset: 2–3 min Duration: 35–45 min t1/2: 22–29 min	• Monitor for bradycardia • Metabolized by Hoffman degradation • NMBA of choice in kidney and liver failure
Rocuronium	Nondepolarizing agent	IV: 0.6–1.2 mg/kg Infusion: 7–12 mcg/kg/min	Onset: 30–60 sec Duration: 30–40 min t1/2: 60 min	• Cardiovascular effects: vagolytic effect (increased heart rate) • May require dose adjustment in liver and kidney dysfunction
Vecuronium	Nondepolarizing agent	IV: 0.08–0.1 mg/kg Infusion: 0.8–1.2 mcg/kg/min	Onset: 1–3 min Duration: 45–65 min t1/2: 40–60 min	• Primary metabolism in liver • May require dose adjustment in liver and kidney dysfunction
Pancuronium	Nondepolarizing agent	IV: 0.05–0.15 mg/kg Infusion: 0.4–1 mcg/kg/min	Onset 2–5 min Duration 22–24 min t1/2: 90–160 min	• Metabolized in the liver and eliminated through the urine • Elimination half-life is doubled in both renal and hepatic failure • Resistance may happen in burn patients (>20%)
Succinylcholine	Depolarizing agent	IV: 1–2 mg/kg IM: 3 mg/kg	Onset: IV: 30–60 sec IM: 2–3 min Duration: IV: 4–6 min IM: 10–30 min	• Bradycardia and cardiac arrest risk; premedicate with atropine • Contraindications include burns, hyperkalemia, neuromuscular disease, kidney failure, patient history or family history of malignant hyperthermia • May result in rhabdomyolysis with hyperkalemia, ventricular arrhythmias, and cardiac arrest in children who have undiagnosed neuromuscular disorders

mg, milligrams; mcg, micrograms; kg, kilograms; IV, intravenous; min, minutes; sec, seconds; PO, oral; t1/2, elimination half-life

TABLE 15-7	Medications for Use During Weaning/for Withdrawal			
Medication	**Type**	**Dosing**	**Onset and Duration**	**Comments**
Methadone	Narcotic analgesic	Iatrogenic narcotic dependency: Dosing must be individualized to the patient IV or PO dosing	Onset IV: 10–20 min PO: 30–60 min Duration: IV: max effect 1–2 hr PO: 6–8 hr	• Life-threatening respiratory depression • Prolonged QT interval or torsade de pointes • Death • Cardiac arrhythmias • Increased intracranial pressure • Histamine release
Clonidine	Sedation, withdrawal control	Iatrogenic dependency: Dosing must be individualized to the patient PO: 1–5 mcg/kg/dose every 6–8 hr	Onset: 30–60 min Duration: 6–10 hr	• May cause hypotension and bradycardia • May convert to transdermal dosing • May also be used as analgesic

mcg, micrograms; kg, kilograms; IV, intravenous; min, minutes; PO, oral; hr, hour

VII. **Monitoring sedation level**
   a. Tools
      i. No adequate scales to measure sedation in children receiving NMBA
      ii. State Behavioral Scale (SBS)
         a. Uses progressive stimuli to evaluate level of sedation
         b. Use in critically ill infants and children ages 6 months to 6 years
      iii. Comfort Scale
         a. Measures postoperative pain, nonpain distress, sedation, and analgesia
         b. No pediatric age restriction
   b. Titration
      i. Evidence supports nurse-led sedation algorithms are safe
      ii. Use minimum effective dose to reduce prolonged sedation
VIII. **Monitoring for withdrawal syndrome**

During the process of weaning from sedation and analgesia, it is important to monitor for signs of withdrawal.

   a. Variables associated with risk of withdrawal syndrome
      i. Duration of medication therapy
      ii. Maximum cumulative dose of medications
      iii. Type of opioid (fentanyl and remifentanil associated with more withdrawal than morphine)
      iv. Type of sedative
      v. Younger age associated with increased risk of withdrawal syndrome

  b. Tools
    i. Withdrawal Assessment Tool (WAT-1)
    ii. Sophia Observation withdrawal Symptoms-scale (SOS)
  c. Strategies for weaning
    i. May transition to alternative medications
    ii. May use enteral forms of currently administered medications if available
    iii. Ensure monitoring and adequate treatment of intolerable symptoms
    iv. Taper one medication class at a time
      a. Taper parenteral narcotic off over 3 days (decrease by 10% every 8 hours)
      b. Then taper sedative off over 5 days (decrease by 20% daily)
    v. Alternate taper (e.g., narcotic taper every Monday and sedation taper every Friday)
    vi. Select a wean plan and evaluate patient tolerance of wean; adjust as needed
  d. Medications (see Table 15-7)

SUGGESTED READINGS

DiGuisto M, Bhalla T, Martin D, Foerschler D, Jones MJ, Tobias JD. Patient-controlled analgesia in the pediatric population: morphine versus hydromorphone. *J Pain Res.* 2014;7:471-475.

Dorfman TL, Schellenberg ES, Rempel GR, et al . An evaluation of instruments for scoring physiological and behavioral cues of pain, non-pain related distress, and adequacy of analgesia and sedation in pediatric mechanically ventilated patients: a systematic review. *Int J Nurs Stud.* 2014;51:654-676.

Kraemer FW, Rose JB. Pharmacologic management of acute pediatric pain. *Anesthesiol Clin.* 2009;27(2):241-268.

Lexicomp Online®, Ann and Robert H. Lurie Children's Hospital of Chicago Formulary, Hudson, Ohio: Lexi-Comp, Inc.; May, 2017.

Monitto CL, Kost-Byerly S, White E, et al. The optimal dose of prophylactic intravenous naloxone in ameliorating opioid-induced side effects in children receiving intravenous patient-controlled analgesia morphine for moderate to severe pain: a dose finding study. *Anesth Analg.* 2011;113(4):834–842. doi:10.1213/ANE.0b013e31822c9a44.

Phelps SJ, Hagemann TM, Lee KR, et al. *Pediatric Injectable Drugs (The Teddy Bear Book)* (10th ed.); American Society of Health Systems Pharmacists; Bethesda, Maryland. 2013.

MICROBIOLOGY

GRAM STAIN EVALUATION

- Rapid preliminary identification by staining, microscopic evaluation (Table 16-1).
- Antibiotic therapy may be initiated or broadened based on Gram stain interpretation. Therapy should NOT be narrowed based on a Gram stain.

TABLE 16-1	Gram Stain Evaluation			
	Gram-Positive Cocci	**Gram-Positive Rods**	**Gram-Negative Cocci**	**Gram-Negative Rods**
Aerobes	Streptococcus	Bacillus	Neisseria meningitidis	E. coli
	Enterococcus	Listeria	Neisseria gonorrhoeae	Klebsiella
	Staphylococcus	Corynebacterium	Moraxella catarrhalis	Enterobacter
		Lactobacillus[a]		Serratia
		Nocardia		Citrobacter
				Morganella
				Proteus
				Salmonella
				Shigella
				Stenotrophomonas
				Pseudomonas
				Pasturella
				Aeromonas
				Alcaligenes
				Burkholderia
			Pleomorphic coccobacilli:	
			Kingella kingae	
			Acinetobacter	
			Haemophilus influenzae	
Anaerobes	Peptostreptococcus	Clostridium spp.	Veillonella spp.	Bacteroides
		Propionibacterium spp.		Prevotella
		Eubacterium		Fusobacterium
		Actinomyces		
		Lactobacillus[a]		

[a]Aerotolerant anaerobe

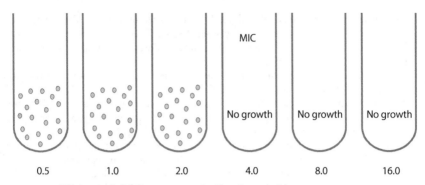

FIGURE 16-1 **Minimum inhibitory concentration (mcg/mL).**

INTERPRETING AND APPLYING MICs

- MIC: minimum inhibitory concentration, or the lowest concentration of an antibiotic that inhibits the growth of a particular bacteria (Figure 16-1).
- Breakpoint: the cutoff that defines susceptibility for an antibiotic and organism pair
  - Breakpoints are determined and updated by the Clinical and Laboratory Standards Institute.[1]
  - Breakpoint cutoffs take into consideration MIC distributions, pharmacokinetics, pharmacodynamics, mechanisms of resistance, and clinical outcome data assessing safety and efficacy.
  - MICs should not be compared across different antibiotics in a susceptibility panel.
  - Antibiotic MICs should only be compared to the breakpoint of the same antibiotic.
  - MIC values are not comparable between different antibiotics. For example, if antibiotic A has a lower MIC compared to antibiotic B, that does NOT necessarily indicate antibiotic A is a better choice.
  - The lower a MIC is from the breakpoint of susceptibility, the more likely that antibiotic will be able to achieve the necessary concentration at the site of action.
  - The intermediate susceptibly category serves as a buffer between the susceptible and resistant categories. Infections due to intermediate susceptible organisms may be treatable if higher doses are used or if the antibacterial is concentrated at the site of infection.
- Limitations and Pearls
  - The choice of antibiotic should be based on the MIC, the breakpoint, and the site of infection.

- Some MIC breakpoints may differ depending on the site of infection. For example, the breakpoint for ceftriaxone susceptibility when treating *Streptococcus pneumoniae* in the bloodstream is ≤ 1, whereas the breakpoint for treating the same organism in the meninges is 0.5.
- Many antibiotics concentrate in the urine and may be used to treat urinary tract infections (UTIs) even when nonsusceptible by in vitro testing.
- A cephalosporin or penicillin derivative should not be used to treat a serious infection caused by an ESBL (extended-spectrum beta-lactamase)–producing gram-negative bacterium even if considered "sensitive" to cephalosporins per MIC breakpoint.
- Isolates initially susceptible may become intermediate or resistant after initiation of therapy. This is most frequently seen when a third-generation cephalosporin is used to treat serious *Enterobacter*, *Citrobacter*, or *Serratia* infections, as a result of inducible amp-C beta-lactamases.
- Interpretation of MICs of organism-antibiotics that do not have a breakpoint is difficult; consult an infectious diseases specialist.

THE ANTIBIOGRAM

- Definition: Summary of antimicrobial susceptibilities of local bacterial isolates.
- Purpose:
  - Guide in selecting empiric antibiotics when susceptibility results are pending.
  - Tool for detecting and monitoring trends in antimicrobial resistance.
- Limitations:
  - Does not take into consideration patient's history of infection/colonization with antibiotic-resistant organisms or past antimicrobial use.
  - MICs are not reported.
  - Interpretation of susceptibility to less common organism (<30 isolates) may be misleading.
  - Data may not be generalizable and may not reflect specific patient populations.
  - Only the first isolate per patient per year is included.

SPECTRUM OF ACTIVITY

ANTIBIOTICS (TABLE 16-2)

NOTE: Refer to your local antibiogram for susceptibility rates in your area.

(continued)

TABLE 16-2 Spectra of Common Intravenous Antibiotics[23]

	Strep	Enterococci	MSSA	MRSA	GNR	Pseudo	B. fragilis (anaerobe)	Atypicals
Penicillins								
Penicillin G	++	+						
Ampicillin	++	++			+/−			
Oxacillin/Nafcillin	+/−		++					
Ampicillin/ Sulbactam	++	++	+		+		++	
Piperacillin/ Tazobactam	++	++	+		++	++	++	
Cephalosporins								
Cefazolin	++		++		+/−			
Cefuroxime	+		+		+			
Cefotetan/Cefoxitin	+		+		+		+/−	
Ceftriaxone/ Cefotaxime	++		+		++			
Ceftazidime	+/−		+/−		++	++		
Cefepime	++		+		++	++		
Ceftaroline	++		++	++	++			
Carbapenems								
Imipenem/ Meropenem	++	+/− (E. faecalis)	+		++	++	++	
Ertapenem	+		+		++		++	

TABLE 16-2 (continued)

	Strep	Enterococci	MSSA	MRSA	GNR	Pseudo	B. fragilis (anaerobe)	Atypicals
Aminoglycosides								
Gentamicin/Tobramycin/Amikacin					++	++		
Fluoroquinolones								
Ciprofloxacin	+/−	+/− (E. faecalis)	+/−	+/−	++	++		++
Levofloxacin	+	+ (E. faecalis)	+	+/−	++	++		++
Moxifloxacin*	+	+ (E. faecalis)	+	+/−	++		+/−	++
Tetracyclines and Glycylcyclines								
Doxycycline	+/−	+/−	+	+	+/−		+/−	+
Tigecycline	+	+	+	+	+		++	+/−
Others								
Aztreonam					++	++		
Trimethoprim/Sulfamethoxazole	+/−		+	+	+/−			
Metronidazole							++	
Nitrofurantoin		+			+/−			
Purely Gram-Positive Agents								
Clindamycin	+		+	+				
Vancomycin	++	++	+	++				
Linezolid	++	++	++	++				
Daptomycin*	++	++	++	++				

Key: ++ = excellent activity; + = good activity; +/− = variable activity.

Strep, Streptococci; MSSA, methicillin-susceptible Staphylococcus aureus; MRSA, methicillin-resistant Staphylococcus aureus; GNR, gram-negative rods; Pseudo, Pseudomonas.

142

ANTIFUNGALS (TABLE 16-3)

TABLE 16-3 Spectra of Common Antifungals[2-5]	Candida albicans, C. parapsilosis, C. tropicalis	C. glabrata, C. krusei	Cryptococcus	Histoplasma/ Blastomyces	Aspergillus fumigatus
Fluconazole	++		++	+/−	
Itraconazole	++	+/−	+/−	++	+/−
Voriconazole	++	+	+	+	++
Posaconazole	++	+	+	+	+
Micafungin/ Caspofungin	++[1]	++			+
Amphotericin	++	++	++	++	++

Key: ++ = excellent activity; + = good activity; +/− = variable activity
[1]C. parapilosis may have reduced susceptibility to micafungin and caspofungin.

ANTIVIRALS (TABLE 16-4)

TABLE 16-4 Therapy for Common Viral Infections	
Virus	**Recommended Therapy**
Herpes Simplex	Acyclovir, valacyclovir
Varicella	Acyclovir, valacyclovir, foscarnet (if acyclovir resistant)
Cytomegalovirus	Ganciclovir, valganciclovir, foscarnet (if ganciclovir resistant)
Adenovirus	Cidofovir
Influenza	Oseltamivir
Respiratory syncytial virus	Supportive care, ribavirin
Enterovirus	Supportive care, IVIG (intravenous immune globulin)*

*Not recommended for routine use; may be useful in selected patients with life-threatening infection

INITIAL EMPIRIC THERAPY FOR COMMON CLINICAL PRESENTATIONS IN THE PICU (TABLE 16-5)

TABLE 16-5 Initial Empiric Therapy for Common Clinical Presentations in the PICU		
Infection	**Common Etiologies**	**Options for Antimicrobial Regimens**
Brain abscess	Streptococci, Enterobacteriaceae, S. aureus, Bacteroides	ceftriaxone + metronidazole ± vancomycin
Encephalitis	N-methyl-D aspartate receptor encephalitis, HSV, Arboviruses, Mycoplasma	acyclovir (add doxycycline if tick-borne infection or mycoplasma suspected)

(continued)

TABLE 16-5 (continued)		
Infection	**Common Etiologies**	**Options for Antimicrobial Regimens**
Bacterial meningitis	Neonate: GBS, E. coli, Listeria	Neonate: ampicillin plus one of the following: cefotaxime OR gentamicin
	Child: S. pneumoniae, N. meningitidis, H. influenzae	Child: ceftriaxone + vancomycin
	Post-neurosurgery: CoNS, S. aureus, GNR	Post-neurosurgery: vancomycin plus one of the following: cefepime OR ceftazidime
Mastoiditis	Acute: S. pneumoniae, GAS, H. influenza	Acute: ceftriaxone
	Chronic: Pseudomonas, other GNR, S. aureus	Chronic: piperacillin/tazobactam ± vancomycin
Jugular vein suppurative thrombophlebitis	Fusobacterium necrophorum	ampicillin/sulbactam
Endocarditis[6]	S. aureus, CoNS, Streptococci, Enterococci	Culture positive: direct therapy against isolated organism and use bactericidal agents according to national guidelines
Community-acquired pneumonia[7]	RSV, influenza, hMPV, S. pneumoniae, H. influenzae, Mycoplasma, S. aureus	ceftriaxone
		Add clindamycin OR vancomycin if MRSA suspected
		Add azithromycin if Mycoplasma or Legionella suspected
		Add oseltamivir if influenza suspected
Sepsis with abdominal source or bowel perforation	Enterobacteriaceae, Streptococci, Enterococci, Bacteroides	ceftriaxone + metronidazole +/− vancomycin
		OR
		piperacillin/tazobactam ± vancomycin
Severe, complicated C. difficile colitis	C. difficile	metronidazole IV + vancomycin (oral or via rectal enema)
Necrotizing fasciitis	Streptococci, S. aureus, Clostridium spp., polymicrobial	vancomycin + piperacillin/tazobactam + clindamycin
Sepsis (community acquired)	Neonate: GBS, E. coli, other GNR, Listeria (rare)	Neonate (early onset <1 week of age): ampicillin plus one of the following: gentamicin OR cefotaxime
		For late-onset neonatal sepsis, consider vancomycin in lieu of ampicillin
	Infant and child: S. pneumoniae, S. aureus, N. meningococcus	Infant and child: vancomycin + ceftriaxone

TABLE 16-5 (continued)

Infection	Common Etiologies	Options for Antimicrobial Regimens
Sepsis with neutropenia	GNR, viridans streptococci, S. aureus	Antipseudomonal antibiotic (ceftazidime OR cefepime OR piperacillin/tazobactam OR carbapenem) + vancomycin ± aminoglycoside ± antifungal
Toxic shock syndrome	S. aureus, GAS	vancomycin + ceftriaxone + clindamycin
		IVIG may be considered for severe or refractory cases
Sepsis with petechial/ purpuric rash	N. meningitides, RMSF	vancomycin + ceftriaxone
		add doxycycline if tick exposure or RMSF suspected
Urosepsis	GNR and Enterococci (less common)	Community acquired: ceftriaxone + vancomycin
		+/− aminoglycosides
		For nosocomial infections can substitute ceftazidime, cefepime, or meropenem for ceftriaxone

NOTE: Empiric therapy should be tailored to local resistance and severity of disease. Broadened antibiotic therapy may be warranted in patients with history of multidrug-resistant infections.

Enterobacteriaceae examples: *E. coli, Klebsiella, Enterobacter, Serratia, Citrobacter, Morganella, Proteus, Salmonella, Shigella;* HSV, herpes simplex virus; GBS, Group B Streptococcus; CoNS, coagulase-negative Staphylococci; GNR, gram-negative rods; GAS, Group A Streptococcus; RSV, respiratory syncytial virus; hMPV human metapneumovirus; IVIG, intravenous immunoglobulin; RMSF, Rocky Mountain spotted fever; CDC, Centers for Disease Control and Prevention

PHARMCOKINETICS AND DRUG INTERACTIONS

PHARMACOKINETICS

- Factors affecting oral absorption:
  - *Absorption improved with food*: posaconazole, itraconazole capsules
  - *Absorption impaired by food*: voriconazole, itraconazole solution, rifampin, isoniazid, pyrazinamide
  - *Absorption impaired by antacids, proton pump inhibitors, and histamine-2 antagonists*: itraconazole, posaconazole
  - *Absorption impaired by calcium (including calcium-rich foods), iron, aluminum, and zinc*: fluoroquinolones, tetracyclines
- Factors affecting distribution
  - *Conditions with potentially altered antibiotic concentrations*: septic shock, abscesses/ walled-off infections
  - *Drugs based on actual body weight in obese children*: most anti-infectives, including vancomycin

TABLE 16-6	Common Antibiotic Drug Interactions	
	Inhibitors	**Inducers**
Anti-infectives	Fluconazole (major)	Rifampin (major)
	Itraconazole (major)	Rifabutin (major)
	Voriconazole (major)	
	Posaconazole (major)	
	Erythromycin (major)	
	Clarithromycin	
	Fluoroquinolones	
	Metronidazole	
	Trimethoprim/sulfamethoxazole	

- *Drugs based on ideal body weight in obese children*: acyclovir
- *Drugs based on adjusted body weight in obese children*: aminoglycosides: dosing based on actual body weight will result in an overdose
- *Protected body sites requiring dose optimization*: cerebrospinal fluid, bone, heart valves
- Metabolism
  - *Substrates*: drugs that undergo extensive metabolism
  - *Inhibitors*: drugs that lead to a decrease in metabolism (increased concentration/toxicity) of a substrate
  - *Inducers*: drugs that lead to an increase in metabolism (decreased concentration/efficacy) of a substrate
  - Examples of anti-infectives with significant drug inhibition/induction (Table 16-6)
- Factors affecting excretion
  - *Renal function*: most anti-infectives are excreted in the urine and require dose REDUCTION in renal insufficiency.

ANTIMICROBIAL STEWARDSHIP

UNINTENDED CONSEQUENCES

- Antibiotic resistance
  - The relationship between antibiotic use and subsequent resistance is well documented.
  - Resistance in children poses a unique challenge, given the paucity of dosing and safety data with newly approved antibiotics.
  - Use the most narrow-spectrum antibiotic for the shortest effective duration of therapy only where a clear indication exists.
- Antibiotic adverse drug effects and allergies
  - Antibiotics are the most commonly prescribed drugs in children and are most likely to be associated with adverse drug reactions (rash, diarrhea, antibiotic-specific toxicities).
  - Clarify the exact nature of every reported allergy: labeling a patient with an allergy can limit future options, possibly leading to selection of inferior antibiotics or more broad-spectrum, expensive alternative options.

- Superinfections
  - Alteration of normal flora by antibiotics can lead to overgrowth of more resistant organisms, such as *Clostridium difficile* and fungi.
  - Superinfections from these pathogens increase morbidity and mortality.

PEARLS

- Common examples of narrowing
  - MSSA (methicillin-sensitive *Staphylococcus aureus*) should be treated with cefazolin or with oxacillin or nafcillin if meningitis is suspected (vancomycin is inferior to cefazolin and oxacillin for treatment of MSSA).
  - Ampicillin/amoxicillin is the empiric drug of choice for *Enterococcus faecalis* infections (vancomycin is inferior to ampicillin for treatment of ampicillin-susceptible *E. faecalis*).
  - *Escherichia coli* and *Klebsiella* species may be treated with cefazolin if susceptible and meningitis is not suspected.
  - *Streptococcus pyogenes* (group A strep) and *S. agalactiae* (group B strep) may be treated with ampicillin.
  - Double covering or addition of anaerobic coverage with metronidazole to piperacillin-tazobactam, ampicillin-sulbactam, or meropenem is generally unnecessary.
- Prophylactic antibiotics
  - If prophylactic antibiotics are continued beyond the operating room, they should be discontinued within 24 hours after the end of surgery in the majority of cases.
  - Prophylactic antibiotics should not be used for chest tubes and indwelling drains.
- Colonization/contamination vs. infection
  - To distinguish infection from contamination or asymptomatic bacteriuria, a positive urine culture must be interpreted in conjunction with a urinalysis and clinical data.
  - Positive growth from endotracheal tube aspirates most often indicates colonization, not infection—clinical correlation is needed.
  - Isolation of coagulase negative Staphylococcus, such as S. epidermidis, from a single blood culture often represents contamination.
  - Isolation of *Candida* from a nonsterile site or urinary culture in a catheterized patient often represents colonization.

REFERENCES

1. Clinical and Laboratory Standards Institute. *Performance Standards for Antimicrobial Susceptibility Testing; Twenty-First Informational Supplement; M100-S25.* Wayne, PA: Clinical and Laboratory Standards Institute; 2015.
2. Kimberlin DW, Brady MT, Jackson MA, Long SA, eds. *Red Book: 2015 Report of the Committee on Infectious Diseases.* 30th ed. Elk Grove Village, IL: American Academy of Pediatrics; 2015.
3. Gilbert DN, Chambers HF, Eliopoulos GM, Saag MS, Pavia AT, eds. *The Sanford Guide to Antimicrobial Therapy 2016.* 46th ed. Sperryville, VA: Antimicrobial Therapy; 2016.
4. Pappas PG, Kauffman CA, Andes D, et al. Clinical practice guideline for the management of candidiasis: 2016 Update by the Infectious Diseases Society of America. *Clin Infect Dis.* 2016;62(4): e1-e50.

5. Patterson TF, Thompson GR, Denning DW, et al. Practice guidelines for the diagnosis and management of aspergillosis: 2016 Update by the Infectious Diseases Society of America. *Clin Infect Dis.* 2016;63(4):e1-e60.
6. Baltimore RS, Gewitz M, Baddour LM, et al. Infective endocarditis in childhood: 2015 update. *Circulation.* 2015;132(15):1487-1515.
7. Bradley JS, Byington CL, Shah SS, et al. The management of community-acquired pneumonia in infants and children older than 3 months of age: clinical practice guidelines by the Pediatric Infectious Diseases Society and the Infectious Diseases Society of America. *Clin Infect Dis.* 2011;52:285-292.

PART 2

Organ Systems

Respiratory

17 Respiratory Formulas and Parameters

PULMONARY VOLUMES

Minute (or Total) Ventilation
- MV = Tidal Volume (V_T) × Respiratory Rate (RR)

Tidal Volume
- $V_T = V_A + V_D$

Alveolar Ventilation (V_A): inversely proportional to $PaCO_2$, doubling of V_A will halve $PaCO_2$
- $V_A = [V_T - \text{Dead Space} (V_D)] \times RR$
  Dead space volume (V_D) — anatomic and physiologic components
  Anatomic dead space is the volume of conducting airways
  Physiologic dead space = Alveolar dead space + Anatomic dead space
  Alveolar dead space is difficult to determine, so use physiologic components as a surrogate
  Approximately 30% of V_T or 2 mL/kg

Dead Space Calculation
- $V_D/V_T = (PaCO_2 - PECO_2)/PaCO_2$
  V_D = Dead space volume
  V_T = Tidal volume
  $PaCO_2$ = Arterial CO_2
  $PECO_2$ = Mean expired CO_2 in a breath (obtain from exhaled CO_2 monitor)

GAS MOVEMENT

Compliance = Change in Volume/Change in Pressure
Static Compliance = $V_T/(P_{plat} - PEEP)$
  P_{plat} – Plateau pressure
  PEEP – Positive end-expiratory pressure
  Nl: 60 to 200 mL/cmH_2O in adults
  >1 mL/cm H_2O/kg in pediatrics
  Reflects pressure to overcome elastic forces of respiratory system
Dynamic Compliance = $V_T/(PIP - PEEP)$
  PIP – Peak inspiratory pressure
  Nl: 50 to 175 mL/cm H_2O (~10%–20% less than static)
  Reflects lung compliance + pressure to overcome airway resistance
  *The difference is an indirect index of flow-resistive properties of the respiratory system
Effective V_T/Kg = $V_T - [(PIP - PEEP) \times \text{tubing compliance factor}]/\text{weight in kg}$
  Typically automatically compensated by ventilator setup parameters
Resistance – (Poiseuille's law) $R = 8 \, nl/\pi r^4$
  Resistance to flow inversely related to the fourth power of the radius.

Mean Airway Pressure:
- $MAP = [I_t/(I_t + E_t)] \times (PIP - PEEP)] + PEEP$

- Correlated to oxygenation, an increase in MAP will improve alveolar volume and improve oxygenation
I_t = Inspiratory time
E_t = Expiratory time
PIP = Peak inspiratory pressure
PEEP = Positive end-expiratory pressure

OXYGEN PARAMETERS AND LUNG INJURY CLASSIFICATIONS

Alveolar gas equation
- $P_AO_2 = (FiO_2 \times (P_{Atm} - P_{H20})) - (P_aCO_2/\text{respiratory quotient})$
FiO_2 = fraction of inspired oxygen
P_{Atm} (sea level) = 760 mmHg
P_{H20} = 47 mmHg
Normal RQ = 0.8
- **Pearls:**
  - Alveolar PO_2 is determined mostly by *level of alveolar ventilation*
  - If FiO_2 is held constant and $PaCO_2$ increases, *PAO_2 and PaO_2 will always decrease*
  - Hypoxia due to hypoventilation is easily overcome by increasing FiO_2

Alveolar-arterial gradient: measure of lung function
- A-a O_2 Gradient= $PAO_2 - PaO_2$
= $[PiO_2 - PaCO_2/RQ] - PaO_2$
= $[(FiO_2 * (P_{Atm} - P_{H2O})) - (PaCO_2/0.8)] - PaO_2$
PAO_2 = Alveolar
PaO_2 = Arterial
RQ = 0.8
P_{Atm} = Atmospheric pressure
P_{H2O} = Water pressure
Nl <10 torr for adults OR age (years)/4 + 4 while breathing room air
A gross approximation of A-a gradient is 5 × FiO_2

PF Ratio = PaO_2/FiO_2
Normal PaO_2/FiO_2 = 100 mmHg/0.21 = approx 500
The lower the ratio, the worse the disease process:
- PF ratio ≤300 mmHg − Acute lung injury (ALI)
- PF ratio ≤200 mmHg − Acute respiratory distress syndrome (ARDS)
      *Beware this does not include any information about amount of pressure being used (e.g., PEEP) so may not be best surrogate

OI (Oxygenation Index) = (MAP * FiO_2 × 100)/PaO_2
- MAP – Mean airway pressure
- If >25 consider the oscillator
- If >30 on 2 Arterial Blood Gases (ABGs), consider extracorporeal membrane oxygenation (ECMO)

Arterial oxygen content of the blood
CaO_2 (mL O_2/dL) = (SaO_2 × Hemoglobin × 1.36) + 0.003*(PaO_2)
0.003*PaO_2 represents the fraction of dissolved oxygen in the blood

Venous oxygen content of the blood:
CvO_2 (mL O_2/dL) = (SvO_2 × Hemoglobin × 1.36) + 0.003*(PvO_2)

Arterial-mixed venous oxygen content difference:

$avDO_2 = CaO_2 - CvO_2$

$CaO_2 \sim 20$ mL/dL

$CvO_2 \sim 15$ mL/dL

Oxygen extraction is approximately 25%; can also be estimated by:

$SaO_2 - SvO_2$

OXYHEMOGLOBIN DISSOCIATION CURVE - SEE FIGURE 17-1

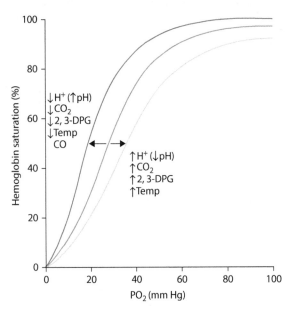

FIGURE 17-1 **Oxyhemoglobin dissociation curve.**

Ways to manipulate oxygen delivery:

Oxygen delivery is dependent on hemoglobin, its dissociation curve, and cardiac output. Increasing hemoglobin does *not* greatly affect SaO_2 or PaO_2, but can increase oxygen delivery substantially by increasing oxygen content of the blood.

Right Shift: Decreased hemoglobin-oxygen affinity; therefore, more oxygen is unloaded to the tissues. Occurs with acidosis and hyperthermia. A good example is exercising when the muscle mass is warm; increased metabolic activity results in acidosis and an increase in 2,3 DPG and benefits from unloading of oxygen from hemoglobin to the tissue.

Left Shift: Increased hemoglobin-oxygen affinity with decreased release to tissues. This occurs with alkalosis, transfused blood, hypothermia, and carbon monoxide poisoning.

Three key points on the oxygen-hemoglobin dissociation curve:

$$PaO_2 \ 100 \ mmHg = SpO_2 \ of \ 97\%$$
$$PaO_2 \ 60 \ mmHg = SpO_2 \ of \ 90\%$$
$$PaO_2 \ 40 \ mmHg = SpO_2 \ of \ 75\%$$

The slope of the curve is flat above **PaO_2 of 60 mmHg**, and becomes very steep below this. Any small drop in PaO_2 below 60 mmHg will cause a precipitous drop in saturation.

SUGGESTED READINGS

Grippi MA, Elias JA, Fishman JA, et al. *Fishman's Pulmonary Diseases and Disorders*.
West JB, Luks AM. *West's Respiratory Physiology: The Essentials*. 10th ed. 2015. Wolters Kluwer, Riverwoods, IL.

18 Respiratory Mechanics and Respiratory Failure

RESPIRATORY MECHANICS

- Developmental considerations
  - Basal metabolic rate is higher in children than in adults, resulting in decreased metabolic reserve in the face of increased oxygen consumption during critical illness
  - More compliant chest wall with decreased elastic recoil
  - Incomplete alveolarization and lack of collateral ventilation (pores of Kohn and canals of Lambert develop at ages 3–4)
  - Airways in children have increased resistance and lack rigid cartilage
    - More susceptible to dynamic compression and airway obstruction
- Compliance: Distensibility of the lung; ease of expansion of the lungs and thorax, determined by pulmonary volume and elasticity; measure of the ratio of change in tidal volume and the pressure it produces:

$$C = \Delta V / \Delta P$$

  - *High compliance* = healthy lung, neuromuscular weakness or paralysis
  - *Low compliance* = acute respiratory distress syndrome (ARDS), pneumonia
- Resistance (Poiseuille's law): Resistance to flow is inversely related to the fourth power of the radius; therefore, if the radius is halved, the resistance is **increased 16-fold.**
  - Results in profound decrease in flow as laminar flow transitions to turbulent flow (see Figure 18-1)

Laminar Flow

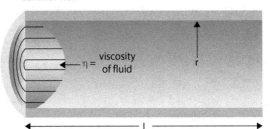

$$\text{Resistance to Flow (R)} = \frac{8\eta L}{\pi r^4}$$

where r = radius of tube
η = viscosity of fluid
L = length of tube

η = viscosity of fluid

r

L

FIGURE 18-1 **Laminar Flow and Poiseuille's Law.**

- Lung volumes (see Figure 18-2)
  - Tidal volume (V_T): volume of air moved during quiet breathing.
  - Vital capacity (VC): maximal volume of air that can be forcibly exhaled after a maximal inspiration.
  - Residual volume (RV): volume of air remaining in lungs after a maximal expiration. It cannot be expired no matter how vigorous or long the effort.
  - Total lung capacity (TLC): volume of air in the lungs at the end of a maximal inspiration.
  - Functional residual capacity (FRC): volume of air remaining in the lungs at the end of a normal expiration.
    - FRC is reduced by supine positioning, abdominal distension, restrictive lung disease, and sedation.

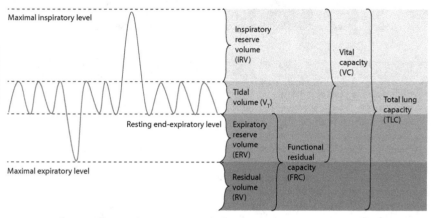

FIGURE 18-2 **Lung volumes.**

- Normal gas exchange requires:
  - Transport of oxygen (O_2) to the alveolus
  - Diffusion of O_2 across the alveolar-capillary membrane
  - O_2 transfer from the blood to the organs
  - Carbon dioxide (CO_2) removal from blood into the alveolus
- Ventilation: Refers to CO_2 exchange at the alveolar level.
  - Determined by <u>minute ventilation</u> and <u>anatomic dead space</u>.

$$\text{Alveolar Ventilation} = [V_T - \text{Dead Space } (V_d)] \times \text{Respiratory Rate (RR)}$$

$$\text{Minute Ventilation} = V_T \times RR$$

$$\text{Dead Space Volume } (V_d) = \text{Anatomic} + \text{Physiologic}$$

  - *Dead space* = the sum of gas volume within the conducting airways that does not reach the alveoli (anatomic) and volume of gas that doesn't participate in gas exchange secondary to inadequate perfusion (physiologic).
  - *Physiologic causes of hypercapnia:*
    - Increased CO_2 production (fever, burns, overfeeding)
    - Decreased alveolar ventilation
      - Decreased V_T
        - Decreased central nervous system (CNS) drive (sedatives)
        - Neuromuscular weakness
        - Flail chest
      - Increased V_d
        - Pulmonary embolus
        - Hyperinflation (asthma, bronchiolitis, cystic fibrosis [CF], excessive positive end-expiratory pressure [PEEP])
        - Decreased cardiac output (dehydration, dysrhythmia, cardiomyopathy, post-cardiopulmonary bypass)
        - Increased pulmonary vascular resistance

- Oxygenation
  - Oxygen content of the blood (CaO_2)

$$CaO_2 = (SaO_2 \times Hgb \times 1.36) + 0.003(PaO_2)$$

  - **Primarily** determined by oxygen saturation (SaO_2) and hemoglobin (Hgb).
  - When hemoglobin content is adequate, patients can have a reduced PaO_2 (defect in gas transfer) and still have sufficient oxygen content for the tissues.
  - Conversely, patients can have a normal PaO_2 and be *profoundly hypoxemic* by virtue of a reduced CaO_2.
    - This paradox (normal PaO_2 and hypoxemia) generally occurs one of two ways:
      - Anemia
      - Altered affinity of hemoglobin for binding oxygen (e.g., carbon monoxide poisoning)
  - Alveolar gas equation (abbreviated)
    - Ideally oxygen that is contained within the alveolus at inspiration equilibrates with arterial blood, as described by the alveolar gas equation:

$$PAO_2 = FiO_2 * (P_B - P_{H20}) - 1.2(PaCO_2)$$

    FiO_2 of air is 21%, P_B (sea level) = 760 mmHg, P_{H20} = 47 mmHg
    - Normal A-a gradient between alveolar (PAO_2) and arterial ($PaCO_2$) is less than 10 mmHg.
    - Alveolar PO_2 is determined primarily by **level of alveolar ventilation**.
    - If FiO_2 is held constant and $PaCO_2$ increases, **PAO_2 and PaO_2 will always decrease**.
    - Conversely, if ventilation falls, PO_2 drops and PCO_2 will rise as well (**i.e., hypoventilation will always lead to high $PaCO_2$**).
    - Hypoxia due to hypoventilation and CO_2 retention is easily overcome by increasing FiO_2.
  - P/F ratio
    - PaO_2/FiO_2 is measure of oxygenation
    - Lower P/F ratio reflective of more impaired oxygenation
    - Does not incorporate mean airway pressure
  - Oxygenation Index (OI)
    - Measure of oxygenation developed for use in neonates with persistent pulmonary hypertension
    - Recommended for use in pediatric ARDS over P/F ratio

$$OI = [\text{mean airway pressure} \times FiO_2 \div PaO_2] \times 100$$

  - *Physiologic causes of hypoxemia*
    - Alveolar hypoventilation
    - Diffusion abnormality
    - Shunt (intracardiac or intrapulmonary)
    - Ventilation/perfusion (V/Q) mismatch
    - Decreased affinity of hemoglobin for oxygen
    - Decreased inspired oxygen content (e.g., high altitude)
- Abnormalities of pulmonary blood flow
  - *Abnormalities of ventilation and perfusion (V/Q mismatch):*
    - Most common cause of hypoxemia in critically ill children.

- V/Q both increase slowly from apex to base of the lung, but blood flow increases more rapidly than ventilation; therefore, V/Q ratio is different as you move from one lung segment to the other.
  - Leads to abnormally high V/Q ratio at the apex of the lung (upright position) and a much lower one at the base.
- Atelectasis exaggerates V/Q mismatch, causing well-oxygenated blood from high V/Q lung units to mix with poorly oxygenated blood from low V/Q units, worsening hypoxemia (asthma, ARDS) and increasing A-a gradient.
  - If there is an oxygen gradient (**i.e., A-a gradient = $[PAO_2 - PaO_2] \geq 30$ mmHg**) then you have V/Q mismatch.
- Hypoxemia caused by V/Q mismatch can be corrected by increasing FiO_2 and providing positive pressure ventilation to recruit consolidated or collapsed lung units.
  - *Shunt*
    - Direct mixing of deoxygenated venous blood that has not undergone gas exchange in the lungs with arterial blood. (e.g., necrotizing pneumonia with significant dead space, pulmonary edema ARDS).
      - Physiologically anatomic shunt (bronchial veins, thebesian veins)
      - Pathologic anatomic shunts (arterial-venous malformation, intracardiac communications)
    - Intrapulmonary shunt occurs as blood perfuses poorly ventilated lung regions; increases A-a gradient.
    - **Clinical tip**: 100% O_2 **does not** resolve hypoxemia.

RESPIRATORY FAILURE IN CHILDREN

- Definition of respiratory failure
  - Inability to provide oxygen and carbon dioxide removal at a rate that matches the body's metabolic demand
- Diagnosis of respiratory failure
  - Physiologic criteria
- Hypoxic respiratory failure: PaO_2 less than 60 mmHg on room air at sea level
- Hypercapnic respiratory failure
  - $PaCO_2$ greater than 50 mmHg with concomitant respiratory acidosis
  - Not strictly defined by set of blood gas values
- Common causes of pediatric respiratory failure (See Figure 18-3)
- Signs and symptoms of respiratory failure
  - *Increased respiratory drive:* increased respiratory rate, anxiety or agitation, dyspnea, accessory muscle use
  - *Respiratory muscle fatigue:* paradoxical "see-saw" breathing, grunting, inability to speak, irregular respirations with apnea
  - *Hypoxemia or hypercapnea:* cyanosis, disordered sleeping, agitation or confusion, obtundation, tachycardia
  - *Evidence of lung disease:* rhonchi, rales, wheezing and poor aeration, asymmetric breath sounds
  - *Loss of protective reflexes:* absent cough or gag, inability to handle secretions
  - *Critical upper airway obstruction:* stridor with severe retractions, drooling, tripod positioning
  - *Decreased respiratory drive (late signs):* bradypnea, shallow breathing, coma, bradycardia, cardiorespiratory arrest

Primary Disorders of the Respiratory Tract

- Upper Airway Obstruction (Croup, epiglottitis, tracheomalacia, adenotonsillar hypertrophy, mass, foreign body, anaphylaxis)
- Lower Airway Obstruction (Asthma, bronchopulmonary dysplasia, bronchiolitis, cystic fibrosis)
- Parenchymal Lung Disease (Pneumonia, bronchiolitis, acute respiratory distress syndrome (ARDS), interstitial lung disease, pulmonary edema)

Disorders Resulting in Mechanical Impairment of Ventilation

- Neuromuscular Disease
- Myopathies
- Spinal Cord Injury
- Chest Wall Abnormalities or Trauma
- Pneumothorax or Large Pleural Effusions
- Abdominal Compartment Syndrome

Failure of Central Nervous System (CNS) to Control Ventilation

- CNS Infections
- Seizures
- Intracranial Injury or Mass
- Metabolic Encephalopathy
- Medications or Intoxications
- Central Alveolar Hypoventilation

Failure to Meet Tissue Oxygen Demands

- Sepsis
- Cardiogenic Shock
- Metabolic Disorders
- Poisoning

FIGURE 18-3 **Common causes of pediatric respiratory failure.**

SUGGESTED READINGS

Cheifetz IM. Year in review 2015: pediatric ARDS. *Respir Care*. 2016;61:980.

Gerhardt T, Hehre D, Feller R, et al . Pulmonary mechanics in normal infants and young children during first 5 years of life. *Pediatr Pulmonol*. 1987;3:309-316.

Grinnan DC, Truwit JD. Clinical review: respiratory mechanics in spontaneous and assisted ventilation. *Crit Care*. 2005;9(5):472-484.

Hammer J. Acute respiratory failure in children. *Paediatr Respir Rev*. 2013;14(2):64-69.

Vo P, Kharasch VS. Respiratory failure. *Pediatr Rev*. 2014;35(11):476-486.

Airway Clearance

AIRWAY CLEARANCE – WHAT ARE THE OPTIONS?

INDICATIONS FOR AIRWAY CLEARANCE

Indications for airway clearance include impaired mucocillary escalator function or impaired cough. According to the American Association for Respiratory Care's Clinical Practice Guidelines for Airway Clearance, it is important to look at the rationale behind your decision to order airway clearance. Is gas exchange being affected by retained secretions? A patient with an increase in secretions may not necessarily need airway clearance when suctioning is all that is needed. With this in mind, the indications for airway clearance are:

1. Evidence of difficulty with secretion clearance
2. Evidence of retained secretions
3. Presence of atelectasis caused by mucus plugging
4. Diagnosis of cystic fibrosis, bronchiectasis, or neuromuscular disease

CHEST PHYSICAL THERAPY (CPT) AKA BRONCHIAL DRAINAGE (BD)

- How it works
  - Percussion to the chest improves air movement and loosens secretions
  - Positioning allows gravity to assist in draining secretions
- Contraindications:
  - Hemoptysis
  - Untreated tension pneumothorax
  - Increased intracranial pressure (ICP)
  - Pleural effusions
  - Brittle bone disease

POSITIVE EXPIRATORY PRESSURE (PEP) DEVICES

- **PEP**
  - How it works:
    - Patient exhales against a fixed orifice, which creates a resistance to flow
    - Airway stability is maintained due to prolonged expiratory time
    - Collateral ventilation allows air to move beyond the obstruction to improve aeration
    - Airflow through device helps move mucus into larger airways
    - Airway clearance is more effective as a result of improved air distribution in the lungs
  - Contraindications
    - Increased work of breathing
    - Increased ICP
    - Hemodynamic compromise
    - Active hemoptysis
    - Untreated tension pneumothorax
    - Recent esophageal surgery
    - Middle ear pathology
- **Flutter**
  - How it works:
    - The patient exhales into the device, which contains a steel ball sitting in a cone

- The patient's expiratory flow causes the steel ball to lift and roll in the cone until the weight of the ball causes it to drop down
    - Movement of the steel ball causes air to oscillate
    - Oscillations of air in the lungs loosens and moves mucus
  ○ Contraindications:
    - Increased work of breathing
    - Increased ICP
    - Hemodynamic instability
    - Active hemoptysis
    - Untreated tension pneumothorax
    - Esophageal surgery
- **Acapella**
  ○ How it works:
    - This therapy combines the effects of PEP and flutter
    - Patient exhales against a fixed orifice, which creates resistance to flow
    - Exhaled air is interrupted by a valve that opens and closes, creating vibrations
    - Adjusting a dial changes the frequency of vibration and resistance to exhalation
  ○ Contraindications:
    - Increased work of breathing
    - Increased ICP
    - Hemodynamic instability
    - Acute sinusitis
    - Active hemoptysis
    - Untreated tension pneumothorax
    - Esophageal surgery

HIGH-FREQUENCY ASSISTED AIRWAY CLEARANCE

- **High-frequency chest wall compression (aka "vest" therapy)**
  ○ How it works:
    - Air inflates a vest or wrap
    - Intermittent pressure pulses create vibrations and air movement throughout the airways ("mini-coughs")
    - Helps loosen and move secretions
  ○ Contraindications:
    - Increased ICP
    - Uncontrolled hypertension
    - Hemodynamic instability
    - Bronchopleural fistula
    - Recent esophageal surgery
    - Active or recent hemoptysis
    - Pulmonary embolism
    - Uncontrolled airway at risk for aspiration
    - Distended abdomen
    - Bronchospasm
    - Suspected tuberculosis (TB)
    - Transvenous pacemaker or subcutaneous pacemaker
- **High-frequency chest wall oscillation**
  ○ How it works:
    - Utilizes a rigid chest cuirass connected to a compressor

- Positive and negative pressure are applied to the chest wall, which is transferred to the airway
- Negative pressure supports lung recruitment
- Vibration mode shakes, thins, and advances secretions to large airways
- Cough mode helps with secretion removal by providing long, deep inspiration immediately followed by sharp, short exhalation
  - Contraindications:
    - >180 kg
    - Burns/skin integrity issues
    - Must have patent airway

INTRAPULMONARY PERCUSSIVE VENTILATION (IPV)

- How it works:
  - Percussive bursts of gas are delivered into the lungs at rates between 100 and 300 breaths per minute
  - These bursts of gas are delivered during inspiration and exhalation to loosen and mobilize secretions
  - High flow rates help patients take a deeper breath, which allows air to get behind trapped mucus
- Contraindications:
  - Untreated tension pneumothorax
  - History of pneumothorax
  - Pulmonary air leak
  - Recent lobectomy
  - Pulmonary hemorrhage
  - Cardiovascular insufficiency/myocardial infarction (MI)
  - Lack of patient cooperation
  - Vomiting

INTRAPULMONARY OSCILLATIONS METANEB

- How it works:
  - Three therapies
    - Aerosol therapy
    - Oscillates the airways with continuous pulses of positive pressure
    - Provides hyperinflation therapy using expiratory pressure to help mobilize secretions and resolve atelectasis
- Contraindications:
  - Active TB
  - Untreated tension pneumothorax or recent history of pneumothorax
  - Recent lobectomy
  - Hemoptysis
  - Cardiovascular instability
  - Vomiting
  - Lack of patient cooperation

COUGH ASSIST

- How it works:
  - Mimics the cough mechanism by providing a positive pressure followed by generating a negative pressure to move secretions forward
  - Inspiratory pressure moves air distal to the mucus

- Inspiratory and expiratory pressures simulate cough
- Fast expiration simulates cough
- Expiratory flow loosens and moves secretions toward the mouth
- Contraindications:
  - History of bullous emphysema
  - Susceptibility to pneumothorax or pneumomediastinum
  - Recent barotrauma

SUGGESTED READINGS

Fink BJ, Hess DR. Secretion clearance techniques. In: Hess DR, MacIntyre NR, Mishoe SC, Galvin WF, Adams AB, Sapsonick AB, eds. *Respiratory Care Principles & Practice*. St. Louis, MO: W.B. Saunders Company; 2002:671-689.

Hayek Medical. *Biphasic Cuirass Ventilation: Training, Identification, and Orientation Guide*. Philadelphia, PA: 2012.

Hill-Rom. *The MetaNeb System User Manual*. Batesville, IN: 2-6.

Strickland SL, Rubin BK, Drescher GS, et al. AARC clinical practice guideline: effectiveness of nonpharmacologic airway clearance therapies in hospitalized patients. *Respir Care*. 2013;58(12):2187-2193.

Vines DL, Gardner DD. Airway clearance therapy (ACT). In: Kacmarek RM, Stoler JK, Heuer AJ, eds. *Egan's Fundamentals of Respiratory Care*. 11th ed. St. Louis, MO: Elsevier; 2016:951-967.

Volsko TA. Airway clearance therapy: finding the evidence. *Respir Care*. 2013;58(10):1669-1678.

Walsh BK. Airway clearance techniques and hyperinflation therapy. In: Walsh BK, ed. *Neonatal and Pediatric Respiratory Care*. 4th ed. St. Louis, MO: Saunders; 2015:199-204.

Pediatric Airway Obstruction 20

AIRWAY PHYSICS

- Poiseuille's law
  - $Q = \dfrac{\Delta P \pi r^4}{8 \eta l}$; r = Radius of airway
  - Flow (Q) is proportional to the radius to the fourth power; incremental changes in the radius cause exponential decreases in airflow
- Bernoulli's principle
  - Increased airflow results in a decrease in pressure
  - Narrowed airway → Increased airflow speed → Decreased intraluminal pressure (vacuum) → Further collapse of walls of lumen
- Stridor – high-speed airflow through collapsed tissues causes vibration and a resonance, resulting in a sound

NOISY BREATHING

- Physical obstruction of the airway is associated with noise on inspiration or expiration, depending on the site and nature of the lesion
- Stridor is not only audible, but also visible
  - Examiner should be able to visualize site of obstruction while noise is being made
  - Requires adequate instrumentation techniques of the airway
- Isolated tachypnea (i.e., without stridor) is not a sign of airway obstruction

SYMPTOMS BY SUBSITE SEE TABLE 20-1

TABLE 20-1 Symptoms by Subsite

Subsite	Hallmark Symptoms
Nasal	Mouth breathing, snoring **Acute respiratory distress in neonates** – obligate nasal breathers
Pharynx	Snoring, **stertor** (pharyngeal resonance, similar to snoring), retractions
Supraglottis	**Pure inspiratory stridor**, **dysphagia in infants**, retractions, pectus excavatum
Glottis	**Biphasic stridor**, retractions, **hoarseness**
Subglottis	Inspiratory or biphasic stridor, retractions, barking cough, **recurrent croup**
Trachea	**Expiratory stridor**, barking cough, poor secretion clearance

Bolded comments highlight findings fairly specific to that subsite, allowing better localization and differential diagnosis.

LESIONS AND TREATMENTS BY SUBSITE

NASAL OBSTRUCTION

- Piriform aperture stenosis
  - Bony narrowing of the anterior nasal vestibule in neonates; results in airway-related respiratory distress and feeding problems
  - Diagnosed by computerized tomography (CT) scan showing <8 mm patency between nasal processes of maxillary bone
  - Can be associated with holoprosencephaly (central incisor) or choanal atresia
  - Treatment: sublabial approach to nasal vestibule with high-powered drill reduction of nasal process of maxillary bone
- Choanal atresia/stenosis
  - Incomplete or uncannulated opening from the nose to the nasopharynx in neonates; results in airway-related respiratory distress
  - CHARGE syndrome (coloboma, heart defects, atresia choanae, growth retardation, genital abnormalities, and ear abnormalities)
  - May go undiagnosed if unilateral
  - Treatment: transnasal or transpalatal resection of posterior obstructive tissues

PHARYNGEAL OBSTRUCTION

- Adenotonsillar disease
  - Most common cause of obstructive sleep apnea (OSA) in children
  - Diagnosed by direct visualization on exam and attended nocturnal polysomnogram
  - Treatment: adenotonsillectomy adequately treats >80% of patients with pharyngeal airway obstruction
- Pharyngomalacia
  - Poor pharyngeal muscle tone, results in collapse of tissues and obstruction with stertor
  - Treatment: noninvasive positive pressure ventilation (continuous or bilevel)
- Glossoptosis/macroglossia (Figure 20-1)

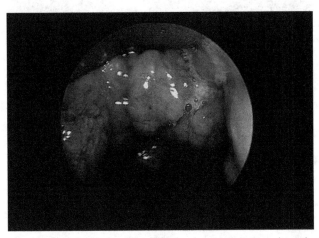

FIGURE 20-1 **Glossoptosis causing upper airway obstruction.** Note how the base of the tongue compresses the epiglottis against the posterior pharynx.

- Tongue and tongue base obstruction of the airway
- Pierre-Robin's sequence, Down's syndrome, lingual tonsil hypertrophy, isolated micrognathia, Ludwig's angina (anterior floor of mouth abscess)
- Treatment: alleviate obstruction by resection, advancement, or bypass (i.e., tracheotomy)
- Pharyngeal obstruction results primarily in sleep apnea symptoms

SUPRAGLOTTIC OBSTRUCTION

- Laryngomalacia
  - Most common cause of stridor in infants, primarily during feeding
    - Generally present from birth
    - Stridor ranges in quality from squeaky to grunting
    - Worse when flat and supine, better when prone
    - Associated with vibratory sensation in the patient's back
    - Strongly associated with gastroesophageal reflux disease
  - Tubular or omega-shaped epiglottis, resulting in partial airway obstruction that is worsened by rapid breaths during suck-swallow-breath cycle
  - Interruption of breaths results in retractions, feeding dyscoordination, dysphagia, and aspiration, as well as increased work of breathing during feeding
    - May cause failure to thrive due to increased caloric output and decreased intake during feeding
    - Decreased laryngeal sensation has also been implicated in contributing to dysphagia in laryngomalacia (either primary or from reflux stimulation)
  - Approximately 15% to 20% of patients require surgical intervention (supraglottoplasty) due to failure to thrive (Figures 20-2 and 20-3)
  - Many patients with moderate symptoms will respond positively to high-dose reflux regimen; the majority may be observed for resolution by 18 to 24 months of age

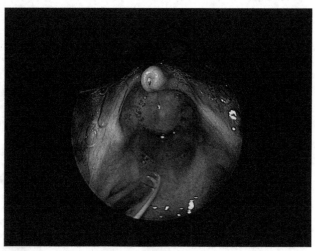

FIGURE 20-2 Laryngomalacia resulting in failure to thrive. The epiglottis is completely curled and fully obstructs the airway on inspiration.

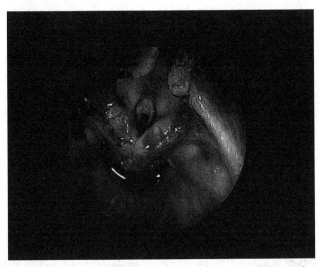

FIGURE 20-3 **The patient in Figure 20-2 immediately after supraglottoplasty.**

- Glottic obstruction
  - Vocal cord paralysis
    - Unilateral – generally acquired, rarely causes airway obstruction
      - Dysphagia/hoarseness
      - Observe for at least 12 months for return of function
    - Bilateral – generally congenital, always causes airway obstruction
      - Dysphagia
      - Airway obstruction with biphasic stridor
      - Observe for return of function, but generally requires tracheotomy for obstructive symptoms
  - Intubation injury – edema, granulation, and granuloma
    - Hoarseness and stridor with failed or difficult extubation
    - Generally requires combined medical/surgical approach
      - Endoscopic debridement/dilation
      - IV steroids, inhaled steroids, racemic epinephrine, reflux management, airway support (O_2, noninvasive positive pressure, Heliox, etc.) to prevent reintubation
- Subglottic obstruction
  - Subglottic stenosis (SGS) (Figure 20-4)
    - Congenital – small, narrow, or misshapen cricoid ring
      - Recurrent croup worsening with age in frequency and severity
      - Increasing exertional dyspnea with age
      - At risk for additional acquired stenosis if intubated with age-appropriate endotracheal tube
    - Acquired – more common than congenital; intubation injury
      - Prolonged intubation $\rightarrow$ tissue erosion $\rightarrow$ inflammatory processes $\rightarrow$ intraluminal scarring
      - **Best treatment is prevention – proper tube sizing and early extubation**
      - SGS in evolution may be treated endoscopically to prevent stenosis

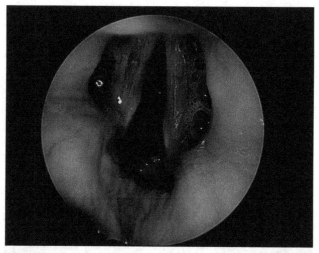

FIGURE 20-4 Grade III subglottic stenosis in an adolescent, visible through the vocal cords.

- In general, grade I to II stenosis can be managed endoscopically; grade III to IV requires open repair
- Endoscopic management
  ○ Radial incisions with serial balloon dilation
  ○ Steroid injection
  ○ Application of mitomycin
- Open management
  ○ Tracheotomy
  ○ Laryngotracheal reconstruction with thyroid or rib cartilage graft
○ Subglottic hemangioma (Figure 20-5)
  ▪ Most common tumor of the pediatric subglottis (but still quite rare)
  ▪ Presentation at 4 to 6 weeks of age
    • Worsening stridor with agitation; improves with calming
    • Improves with steroid therapy
    • Often misdiagnosed as croup
    • Associated with dermal hemangioma of the head and neck, particularly in the "beard" distribution (cheek, lips, mandible, upper neck)
  ▪ Typical natural history
    • Rapid growth phase, 9 to 12 months
    • Slow resolution phase, 5 to 10 years
      ○ 50% resolved by age 5
      ○ 70% resolved by age 7
      ○ 90% resolved by age 9
  ▪ Treatment: propranolol has quickly become first-line therapy
    • Other options or adjuvants include intralesional or IV steroids, interferon, endoscopic CO_2 laser resection, and open resection
    • Tracheotomy is rarely necessary in the modern era

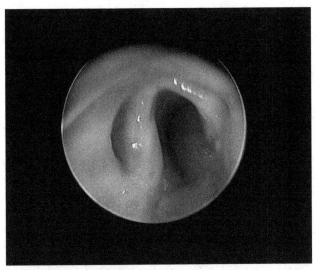

FIGURE 20-5 **Subglottic hemangioma in a neonate.** Smooth and round, posteriorly based, and causing near-complete obstruction.

- ○ Croup
  - ▪ Acute laryngotracheobronchitis – focus of narrowing is at the smallest part of the airway in children (the subglottis)
  - ▪ Inspiratory stridor, retractions, and barking cough associated with typical upper respiratory tract (URI) symptoms (fever, rhinorrhea, congestion)
    - • Steeple sign on airway film (Figure 20-6)
    - • Avoid instrumentation if possible (i.e., laryngoscopy or intubation)
  - ▪ Oral steroids with or without nebulized racemic epinephrine for control of airway symptoms
  - ▪ Recurrent croup may be a sign of congenitally narrowed airway predisposing to croup with URI
- • Tracheal obstruction
  - ○ Tracheal stenosis (Figure 20-7)
    - ▪ Similar pathogenesis to subglottic stenosis: intubation injury with resultant scarring
    - ▪ Treatment different due to lack of stable cartilage structure (cricoid cartilage in subglottis)
      - • Endoscopic – balloon dilation, steroid injection, mitomycin
      - • Open – cartilage graft is ineffective, requiring tracheal resection with reanastomosis vs. slide tracheoplasty
  - ○ Tracheomalacia (Figure 20-8)
    - ▪ Misshapen tracheal cartilage rings provide poor anteroposterior support of the airway, resulting in collapse of the airway from positive intrathoracic pressure (i.e., cough)
    - ▪ Expiratory stridor, barky cough, poor clearance of lower airway secretions, prolonged recovery post-URI
    - ▪ Severe tracheomalacia may require tracheostomy tube until older age to stent the airway open

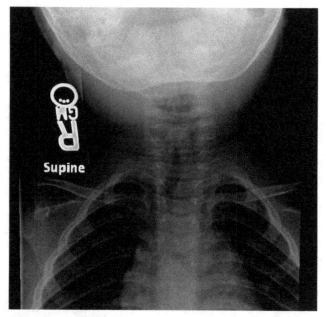

FIGURE 20-6 **Steeple sign during croup.**

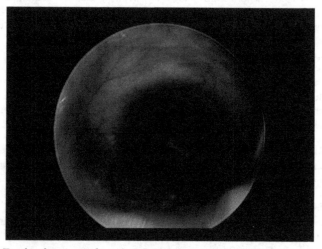

FIGURE 20-7 **Tracheal stenosis from intubation injury in a 4-year-old.**

- Complete tracheal rings
  - Congenital malformation of the trachea, with circular tracheal cartilage rings instead of horseshoe shaped
    - Small diameter with poor elasticity (rigid)

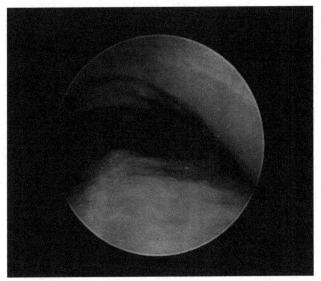

FIGURE 20-8 Tracheomalacia in an 18-month-old. Note the anteroposterior compression of the trachea.

- Can be one tracheal ring or include the entire trachea, including bronchial cartilage rings
- Strongly associated with other intrathoracic abnormalities (especially pulmonary artery sling)
- Minimizing instrumentation prior to repair is critical
- Slide tracheoplasty has revolutionized treatment of this airway lesion and improved airway-specific survival dramatically

MANAGING AIRWAY EMERGENCIES

INITIAL RESPONSE

- Assess situation and call for appropriate support – supervising physician, anesthesiology or otolaryngology, or full code
- Understanding the lesions described earlier and the patient's most likely cause/site of lesion is critical in understanding techniques that can bypass or alleviate the obstruction
- Utilize the airway support ladder:
  - Supplemental O_2 via nasal cannula, simple mask, nonrebreather mask
  - Add Heliox for increased O_2-carrying capacity of blood
  - Manual maneuvers for improved airway patency – chin lift, jaw thrust, bag-mask ventilation
  - Pharyngeal obstruction can be stented by noninvasive positive pressure ventilation or bypassed by oral airway device, nasopharyngeal airway/nasal trumpet, or laryngeal mask airway (LMA)
  - Intubation with rapid sequence technique, through an intubating laryngeal masking device, or utilizing flexible bronchoscope or indirect visualization guidance (video laryngoscope)

- ○ In situations where the airway lesion is unknown or intervention poses further risks, then evaluation by an airway surgeon is appropriate with possible rigid laryngoscopy/bronchoscopy for diagnosis and management
- ○ Inability to intubate can require an emergent airway insertion, like cricothyroidotomy or tracheotomy
- Always remember, the airway is critical: do what it takes to establish and maintain a safe airway

SUGGESTED READINGS

Darrow DH. Surgery for pediatric sleep apnea. *Otolaryngol Clin North Am.* 2007;40(4):855-875.

Ida JB, Thompson DM. Pediatric stridor. *Otolaryngol Clin North Am.* 2014;47(5):795-819.

Richter GT, Thompson DM. The surgical management of laryngomalacia. *Otolaryngol Clin North Am.* 2008;41(5):837-864.

21 Asthma and Status Asthmaticus

Asthma is a heterogeneous disease of bronchial inflammation and bronchospasm. Status asthmaticus is a state of respiratory compromise characterized by bronchial inflammation and bronchospasm secondary to asthma with resultant prolonged expiratory phase, tachypnea, dyspnea, and work of breathing; it does not respond to conventional therapy and may lead to respiratory failure.[1,2]

EPIDEMIOLOGY

Asthma affects 8.7 million children in the United States with the highest prevalence in children 5 to 17 years of age.[3]

- Blacks are disproportionately affected, and there is no gender predilection.
- Seventy to eighty percent of children have allergic symptoms.
- There are familial links, but asthma is more likely to develop if the mother has allergies or asthma rather than the father.[3]

PATHOPHYSIOLOGY

Asthma and status asthmaticus are due to increased inflammation of the lower airway leading to:

- Airway irritability and bronchospasm
- Overproduction of mucus
- Mucosal edema

Combined, these lead to airway obstruction via bronchoconstriction and mechanical obstruction.[1]

RESPIRATORY MECHANICS IN ASTHMA

PULMONARY CHARACTERISTICS OF ASTHMA

- Hyperinflation and increased functional residual capacity
- Heterogeneous lung parenchyma
- Airways can be affected in multiple ways[2]:
  - Complete obstruction of the airway (i.e., mucus plugging)
  - Partial obstruction present throughout the respiratory cycle
  - Partial obstruction present throughout expiration → prone to air trapping
  - No bronchial obstruction → prone to overdistention during an asthma exacerbation
  - V/Q mismatch occurs due to shunt physiology and increased dead space ventilation[1]
  - Areas of atelectasis secondary to mucus plugging lead to intrapulmonary shunt physiology
  - Areas of hyperinflation can lead to pulmonary blood flow obstruction and increased dead space ventilation

CARDIOPULMONARY INTERACTIONS

- Extreme fluctuations in intrathoracic pressures during an acute asthma exacerbation can affect both the preload and the afterload on the heart.
- High lung volumes and intrathoracic pressures increase the pulmonary vascular resistance.

- High intrathoracic pressures decrease blood return to the right atrium (i.e., preload).
- Negative inspiratory pressures increase afterload on the left ventricle.
- These changes lead to pulsus paradoxus.
- Changes in systolic blood pressure of more than 10 to 15 mmHg between inhalation and exhalation may be an indicator of impending respiratory failure.[1]

DIAGNOSTIC CONSIDERATIONS

DIFFERENTIAL DIAGNOSIS[1,3]

Pneumonia – viral or bacterial, allergic bronchopulmonary aspergillosis, foreign body aspiration, cardiogenic pulmonary edema, anatomic lesions that may be fixed (e.g., airway web or hemangioma) or dynamic (tracheomalacia), immunodeficiency, bronchopulmonary dysplasia, vocal cord paralysis

HISTORY AND PHYSICAL

- History
  - Acuity of symptoms, presence of fever, upper respiratory symptoms, exposures to allergens, personal or family history of asthma, allergies, eczema
  - **Red flags:** intensive care unit (ICU) admissions for asthma, history of mechanical ventilation, frequent emergency room visits[1]
- Physical exam
  - Respiratory effort (i.e., accessory muscle use), dyspnea, breath sounds
  - Mental status, perfusion (e.g., capillary refill), liver edge
  - **Ominous signs:**
    - Lethargy, altered mental status
    - The silent chest – severe airway obstruction vs. pneumothorax
    - Paradoxical thorcoabdominal breathing
    - Severe dyspnea or inability to phonate[1]
    - Altered mental status, poor perfusion, and tachycardia can be signs of hypercarbia
- Laboratory workup
  - Complete blood count: an elevated white blood cell count may raise suspicion for infection; however, could also be secondary to stress response or administration of steroids[1]
  - Electrolytes and metabolic profile:
    - Elevated blood urea nitrogen (BUN) and creatinine may indicate level of dehydration
    - Prolonged β-agonist therapy can decrease extracellular potassium concentration
- Arterial blood gas
  - Initial – hypoxemia and hypocarbia can be seen due to V/Q mismatch and hyperventilation.
  - Normal or high PCO_2 in a tachypneic patient is a concerning finding and may indicate impending respiratory failure.[1]
  - Lactatemia or lactic acidosis is a common finding in status asthmaticus
    - Mostly type B acidosis – not associated with tissue dysoxia but rather secondary to β-adrenergic therapy, leading to derangements in glucose metabolism
    - Can lead to tachypnea to achieve a compensatory respiratory alkalosis and can lead to a confounding picture for the clinician treating status asthmaticus[4,5]
    - Type A acidosis can be due to impaired oxygen delivery in a setting of shock, overloaded respiratory muscles, or poor clearance[5]
- Chest x-ray
  - Recommended for initial presentations and all ICU admissions
  - Typically hyperinflated with flattened diaphragms

○ Look for pneumothorax, foreign body (could manifest as asymmetry), cardiomegaly, pulmonary edema, chest mass, and infectious infiltrate[1]

TREATMENTS

CORTICOSTEROIDS

- Break the cycle of inflammation that underlies an asthma exacerbation
- Must be systemic, and IV steroids are preferred in status asthmaticus
- Methylprednisolone is potent and has a low mineralocorticoid effect
- Treatment duration depends on the severity of the asthma exacerbation, but should continue until symptoms are resolved at minimum
- Dose: loading dose is 2 mg/kg, then 0.5 to 1 mg/kg every 6 hours (maximum dose 60 mg)
- Side effects: hyperglycemia, hypertension, rarely agitation/psychosis[1]

INHALED β-AGONIST

- Inhaled β-agonists (e.g., albuterol) are the initial therapy in status asthmaticus.
- β-adrenergic effect on the β2 receptor causes bronchodilation.[1]
  ○ Dose: Starting dose 0.15 to 0.5 mg/kg/hr up to 20 mg/hr continuously via nebulization
  ○ Side effects:
    - Tachycardia, palpitations, diastolic hypotension
    - Hypokalemia, hyperglycemia, lactemia (see earlier)[1,3]
- Hypoxemia due to worsening V/Q mismatch can also be seen with initiation of β-agonist therapy. Pulmonary blood vessels that are naturally shunting away from lung zones with poor ventilation due to hypoxic vasoconstriction will begin to vasodilate from the β-adrenergic effect. This leads to increased blood flow in areas of poor lung ventilation.[1]

SYSTEMIC β-AGONISTS

- Systemic β-agonists are beneficial in severe status asthmaticus, as inhaled therapies may not reach all lung zones.
- IM epinephrine is a nonselective β-agonist with a high side effect profile.
- Terbutaline is a fairly selective β2-agonist used frequently in status asthmaticus.
  ○ Can be given subcutaneously if no IV access is available.
  ○ Dose: subcutaneously 0.01 mg/kg/dose up to 0.3 mg.
  ○ Intravenous loading dose: 10 mcg/kg with continuous infusion at 0.1 to 10 mcg/kg/min.
  ○ Side effects: similar to those of inhaled β-agonist. Chest pain and an increase in troponins have been reported with the use of terbutaline; thus, this medication warrants close cardiac monitoring.[1]

ADJUVANT THERAPIES

- Anticholinergics (e.g., ipratropium) are parasympatholytics and cause bronchodilation with minimal side effects.
  ○ Dose of ipratropium: 125 to 500 micrograms inhaled every 4 to 6 hours[1]
- Magnesium sulfate causes bronchodilation as a calcium channel blocker. Its efficacy in the setting of status asthmaticus is controversial and appears most effective when magnesium levels of 4 mg/dL are targeted.[1]
  ○ Dose: 25 to 50 mg/kg/dose or as continuous infusion 10 to 20 mg/kg/hr
  ○ Side effects: Hypotension, central nervous system (CNS) depression, muscle weakness

- Helium-oxygen allows for less turbulent flow through narrow airways; it is most efficacious as an 80/20 mixture, limiting its use to patients with normoxemia on an FiO_2 of 0.21.[1]
- Methylxanthines (theophylline, aminophylline) cause bronchodilation by inhibiting phosphodiesterase; not generally recommended but may consider in very critically ill children[3]
  - Have narrow therapeutic ranges
  - Side effects: seizures, cardiac arrhythmias

NONINVASIVE MECHANICAL VENTILATION

Noninvasive ventilation with continuous or bilevel positive pressure (CPAP or BiPAP) can improve work of breathing and asthma scores when used with corticosteroids and β-agonists.

- May facilitate delivery of inhaled β-agonist.
- Alleviates work of breathing by maintaining small airway patency.
- Associated with use of fewer adjuvant therapies.
- Side effects are minimal and include redness of the face and agitation with application of the mask in small children.[4]

MECHANICAL VENTILATION

Mechanical ventilation in children with status asthmaticus can be challenging and is reserved for those that present following cardiopulmonary arrest, persistent hypoxemia, or those with a severe respiratory acidosis not responsive to medical therapies.[1,2]

- Intubation may be associated with hypotension and even cardiac arrest as venous return decreases when transitioning to positive pressure ventilation.
- High risk of barotrauma, pneumothorax, and air leak syndrome.
- Concern for myopathy with prolonged steroid and paralytic use.
- Risk of a secondary ventilator-associated pneumonia.[1]

VENTILATORY STRATEGIES

- Mechanical ventilation in the patient in status asthmaticus should aim to utilize the lowest pressure possible and avoid further hyperinflation.[1] Patients often worsen initially due to addition of positive pressure to a system of high pressure.
- Permissive hypercapnia
  - Aim for a pH >7.2, or allow for "permissive hypercapnia"
  - Ensure early volume resuscitation
  - Use low tidal volumes with adequate exhalation time
    - Increase exhalation time by decreasing respiratory rate and inspiratory time
    - Low tidal volumes allow for complete exhalation after each breath[1,2]
- Mode of ventilation
  - Volume control is preferable mode of ventilation compared to pressure control, as the airway resistance and lung compliance can vary dramatically and change rapidly in status asthmaticus.[1,2]
  - Pressure-regulated volume control offers additional advantage of decelerating flow pattern, which allows for lower peak pressures and more even distribution of tidal volume.[1]
- Plateau pressure
  - Assessing the plateau pressure in mechanically ventilated patients in status asthmaticus allows the clinician to assess the severity of airway obstruction and the extent of barotrauma.[2]

- ○ The peak inspiratory pressure does not reflect the pressure seen in most of the alveoli in obstructive lung disease.
- ○ Plateau pressure is measured by holding the patient at the end of inspiration (end inspiratory pause) for several seconds and allowing pressures to equilibrate.
- ○ Plateau pressure can estimate the degree of hyperinflation.
- o The difference in peak inspiratory pressure to plateau pressure (peak to plateau difference) can give the clinician a sense of the degree of airway obstruction.[2]
- Positive end-expiratory pressure
  - ○ The role of extrinsic positive end-expiratory pressure (PEEP) remains controversial. Matching extrinsic PEEP to the patient's own PEEP is a commonly used strategy.[1,2]
  - ○ Patients with asthma already have a high intrinsic PEEP due to air trapping.[1]
  - ○ Extrinsic PEEP > intrinsic PEEP could prohibit full exhalation and worsen hyperinflation.[2]
  - ○ Matching PEEP set on the ventilator to the intrinsic PEEP prevents airway collapse and promotes full exhalation.[1]
  - ○ Intrinsic PEEP can be measured with an end-expiratory hold in the mechanically ventilated and paralyzed patient.

SEDATING THE INTUBATED AND MECHANICALLY VENTILATED PATIENT

- Intubation
  - ○ IV fluids should be available when intubating to increase preload to the right heart when transitioning from negative to positive pressure ventilation.
  - ○ Ketamine is a good choice for induction, as it acts as a bronchodilator, allows for some spontaneous breathing, and is hemodynamically fairly neutral.
  - ○ Ketamine is a sialagogue, and the use of glycopyrrolate should be considered.
  - ○ Avoid morphine, as it can release histamines, causing hypotension and worsening bronchospasm. Fentanyl is preferred.
  - ○ A paralytic agent such as rocuronium or vecuronium should be used to prevent or minimize laryngospasm and bronchospasm.[1]
- Sedating the ventilated patient
  - ○ Asthmatics should be well sedated to avoid the patient competing with the ventilator and to suppress coughs and gags, which can lead to complications such as pneumothorax.
  - ○ Fentanyl is preferred over morphine for sedation in status asthmaticus due to its hemodynamic profile and absence of histamine release.[1]
  - ○ Dexmedetomidine is another useful agent in the prolonged sedation of an asthmatic.
- Paralytic use
  - ○ Paralytics may have to be used to suppress intrinsic effort to breath and the cough and gag reflexes.
  - ○ Prolonged used of paralytics can lead to myopathy, especially with concomitant steroid use.
  - ○ Train of fours should be monitored at least daily along with daily breaks in paralytic infusions to avoid myopathy.[1]

RESCUE THERAPY

Anesthetics – have limited data but have bronchodilatory properties, may reduce work of breathing, decrease metabolic demand, and improve patient synchrony with the ventilator[8]

- IV anesthetics – ketamine and propofol
- Inhaled anesthetics – halothane, enflurane, and isoflurane (sevoflurane may have bronchoconstrictive effects)

Extracorporeal membrane oxygenation – may be considered when all other therapies have failed

REFERENCES

1. Bigham MT, Brilli RJ. Status asthmaticus. In: Nicols DG. Shaffner DH, eds. *Rogers' Textbook of Pediatric Intensive Care*. 5th ed. Philadelphia, PA: Wolters Kluwer; 2016:710-719.
2. Oddo M, Feihl F, Schaller MD, et al. Management of mechanical ventilation in acute severe asthma: practical aspects. *Intensive Care Med*. 2006;32:501-510.
3. Wade A, Chang C. Evaluation and treatment of critical asthma syndrome in children. *Clin Rev Allergy Immunol*. 2015;48(1):66-83.
4. Meert KL, McCaulley L, Sarnaik AP. Mechanism of lactic acidosis in children with acute severe asthma. *Pediatric Crit Care Med*. 2012;13(1):28-31.
5. Manthous CA. Lactic acidosis in status asthmaticus: three cases and review of the literature. *Chest*. 2001;119(5):1599-1602.
6. Basnet S, Mander G, Andoh J, et al. Safety, efficacy, and tolerability of early initiation of noninvasive positive pressure ventilation in pediatric patients admitted with status asthmaticus: a pilot study. *Pediatr Crit Care Med*. 2012;13(4):393-398.
7. Shivo M, Phan C, Louie S, et al. Critical asthma syndrome in the ICU. *Clin Rev Allergy Immunol*. 2015;48(1):31-44.
8. Tobias JD. Therapeutic applications and uses of inhalational anesthesia in the pediatric intensive care unit. *Ped Crit Care Med*. 2008; (9):169-179.

22 Blood Gases and Acid-Base Disorders

DEFINITIONS

- **pH** = power of Hydrogen defined by the Henderson-Hasselbalch equation:

$$pH = pK + \log([HCO_3^-]/0.03\,PCO_2)$$

- **Acidosis** = decrease in arterial pH
  - Respiratory acidosis – caused by CO_2 retention. This increases the denominator in the Henderson-Hasselbalch equation and depresses the pH.
    - Hypoventilation and ventilatory failure can cause respiratory acidosis.
  - Metabolic acidosis – reduced pH not explained by increased PCO_2. Caused by a primary fall in the numerator [HCO_3^-] of the Henderson-Hasselbalch equation.
    - It is usually associated with an increased anion gap (see later).
- **Alkalosis** = increase in arterial pH
  - Respiratory alkalosis – the decreased PCO_2 explains the increased pH.
    - Seen in alveolar hyperventilation.
  - Metabolic alkalosis – raised pH out of proportion to changes in PCO_2.
    - It is associated with hypokalemia, exogenous alkali administration, or volume contraction (e.g., severe prolonged vomiting) when the plasma bicarbonate concentration rises.
- **Anion gap:** helps differentiate between acid gain and HCO_3^- loss.

$$\text{Anion gap} = [Na^+] - ([Cl^-] + [HCO_3^-])$$
$$\text{Normal gap } 8 - 12\,mEq/L$$

- See Figure 22-1.
- Anion gap acidosis: gap >12 mEq/L
  - Caused by decrease in HCO_3^- balanced by an increase in unmeasured acid ions, not by an increase in chloride.
  - Causes include salicylates, methanol, paraldehyde, ethylene glycol, lactic acidosis, ketoacidosis (from diabetes or starvation), and uremia.
- Non–anion gap acidosis: gap 8 to 12 mEq/L
  - Caused by a decrease in HCO_3^- balanced by an increase in chloride.
  - Causes include renal tubular acidosis, carbonic anhydrase inhibitor, and diarrhea.

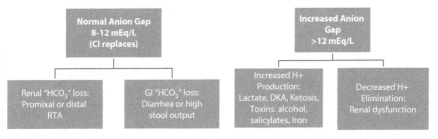

FIGURE 22-1 **Anion gap.**

- Table 22-1 gives normal values for infants and children.
- **Fencl-Stewart approach to understanding acid-base balance:** looks for unmeasured anions, which could contribute to a pH disturbance.

$$BE_{explained} = H_2O + Cl^- + albumin$$

H_2O contribution = 0.3 (Na^- + 140)
Cl^- contribution = 102 − (Cl^- × 140/Na)
Albumin contribution = 3.4 (4.5-albumin)
BE: base excess

$$BE_{unexplained} = {}^*BE_{measured} - BE_{explained}$$

*Get $BE_{measured}$ from blood gas

CLINICAL APPROACH TO BLOOD GAS INTERPRETATION

- Blood gases provide measurements of pH, PCO_2, PO_2, total hemoglobin, and derivation of indices such as oxygen content, HCO_3^-, base deficit/excess, and oxyhemoglobin saturation.
- Blood gases allow for the determination of pathologic states and whether the abnormalities are primarily respiratory or metabolic.

  When evaluating acid-base disorders, it is best to take a stepwise approach (see Figure 22-2).

1. Determine whether the patient is acidotic or alkalotic.
2. Determine whether the primary process is respiratory or metabolic.
   - If respiratory, is it acute or chronic?
   - If metabolic, is there an anion gap?
3. Determine the primary disturbance and then evaluate for mixed disorder by the degree of compensation (see the following formulas and Tables 22-1 and 22-2).
   - A simple disturbance should have one acid-base disorder.
   - A mixed disorder can be detected by calculating the expected compensation and then comparing that to the actual value.

TABLE 22-1	Normal Values	
Measurement	**Newborn Infant**	**Infant and Child**
Rate (bpm)	40–60	20–30 <6 yr
		15–20 >6 yr
pH	7.3–7.4	7.3–7.4 <2 yr
		7.35–7.45 >2 yr
PCO_2 mmHg	30–35	30–35 <2 yr
		35–45 >2 yr
HCO_3^- (mEq/L)	20–22	20–22 <2 yr
		22–24 >2 yr
O_2 saturation (%)	≥95	>95
PO_2 mmHg	60–90	95

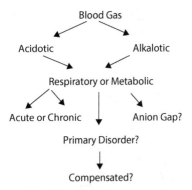

FIGURE 22-2 **Stepwise approach to blood gas interpretation.**

TABLE 22-2		Expected Compensatory Changes	
Disorder	**pH**	**Primary Change**	**Expected Compensation**
Acidosis			
Metabolic	↓	↓ HCO_3^-	↓ PCO_2 by 1–1.5 × fall in HCO_3^-
Acute Respiratory	↓	↑ PCO_2	↑ HCO_3^- by 1 mEq/L for each 10 mmHg rise in PCO_2
Chronic Respiratory	↓	↑ PCO_2	↑ HCO_3^- by 3.5 mEq/L for each 10 mmHg rise in PCO_2
Alkalosis			
Metabolic	↑	↑ HCO_3^-	↑ PCO_2 by 0.25–1 × rise in HCO_3^-
Acute Respiratory	↑	↓ PCO_2	↓ HCO_3^- by 1–3 mEq/L for each 10 mmHg fall in PCO_2
Chronic Respiratory	↑	↓ PCO_2	↓ HCO_3^- by 2–5 mEq/L for each 10 mmHg fall in PCO_2

EXPECTED COMPENSATORY CHANGES IN pH AFTER A PRIMARY DERANGEMENT

- Metabolic acidosis: Expected $PCO_2 = 1.5 \times [HCO_3^-] + 8$
- Metabolic alkalosis: Expected $PCO_2 = 0.7 \times [HCO_3^-] + 20$
- Acute metabolic changes will have a change in pH by 0.15 for every change in $[HCO_3]$ of 10 mmHg.
- Acute respiratory changes will have a change in pH by 0.08 for every change in PCO_2 of 10 mmHg.

OXYHEMOGLOBIN DISSOCIATION CURVE

- Oxyhemoglobin dissociation curve: relates O_2 saturation to PO_2. See Figure 22-3.
  ○ Curve shifted to the left (increased hemoglobin affinity for oxygen): alkalosis, hypothermia, hypocarbia, decreased 2,3-diphosphoglycerate (2,3-DPG), increased fetal hemoglobin, carbon monoxide poisoning, and anemia

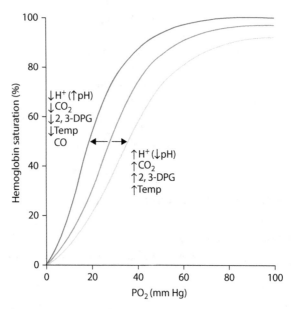

FIGURE 22-3 Oxyhemoglobin dissociation curve.

○ Curve shifted to the right (decreased hemoglobin affinity for oxygen): acidosis, hyperthermia, hypercarbia, and increased 2,3-DPG

SUGGESTED READINGS

Grippi MA, Elias JA, Fishman JA, et al. Fishman's Pulmonary Diseases and Disorders. www.accessmedicine.com. Mcgraw Hill Education (this is the reference for figure 22-3)

Rozenfeld RA. Acid-base balance. In: Green TP, Franklin WH, Tanz RR, eds. *Pediatrics: Just the Facts.* New York: McGraw Hill; 2005:151-152.

West JB. *Pulmonary Pathophysiology - The Essentials.* 8th ed. Wolter, Kluwer, Lippincott, Williams & Wilkins; 2012, Riverwoods, IL.

Williams AJ. Assessing and interpreting arterial blood gases and acid-base balance. *BMJ.* 1998;317:1213-1216.

PATHOPHYSIOLOGY OF ACUTE RESPIRATORY DISTRESS SYNDROME (ARDS)

- Acute inflammation occurring as a result of either direct or indirect injury
- Hallmark of acute phase is diffuse alveolar damage via altered permeability of pulmonary endothelial and epithelial cells
  - Leads to accumulation of protein-rich fluid in alveoli
  - Inactivates surfactant
  - Leads to hypoxia and impaired lung compliance

DEFINITIONS

- P/F Ratio
  - PaO_2/FiO_2 is a measure of oxygenation
  - A lower P/F ratio is reflective of more impaired oxygenation
  - Does not incorporate mean airway pressure
- Oxygenation Index (OI)
  - Measure of oxygenation developed for use in neonates with persistent pulmonary hypertension
  - Recommended for use in pediatric ARDS over P/F ratio

$$OI = [\text{mean airway pressures} \times FiO_2 \div PaO_2] \times 100$$

DIAGNOSTIC CRITERIA

HISTORICAL DEFINITION

- Acute lung injury (ALI)
  - Acute onset of respiratory failure
  - Bilateral infiltrates on chest x-ray (CXR)
  - $PaO_2/FiO_2 < 300$
  - Absence of left ventricular failure
- Acute respiratory distress syndrome (ARDS)
  - Acute onset of respiratory failure
  - Bilateral infiltrates on CXR
  - $PaO_2/FiO_2 < 200$
  - Absence of left ventricular failure

BERLIN DEFINITION OF ARDS (2012)

- Respiratory failure within one week of a known clinical insult OR new or worsening respiratory symptoms
- Bilateral opacities on CXR not explained by effusions, collapse, or nodules
- Respiratory failure not fully explained by cardiac failure or fluid overload
- Impaired oxygenation with positive end-expiratory pressure (PEEP) ≥5 cm H_2O
  - Mild: P/F ratio 200 to 300
  - Moderate: P/F ratio 100 to 200
  - Severe: P/F ratio <100

PEDIATRIC ACUTE LUNG INJURY CONSENSUS CONFERENCE (2015)[1] (TABLE 23-1)

- Excluded patients with perinatal lung disease
- Recommendation to use OI preferentially over P/F ratio as metric of severity of lung disease
- Provision for noninvasively ventilated patients

TABLE 23-1	PALICC Definition of ARDS			
Age	Exclude patients with perinatal-related lung disease			
Timing	Within seven days of known clinical insult			
Origin of Edema	Respiratory failure not fully explained by cardiac failure or fluid overload			
Chest Imaging	Chest imaging findings of new infiltrate(s) consistent with acute pulmonary parenchymal disease			
Oxygenation	**Noninvasive mechanical ventilation**	**Invasive mechanical ventilation**		
	PARDS (No severity satisfaction)	Mild	Moderate	Severe
	Full face mask bilevel ventilation or CPAP ≥5 cm H_2O	$4 \leq OI < 8$	$8 \leq OI < 16$	$OI \geq 16$
	PF ratio ≤ 300	$5 \leq OSI < 7.5$	$7.5 \leq OSI < 12.3$	$OSI \geq 12.3$
	SF ratio ≤ 264			
Special Populations				
Cyanotic Heart Disease	Standard criteria as noted earlier for age, timing, origin of edema, and chest imaging with an acute deterioration in oxygenation not explained by underlying cardiac disease.			
Chronic Lung Disease	Standard criteria as noted earlier for age, timing, origin of edema with chest imaging consistent with new infiltrate, and acute deterioration in oxygenation from baseline that meet oxygenation criteria noted previously.			
Left Ventricular Dysfunction	Standard criteria as noted earlier for age, timing, and origin of edema with chest imaging changes consistent with new infiltrate and acute deterioration in oxygenation that meets previous criteria not explained by left ventricular dysfunction.			

CAUSES OF ARDS (TABLE 23-2)

- Direct or indirect lung injury

TABLE 23-2	Causes of ARDS
Direct Lung Injury	**Indirect Lung Injury**
Pneumonia	Sepsis
Pneumonitis (e.g., aspiration, inhalational injury)	Pancreatitis
Trauma (e.g., pulmonary contusion)	Burns
Submersion Injury	Transfusion-Related Lung Injury (TRALI)
Fat Embolism	Cardiopulmonary Bypass

PRINCIPLES OF MANAGEMENT

- Management of invasive ventilatory support: Lung-protective ventilation
  - ARDSNET trial[2] showed survival benefit in targeting V_T 6 mL/kg vs. 12 mL/kg in adults with ARDS
  - PALICC group[1] recommends:
    - V_T 5 to 8 mL/kg for all intubated children with ARDS
    - With poor compliance, target 3 to 6 mL/kg instead
  - Permissive hypercapnia/pH goal:
    - PALICC group[1] suggests maintaining pH >7.20 to 7.30
      - Exceptions include patients with elevated intracranial pressure (ICP), pulmonary hypertension, hemodynamic instability, or left ventricular dysfunction for whom acidemia confers an additional risk of decompensation
      - Insufficient data to recommend a lower limit; may consider pH >7.15 in severe disease
  - Oxygenation goals:
    - No mortality increase with liberalization of SaO_2 goal to >87% in ARDSNET
    - PALICC suggests SaO_2 92% to 97% in mild ARDS, 88% to 92% in severe ARDS
      - If goal SaO_2 88% to 92%, consider monitoring lactate/MVO_2
      - Recruit lung volume with increasing PEEP as tolerated to facilitate weaning of FiO_2 to a goal of <60%
- Management of nonpulmonary support
  - *Sedation:* target sedation to safe tolerance of mechanical ventilation, optimization of oxygen delivery (DO_2), minimization of oxygen consumption (VO_2), work of breathing
  - *Neuromuscular blockade:* if unable to achieve targeted pH/SaO_2 goals, consider neuromuscular blockade to further enhance DO_2/VO_2
  - *Fluid management:* following any necessary initial fluid resuscitation and stabilization of hemodynamic status, aim to avoid positive fluid balance and consider diuresis if evidence of volume overload
  - *Nutrition:* as in all critically ill children, whenever safe, the enteral route for provision of nutrition is preferred over parenteral nutrition
  - *Transfusion:* if DO_2 appears to be adequate, as assessed clinically and by laboratory evidence (normal lactate, MVO_2), PALICC recommends a transfusion threshold of Hgb <7.0 g/dL

REFERENCES

1. Pediatric Acute Lung Inury Consensus Conference Group. Pediatric acute respiratory distrses syndrome: Consensus recommendations from the Pediatric Acute Lung Inury Consensus Conference. *Pediatr Crit Care Med.* 2015;16(5):428-439.
2. Brower RG, Matthay MA, Morris A, et al. Ventilation with lower tidal volumes as compared with traditional tidal volumes for acute lung injury and the acute respiratory distress syndrome. *N Engl J Med.* 2000;342(18):1301-1308.

Mechanical Ventilation

Mechanical ventilation is provided to ensure adequate oxygenation and minute ventilation. The means to achieve these goals will vary depending upon the lung pathophysiology. Indications to improve oxygenation include pneumonia, pulmonary edema, and acute respiratory distress syndrome. Clinical situations requiring maintenance of minute ventilation include postoperative patients, asthma, and bronchiolitis. Several modes of mechanical ventilation are available to optimize patient recovery by normalizing pulmonary gas exchange while minimizing lung disease.

CONVENTIONAL MECHANICAL VENTILATION (SEE TABLE 24-1)

- There are various ways to deliver a tidal volume to the patient, but understanding the basic terminology helps to understand the benefits or pitfalls of a particular mode.
  - Breaths are either mandatory and triggered by the machine (control mode) or on demand and triggered by the patient (assist mode).
  - Variables determining the breath
    - Trigger: the variable starting the breath. In a spontaneously breathing patient, a change in flow or pressure with an effort can trigger a breath; if the patient becomes apneic, the machine can deliver the breath based on a timed interval.
    - Cycle: the variable stopping the breath. In a volume mode of ventilation when the volume is delivered, the inspiratory phase will stop—it is volume cycled. In a pressure mode, the time the pressure is maintained will cycle the breath off—it is time cycled. The pressure support mode is flow cycled.
    - Limit: the goal of the delivered gas flow, either volume or pressure.

VOLUME VENTILATION

- The primary input is volume to be delivered from the ventilator. Airway and alveolar pressures generated as a result of the volume delivered will vary depending upon the resistance to flow and the compliance of the respiratory system.

TABLE 24-1 Ventilator Modes

Variable	Ventilator Mode		
	Volume Control	**Pressure Control**	**PRVC**
Tidal Volume	Constant	Variable	Constant
Peak Airway Pressure	Variable	Constant	Variable (based on compliance and resistance)
Peak Alveolar Pressure	Variable	Constant	Variable (based on compliance)
Flow Pattern	Decelerating or Constant	Decelerating	Decelerating
Peak Flow	Constant	Variable	Variable
Inspiratory Time	Measured value, based on peak flow and RR	Preset	Preset
Respiratory Rate	Preset	Preset	Preset

- SIMV: synchronized intermittent mandatory ventilation (flow/pressure initiated, volume limited, volume/time cycled)
  - The volume set can be delivered in synchrony with a patient effort, decreasing the work of breathing.
  - With apnea, the rate set and the volume delivered will result in the minute ventilation the patient receives.
- Assist control (flow/pressure/time initiated, volume limited, volume/time cycled)
  - Volumes delivered are consistent and synchronized with patient effort.
  - If there is no patient effort, the rate set and volume delivered determine the minute ventilation.
  - In contrast to SIMV, every patient effort results in the entire delivered tidal volume with each breath.
- IMV: intermittent mandatory ventilation (time initiated, volume limited, volume/time cycled)
  - Rarely used pediatric mode delivering a volume of breath regardless of patient effort.

PRESSURE VENTILATION

- Primary input is a pressure limit. Variable tidal volumes will result based on the respiratory system compliance and resistance.
  - Pressure control
    - SIMV-PC (flow/pressure/time initiated, pressure limited, time cycled) is a synchronized mode of ventilation delivering flows as in IMV-PC, but can be triggered by patient effort.
    - IMV-PC (time initiated, pressure limited, time cycled) is a control mode of ventilation in which gas flow is rapid at initiation of breath but decreases when the pressure limit is reached, resulting in a constant airway or alveolar pressure during the inspiratory cycle, in turn resulting in higher mean airway pressures than volume modes achieving similar peak inspiratory pressure.
  - Pressure support (flow/pressure initiated, pressure limited, flow cycled)
    - Flow from the ventilator will generate the pressure level set. Tidal volume will vary, and each respiratory effort will be supported when triggered. The pressure is maintained until the inspiratory flow decreases to preset levels designed by the ventilator software.
    - There is no backup respiratory rate; thus, the patient must have an adequate respiratory rate and drive to breathe. This mode is best used as a weaning method from support.

PRVC

- Pressure regulated volume control (flow/time initiated, pressure limited, time or flow cycled)
  - A mode combining volume ventilation and pressure ventilation
  - Minute ventilation is guaranteed with set tidal volume and rate
  - Decelerating inspiratory flows like pressure control apply consistent airway pressures, minimizing peak pressures based on the machine's algorithm
  - Can be used in control or assist mode

SETTING UP THE VENTILATOR (SEE FIGURE 24-1)

- Adequate minute ventilation is required to meet metabolic demands by having an appropriate respiratory rate and tidal volume (MV = RR × TV)
  - Rate
    - Respiratory rate is set initially for physiologic normative rate for the patient's age; rates generally are higher for younger children. Inspiratory time (iT) defines the time allowed for gas to flow and is lower in infants and children than for adults; times vary from 0.4 to 1 second.

Initial Ventilator Settings:

A. Volume Control or PRVC:

<u>Rate:</u> normal range for age

<u>TV</u>: 6-8 mL/kg (4-6 mL/kg in some disease states e.g. ARDS)

<u>PEEP:</u> Start with 5 cm H_2O and increase clinically as indicated

<u>I-Time:</u> 1:2 (must increase E-time in obstructive disease to avoid air trapping)

**Make sure PIP not too high

B. Pressure Control:

<u>Rate:</u> normal range for age

<u>PEEP:</u> Start with 5 cm H_2O and increase clinically as indicated

<u>PC:</u> Set pressure to produce adequate chest rise and TV's (6-8 mL/kg unless ARDS)

**Make sure TV's are adequate

FIGURE 24-1 **Initial ventilator settings.**

- With higher rates, short iT is necessary to allow for exhalation time and avoiding breath stacking. When exhaled time is prolonged such as in acute asthma, the iT may again be shortened to allow complete exhalation.
  - ○ Tidal volume
    - Volume mode
      - Volumes generally delivered are 6 to 10 mL/kg of body weight. Ideal body weight calculations may be necessary in very obese patients, as the tidal volumes used based on actual weight will result in overdistension of the lungs and high peak inspiratory pressure.
      - Peak inspiratory pressure and plateau pressure are monitored closely with this mode of ventilation, as they may increase greatly with decreased lung compliance.
      - High peak pressure (greater than 30 cm H_2O) is associated with alveolar overdistention and lung damage. Illnesses such as ARDS and poor lung compliance frequently result in high peak pressure. Strategies for volume ventilation in this instance include using small tidal volumes, 4 to 6 mL/kg, and increased frequency to achieve the desired level of gas exchange.
    - Pressure mode
      - Pressure input limits peak pressures and generally will be limited to less than 30 cm H_2O.
      - Tidal volumes in this mode are variable based on resistance to flow and compliance of the respiratory system. Pressure limits for neonates are lower than for children.
      - Limited pressures above the end-expiratory pressure are set from 12 to 30 centimeters of water.

- Oxygenation goals are primarily met by adjusting inspired oxygen concentration and positive end-expiratory pressure (PEEP). Subtle adjustments in inspiratory flows will alter mean airway pressure—adjustments that may alter oxygenation.
  - Supplemental oxygen can be supplied from 21% to 100% oxygen. Many newer-generation ventilators can substitute gases other than nitrogen, such as helium, for therapeutic use while maintaining appropriate tidal volumes.
  - PEEP is maintained by flow through the ventilator circuit to keep alveolar pressures at set levels. With minimal lung disease, PEEP is set at 3 to 5 cm H_2O. Increasing PEEP increases alveolar surface area, thereby increasing functional residual capacity and improving oxygenation. With ARDS, PEEP levels are higher and are not uncommonly 15 to 20 cm H_2O. Higher levels of PEEP may lead to interstitial emphysema, pneumothorax, and pneumomediastinum, as well as alveolar overdistention and worsened perfusion and ventilation mismatch.

HIGH-FREQUENCY MECHANICAL VENTILATION

HIGH-FREQUENCY OSCILLATORY VENTILATION (HFOV) (SEE TABLE 24-2)

- Electrically powered, electronically controlled piston-diaphragm with active inhalation and exhalation primarily used to improve oxygenation in patients with ARDS. Conceptually, there is less phasic volume and pressure changes to the alveolus, reducing ventilator-associated lung injury.
  - Ventilator settings
    - Oxygenation
      - Mean airway pressure (MAP): in conjunction with FiO_2, used to adjust oxygenation
      - Initial settings
        - 5 cm H_2O greater than MAP for conventional mechanical ventilaiton (CMV) (high-volume strategy)
        - 2 cm H_2O less than CMV for air leak syndromes (low-volume strategy)
  - Ventilation, CO_2
    - Amplitude: set by power control
      - *Increase* will increase TV and *reduce* CO_2
      - Changes in amplitude will change MAP
      - *Primary* control parameter for CO_2 management
  - Hertz
    - *Increase* Hz will *increase* CO_2
    - Babies Hz typically 8 to 12

TABLE 24-2	HFOV Settings and Adjustments			
Starting Amplitude			**Starting Frequency**	
Infant	40–50 cm H_2O	<2 kg	15 Hz	
Child	50–60 cm H_2O	2–12 kg	10 Hz	
Adult	60–100 cm H_2O	13–20 kg	8 Hz	
		21–30 kg	7 Hz	
		>30 kg	6 Hz	

Decrease CO_2	**Increase O_2**
Decrease Frequency (Hz)	Increase FiO_2
Increase Amplitude (ΔP)	Increase Bias Flow
Adjust Bias Flow	Increase MAP
Reduce ETT Cuff Pressure	

- Children and adults >40 kg Hz 3 to 6
- Ensure minimal leak from cuffed endotracheal tube (ETT); increased air leak around ETT allows for improved CO_2 clearance, but may be at the expense of losing MAP and worsening oxygenation
  - ○ Adjustments
    - MAP
      - Increase in 1- to 2-cm H_2O increments to improve oxygenation
      - Slowly decrease in 1-cm H_2O increments to wean, often one or two times daily
      - Consider recruitment of alveolar units with initial MAP setup
        - ○ First 30 to 60 seconds set MAP at peak inspiratory pressure (PIP) of CMV then reduce to goal MAP if hemodynamics allow.
        - ○ Consider recruitment maneuver with incremental increase in MAP or loss of MAP as in suctioning.
    - Amplitude
      - Clinically adjusted to obtain chest "wiggle." Correlating wiggle to arterial blood gases (ABG) may help evaluate changes in lung compliance or airway resistance.
      - In the weaning phase, changes in amplitude are made in increments of 2 to 4 cm H_2O.
  - ○ Ensure adequate intravascular volume and cardiac output.
    - The higher intrathoracic pressure may adversely affect cardiac preload.
    - Consider volume loading (~5 mL/kg) or initiating inotropes.
  - ○ Overdistention with increased MAP will result in alveolar damage, increased pulmonary vascular resistance (PVR), and desaturation

HIGH-FREQUENCY JET VENTILATION (HFJV) (SEE TABLE 24-3)

- Delivers a pulse of gas into the ETT via a special adapter and pinch valve mechanism and is used in tandem with a conventional ventilator. Often used for air leak syndromes due to very small volumes used in bulk flow and reliance on alveolar oxygen diffusive properties.
  - ○ Ventilator settings
    - Oxygenation
      - PEEP set by conventional ventilator is adjusted to optimize oxygenation in conjunction with FiO_2.
      - PEEP is started at conventional ventilator setting and adjusted up until there is consistent oxygenation.
    - Ventilation
      - The delta P (PIP-PEEP) is proportional to tidal volume and is the *primary* determinate of ventilation
        - ○ PIP is usually set around CMV PIP
        - ○ PIP adjustments by 2 to 6 cm H_2O
        - ○ Pressure-limited ventilator; changing PIP or PEEP independently will change delta P
      - HFV rate is secondary adjustment for ventilation
        - ○ Range 4 to 11 Hz, usually starting at 7 Hz or 420 bpm
        - ○ *Increase* in rate, *decreases* CO_2
        - ○ Lower rates for air leaks to reduce air trapping
        - ○ If jet PEEP is higher than CMV PEEP set, lower rate
    - IMV rate set on conventional ventilator is generally 0 to 4 with inspiratory time of 0.4 to 0.6 and tidal volumes of 6 mL/kg to provide breaths to prevent or treat atelectasis
  - ○ Mean airway pressure limited to conventional ventilator capabilities

TABLE 24-3 Troubleshooting the Jet Ventilator (HFJV)

Objective	Circumstances	Actions to Take
Lower PCO_2	Hypercapnea	Raise HFJV PIP
		Raise HFJV rate
		Note: Watch for elevated PEEP
Raise PO_2	Atelectasis on CXR	Raise the following in this order:
		1. PEEP/CPAP
		2. CV rate (max = 10 bpm)
		3. CMV PIP
		4. CMV I-Time
		These increases are temporary; discontinue as soon as process has reversed.
Raise PO_2	Overdistension on CXR	Repeat the earlier actions at a higher PEEP/CPAP
		Reduce MAP by decreasing CMV support
		1. CMV rate <10 BPM
		2. CMV I-Time <0.5 sec
		3. PEEP < 6 cm H_2O
		4. Raise Jet PIP to maintain PO_2
Raise PCO_2	PO_2 drops every time HFJV PIP is dropped	Lower HFJV PIP and/or raise PEEP
		Raise PEEP before dropping HFJV PIP
Lower PO_2	PCO2 is also low	Lower the following in this order as necessary:
		1. FiO_2
		2. CV PIP and/or rate
		3. PEEP
		Lower HFJV PIP
Lower PEEP	PEEP on CV has been turned down to minimum	Lower the following in this order as necessary:
		1. HFJV on time to 0.02 sec
		2. HFJV rate
		3. IMV flow rate, if appropriate

Parameter	Typical Setting	When to Raise	When to Lower
HFJV PIP	20 cm H_2O	To lower PCO_2	To raise PCO_2
HFJV Rate	420 bpm	To increase MAP and PO_2	Lengthen expiratory time (E-time); reduce unintentional PEEP in larger patients or when weaning
		To decrease PCO_2 in smaller patients	To increase PCO_2
HFJV I-Time	0.02 sec	To reach PIP at low HJFV rates (larger patients)	Keep at minimum of 0.02 in almost all cases.
CV Rate	0–3 bpm	To reverse atelectasis	Concern for air leak
			Hemodynamic compromise

(continued)

TABLE 24-3	(continued)		
Parameter	Typical Setting	When to Raise	When to Lower
CV PIP	15–20 cm H_2O	To reverse atelectasis	When air leak is present
			When not recruiting alveoli
CV I-time	0.4 sec	To reverse atelectasis	When air leak is present
			When not recruiting alveoli
PEEP	4–8 cm H_2O	To improve oxygenation	Usually when air leaks present
			When not recruiting alveoli

http://www.bunl.com/

TABLE 24-4	VDR Adjustments
Decrease CO_2	**Increase O_2**
↑ PIP by 2–3 cm H_2O (maximum around 40 cm H_2O)	↑ PIP by 2–3 cm H_2O
If PIP at max, ↓ Frequency rate by 50	↑ Frequency rate by 50
↓ Oscillatory CPAP (increases delta P)	↑ Oscillatory CPAP by 1–2 cm H_2O (maximum around 20 cm H_2O)
Ensure leak around ETT balloon	↑ Supplemental oxygen
↑ Inspiratory time	↑ Inspiratory time

- ○ Servo pressure: an important monitoring parameter reflecting the driving pressures required to maintain desired PIP
  - ▪ Increase in servo pressure is seen in improved compliance and resistance of respiratory system. It will also occur with increase in ETT leak and leak in ventilator circuit.
  - ▪ Decrease in servo pressure reflects worsening compliance, increased resistance such as in bronchospasm, obstruction of ETT, and increase in intrathoracic pressure as seen in tension pneumothorax.

HIGH-FREQUENCY PERCUSSIVE VENTILATION (HFPV) (SEE TABLE 24-4)

- A hybrid approach to ventilation combining phasic pressure control with high frequency and used for both hypoxemia and hypercarbic respiratory failure. Felt to be particularly indicated for patients with excessive pulmonary secretions such as bronchiolitis and patients with cystic fibrosis.
  - ○ Ventilator settings
    - ▪ Oxygenation
      - PEEP: two settings on the VDR, a demand PEEP and oscillatory PEEP. Demand PEEP is typically set at 2 cm H_2O, and adjustable PEEP is the oscillatory setting. The sum of demand and oscillatory PEEP will equal the desired PEEP for the patient. The desired PEEP is rarely less than 8 cm H_2O (2 cm H_2O from demand and 6 cm H_2O from oscillatory). Total PEEP is generally less than 20 cm H_2O.
      - MAP: increased by increased PIP, increased PEEP, or increase in inspiratory time.
      - Inspired supplemental oxygen.
    - ▪ Ventilation
      - PIP: peak pressures are not PEEP compensated and are pressure limited. An increase in the PEEP will reduce the PEEP to peak pressure difference (delta P) reducing the effective tidal volume.

- Convective rate: set at typical physiologic rate for age.
- Percussive rate: 500 to 700 bpm provides the oscillatory compo[...]
  runs through the entire respiratory cycle.
- Ensure minimal leak from ETT.
  - Adjustments
    - PEEP
      - Demand PEEP is maintained at 2 cm H_2O
      - Adjust oscillatory PEEP by 1 to 2 cm H_2O to improve oxygenation and reduce by 1 to 2 to a minimum of 6 cm H_2O
    - Percussive rate
      - 500 to 700 bpm, typically starting at 600
      - Adjustments are made in increments of 50
      - Decrease frequency for hypercarbia (similar to HFOV, this decreases effective pressure changes, reducing CO_2 clearance)
    - Inspiratory time (iT)
      - Maintain I:E ratio of 1:1
      - Increase iT may increase MAP, improving oxygenation and increasing CO_2 clearance
    - PIP (pulsatile flow rate)
      - Typically set at CMV PIP
      - To improve CO_2 clearance, increase by 2 to 3 cm H_2O. An increase in PEEP requires an increase in PIP to maintain the same delta P and ventilation parameters.

AIRWAY PRESSURE RELEASE VENTILATION (APRV)

- A pressure mode based on reverse I:E physiology. The work of breathing to perform inflation, overcoming air flow resistance and elastic forces, is reduced by the constant inflation pressure. The expiratory phase is reliant upon lung recoil with high expiratory flow rates in ARDS. Spontaneous respiratory effort is encouraged and may result in improved dependent gas distribution recruiting dependent areas without elevated airway pressure
  - Ventilator settings: there are two pressure settings and two time settings
    - P_{High}: upper pressure limit of inflation, similar to mean airway pressure is important determinate of oxygenation
    - P_{Low}: analogous to PEEP, change in pressures determines released volume and thus ventilation
    - T_{High}: the time allowed for the P_{High} to be maintained
    - T_{Low}: the time allowed for P_{Low} to be maintained
  - Parameters: pressure
    - High pressure: set at *plateau* pressure, somewhat higher than MAP on conventional ventilation
      - Small babies: 10 to 25 (cm H_2O)
      - Children: 20 to 30 (cm H_2O)
      - Adults: 20 to 35 (cm H_2O)
      - Low pressure: 0 (cm H_2O)
  - Parameters: time
    - Babies
      - 2 to 3 seconds T_{High}
      - 0.2 to 0.4 seconds T_{Low}
    - Children
      - 3 to 5 seconds T_{High}
      - 0.2 to 0.8 seconds T_{Low}

- 4 to 6 seconds T_{High}
  - 0.2 to 0.8 seconds T_{Low}
  - Oxygenation
    - Alveolar recruitment is important for improving oxygenation and is achieved by adjusting P_{High} and T_{High}
    - P_{High} adjusted in increments of 1 to 2 cm H_2O to improve oxygenation
    - T_{High} increase by 0.5 seconds per change may increase alveolar recruitment and will affect ventilation
    - P_{Low} increase will increase intrinsic PEEP but will reduce ventilation at the same time; P_{Low} is adjusted in 0.1-second increments
    - Inspired supplemental oxygen
  - Ventilation
    - Increasing alveolar ventilation: increased high pressure increases the volume in the lung; increasing the time at the high pressure may allow more diffusive CO_2 exchange. Minimizing P_{Low} will increase the pressure changes and maximize the volume exchanged.
      - Increase P_{high} and T_{high}
    - Increasing minute ventilation: a decrease in the time at high pressure results in more releases per minute; a T_{high} of 4 seconds will have a release 15 times a minute, whereas a T_{high} of 3 seconds will increase to 20 times a minute.
      - Increase P_{high} and decrease T_{high}
    - Pressure support in the acute phase of ARDS is not necessary with APRV, as the work of overcoming the resistance to flow has already been achieved; the added pressure from pressure support only will increase peak alveolar pressure. In the weaning phase, however, as P_{high} is reduced, the addition of pressure support is indicated.

NONINVASIVE POSITIVE PRESSURE VENTILATION (NIPPV)

- NIPPV is mechanical ventilator support that does not bypass the upper airway (as does an endotracheal tube) and is provided by a mask, typically nasal or full face.
- Contraindications
  - Life-threatening hypoxemia
  - Increasing $PaCO_2$
  - Reduced Glasgow Coma Score (GCS), impaired ability to clear secretions and protect airway
  - Hemodynamic instability
  - Postoperative facial, tracheal, esophageal, or gastric surgery
- Common pediatric uses
  - Asthma
  - Bronchiolitis
  - Neuromuscular disorders
  - Pediatric obstructive sleep apnea (OSA)
  - Postoperative, postextubation
- NIPPV modes
  - Continuous positive airway pressure (CPAP)
    - Positive pressure is applied throughout the respiratory cycle
    - Typically used for OSA; airway obstruction relieved by CPAP after extubation and recruitment of functional residual capacity (FRC), maintaining airway patency and opening collapsed alveoli.
    - Pressures range from 5 to 15 cm H_2O

- Bilevel support
  - Provides inspiratory flows, decreasing inspiratory muscle work.
  - Inspiratory pressures provide a tidal volume, increasing alveolar ventilation.
  - Increased inspiratory pressures will help recruitment of FRC and collapsed alveolar units.
  - Pressures above expiratory pressure (EPAP) are usually 5 to 20.
  - Inspiratory support is triggered by a flow change in the circuit.
  - Pressure is limited to set pressure; a setting of IPAP 10/EPAP 5 cm H_2O will provide a delta pressure for ventilation of 5 cm H_2O. Tidal volume goals are then evaluated to ensure minute ventilation, generally achieving 6 to 8 mL/kg per breath.
  - Rate can be delivered in timed mode.

SUGGESTED READINGS

Jet ventilation. http://www.bunl.com/.

Mechanical ventilation. In: MJ Tobin, ed. *Principles and Practice of Mechanical Ventilation.* 3rd ed. New York: The McGraw-Hill Companies, Inc.; 2013.

VDR. https://percussionaire.com/critical-care/.

Extracorporeal Membrane Oxygenation (ECMO)

25

BACKGROUND

Extracorporeal membrane oxygenation (ECMO) is a form of modified cardiopulmonary bypass that has evolved since the beginnings of bypass in the 1950s.[1] It can be used for days to weeks to support patients with severe cardiac or respiratory failure. Since the first successful use of ECMO in the 1970s, several developments have been made related to cannulation strategies and machinery. However, several topics related to ECMO remain controversial and ill defined, including patient selection ("ECMO candidacy"), timing of ECMO initiation, and proper anticoagulation.[2]

PATIENT SELECTION

Although the Extracorporeal Life Support Organization (ELSO) and several other groups have attempted to standardize guidelines for patient selection, no set of inclusive guidelines exists. General guidelines for patient selection can be found on the ELSO website or within the text published by the organization.[3]

Despite the lack of inclusive guidelines, patients who are admitted to the pediatric intensive care unit or cardiac intensive care unit with respiratory failure, cardiac failure, or high likelihood of sudden cardiac death should be assessed for ECMO candidacy early in their hospital course. This status may change as patient disease status and chance of survival changes. Patient selection and timing of initiation of ECMO will generally depend on the expertise and experience of individual centers.[2]

GENERAL INDICATIONS

- Acute, reversible disease
- Respiratory and/or cardiac failure
- Postoperative cardiac surgery patient with inability to separate from mechanical circulatory support/cardiac bypass
- Weight >2.0 kg
- Gestational age >35 weeks

GENERAL CONTRAINDICATIONS

- Intraventricular hemorrhage > grade II in neonates or intracranial hemorrhage in older children
- Irreversible disease state
  ○ Defining irreversible conditions may be difficult
- Fatal congenital diseases

MODES OF ECMO

In general, two basic modes of ECMO exist, and they are defined by their site of cannula placement: venoarterial (VA) or venovenous (VV). Although a few physiologic differences exist between the two modes, the basic principles and circuit design are similar.[2] Sites of cannulation, advantages, and disadvantages can be seen in Table 25-1.

TABLE 25-1	Modes of ECMO: Venoarterial versus Venovenous		
ECMO	Site	Advantages	Disadvantage
VA	1. Right carotid artery and right internal jugular vein	Full support	May require ligating the carotid artery, resulting in decreased cerebral perfusion in patients without adequate collateral circulation
		Higher oxygenation	
	2. Femoral vein and artery	Decreases pulmonary arterial pressure	
	3. Right atrium and aorta (central cannulation)	Venous saturations can be measured	
VV	1. Internal jugular vein (double-lumen cannula)	Avoids carotid artery ligation	Only supports lungs; no cardiac support
		Perfusion of lungs	
	2. Internal jugular vein and femoral vein	Perfusion of myocardium with oxygenated blood	May elevate mixed venous saturation via recirculation in double-lumen cannula
	3. Bilateral femoral veins	Faster cannulation	
		Safety – fewer emboli	

ECMO SETTINGS

INITIAL PUMP SETTINGS

Flow
- The ability to "flow" well on ECMO depends on the size of the venous cannula(e)
- In general, start the flow at 50 mL/kg/min and increase by 50- to 100-mL increments
- Full pediatric ECMO flow = 90 to 100 mL/kg/min
  - Single-ventricle patients with shunted physiology (e.g., Blalock-Taussig shunt, etc.) may require flows of 150 to 200 mL/kg/minute to achieve adequate perfusion and oxygenation
  - Patients with sepsis or multisystem organ failure may require higher flows[2]
- Goals: SVO_2 ~70% to 75%, adequate perfusion

Oxygenation
- Pump FiO_2 is generally kept at 100%, and ventilator FiO_2 is weaned
  - May decrease pump FiO_2 as saturations or patient's disease status improves

Ventilation
- ECMO pump sweep gas generally starts at 0.5 to 0.8 L/min
  - Sweep gas flow is adjusted up or down to achieve adequate ventilation.
- "Rest" ventilator settings
  - Ventilation strategies on ECMO have evolved over time. In general, it is recommended to use the lowest ventilator settings possible that will prevent atelectasis without using large tidal volume (TV) or high peak inspiratory pressure (PIP). The goal of this strategy is to minimize additional lung injury while on ECMO. Patients with severe respiratory failure may require higher settings.
  - General strategies:
    - Low FiO_2 21%
    - Low TV ~3 to 4 cc/kg
    - Low Rate ~10
    - High PEEP – 7 to 10

TROUBLESHOOTING

In general, problems with the ECMO circuit reflect changes in your patient. Be sure to assess the patient prior to adjusting ECMO settings (especially the flow).

- To increase oxygenation:
  - Increase ECMO FiO_2 (if not 100%)
  - Change FiO_2 on ventilator
  - Transfuse (if anemia/relative anemia) to increase arterial O_2 content
  - Increase ECMO flow (on VA ECMO)
    - Generally a last resort unless perfusion is compromised by lower flow
- To increase ventilation:
  - Increase ECMO sweep gas
  - Consider increasing ventilator settings
    - Be cautious about increasing ventilator settings in order to minimize additional lung injury.
- Collapsed bladder or "chattering":
  - Give volume
    - This problem occurs when there is inadequate volume flowing to the ECMO circuit from the patient. Improving overall volume status increases circulating blood volume, restoring adequate flow to the circuit.
- Declining mixed venous oxygen saturation (SvO_2):
  - Transfuse if anemia or relative anemia
  - Consider increasing ECMO flow
    - Do this only after ensuring adequate hemoglobin, etc.
    - This is more reliable in VA ECMO. It may increase recirculation in VV ECMO.
- Air in line:
  - Clamp arterial and venous lines
  - Use emergency ventilation (above rest settings)
  - CPR until air cleared
- Power failure:
  - Hand-crank the circuit or perform CPR and hand-ventilate
- Sudden negative pressure:
  - Give volume; check patient and cannula position
    - Evaluate cannula position *carefully*, preferably with a surgeon present
- Low saturations +/− high CO_2:
  - Check pump flow (increase)
  - Evaluate membrane oxygenator
  - Check for sweep gas disconnection
  - Treat anemia
  - Consider pneumothorax

REFERENCES

1. Hill JD, Gibbon JH. Development of the first successful heart lung machine. *Ann Thoracic Surg.* 1982;34:337.
2. Dalton HJ, Mennon S. Extracorporeal life support. In: Fuhrman and Zimmerman, eds. *Pediatric Critical Care.* Elsevier, Philadelphia, PA, 2011:717-737.
3. Van Meurs K, Lally KP, Peek G, et al., eds. *ECMO: Extracorporeal Cardiopulmonary Support in Critical Care.* 3rd ed. Ann Arbor, MI: Extracorporeal Life Support Organization; 2005.

26 Chronic Ventilation

RESPIRATORY PHYSIOLOGY IN THE DEVELOPING CHILD

Spontaneous ventilation requires adequate function of the central control of breathing, ventilator muscle function, and lung mechanics.

Respiratory failure occurs when the central respiratory drive and/or power are inadequate to overcome the respiratory load. When the cause of this imbalance is irreversible, the condition becomes chronic respiratory failure.

Developmental factors that affect breathing in the infant and young child may include soft thoracic cage, poorly developed intercostal muscles, lack of bucket-handle motion in the rib cage because of the horizontal alignment of the ribs, short diaphragm, fewer type I muscle fibers, smaller airways and increased resistance, and fewer air-exchange units. Less collateral ventilation and decreased stability of the air-exchange units increase likelihood of collapse.

INTRODUCTION

Improvements in the treatment of acute respiratory failure, the development of subspecialties such as pediatric critical care and neonatology, and advancements in invasive (e.g., tracheostomy and positive pressure ventilation) and noninvasive (mask continuous positive airway pressure [CPAP] or bilevel positive airway pressure [BiPAP]) ventilation have led to an increase in the survival of pediatric patients with chronic respiratory failure.

Infants, children, and adolescents with disorders of central control of breathing, disease of the airways, residual lung disease after severe respiratory illness, persistent pulmonary hypertension, and neuromuscular disorders may experience hypercarbic and/or hypoxemic chronic respiratory failure. Although it is generally possible to identify a primary cause for the respiratory failure, many children have multiple causative factors.

Chronic respiratory failure is pulmonary insufficiency for a protracted period, usually 28 days or longer. The goals of long-term mechanical ventilation are to sustain and extend life, to enhance the quality of life, to reduce morbidity, to improve physical and psychological function, and to enhance growth and development. Patients with reversible neuropathies (e.g., Guillain-Barre syndrome, neuropathy of critical illness), bronchopulmonary dysplasia, pulmonary hypertension, airway abnormalities, and congenital heart disease before or after surgical intervention are on long-term ventilation as a bridge for full recovery. Patients are maintained on long-term ventilation until they recover from the initial insult. Patients with conditions such as central hypoventilation, progressive neuromuscular disease, and high quadriplegia may require ventilatory support indefinitely.

The preferred site for a patient's care after initial discharge with a ventilator is within the family home. When social circumstances do not allow this placement, patients may be placed in a highly skilled nursing facility.

Less than 1% of patients admitted to pediatric intensive care units require long-term non-invasive or invasive ventilatory assistance. The polio epidemic in the 1930s through 1950s led to widespread need of respiratory support for children. At that time a negative pressure ventilation device such as the iron lung was used.

The causes for long-term dependency on chronic ventilation or supplemental oxygen may be categorized as follows:

- Respiratory pump: respiratory muscles, rib cage, ventral abdominal wall (neuromuscular disease, chest wall deformity, spinal cord injury, prune belly syndrome)
- Respiratory drive: congenital central hypoventilation, brain or brainstem injury, central nervous system (CNS) tumors, metabolic disorders
- Airway: obstructive sleep apnea, tracheomalacia, bronchomalacia
- Pulmonary parenchymal or vascular issues: bronchopulmonary dysplasia (BPD), lung hypoplasia, recurrent aspiration, cystic fibrosis (CF), congenital heart disease prior to or following cardiac surgery, pulmonary hypertension

The goals of long-term ventilation are to sustain and extend life, enhance the quality of life, reduce morbidity, improve physical and psychological function, and enhance growth and development. This is achieved by maintaining normal oxygenation and ventilation and minimizing the work of breathing.

Chronically ventilated infants and children recovering from severe illness may benefit from normal family interactions. Whenever possible, home discharge on mechanical ventilation is preferred over long-term hospitalization.

Caring for a child on long-term ventilator support in the home is a complex, physically demanding, emotionally taxing, and expensive process. It changes the family routines, priorities, and lifestyle and may adversely affect family relationships.

The discharge process for a child likely to require long-term ventilator support should start early in the hospital, before stabilization and transition to a portable ventilator.

The decision to initiate long-term ventilation also depends on the disease process and prognosis. Children with degenerative neuromuscular disease such as spinal muscular atrophy (SMA) type I may present with respiratory failure very early in life, often triggered by the first episode of respiratory illness. Although some parents of infants with SMA may decide to limit treatment to palliative care, others choose noninvasive or invasive ventilator support.

Infants and young children with chronic lung disease or airway malacia may improve their respiratory function and wean off ventilator support with adequate ventilation, good nutrition, and measures that promote development and prevent further injury.

Successful home discharge depends also on the presence of adequate resources in the community to support the family. Some programs recommend professional nurses in the home to assist with around-the-clock home care. The level of care depends on adequate funding and the availability of nursing agencies with skilled nurses. Housing may also present a significant barrier to home discharge. Adequacy of access, space for the child, caretakers, equipment, and supplies are other variables. Environmental safety issues include building and electrical code violations and the need for ramps or lifts. Funding for home care for children is challenging and varies across the country.

RESPIRATORY EQUIPMENT FOR HOME CARE

NONINVASIVE

Supplemental oxygen and positive pressure support can be administered by nasal cannula. The nasal cannula system can also deliver heated, supersaturated, high-flow gases. A number of devices are available for CPAP and BiPAP. These devices attach to nasal pillows, nasal mask, or full face mask. They are best suited for the management of obstructive sleep apnea.

Long-term use of a facial mask in small children may result in midface dysplasia. This type of ventilation may also be used in children with mild respiratory insufficiency, recurrent atelectasis, or nocturnal hypoventilation.

Other noninvasive respiratory devices are the cuirass ventilator and the iron lung, both of which are negative pressure devices. The rocker bed may also be used for mild respiratory insufficiency due to muscular weakness.

Diaphragmatic pacing may be used for congenital central hypoventilation syndrome (CCHS) or in older children with high-level quadriplegia. Many patients on diaphragmatic pacing will require tracheostomy because of lack of coordination between diaphragmatic contraction and opening of the glottis.

POSITIVE PRESSURE VENTILATION

A ventilator used in the home should be small, lightweight, and quiet; be able to entrain ambient air; provide continuous flow; and be able to accommodate a wide range of settings: pressure, volume, pressure support, and rate in order to satisfy needs from infancy to adulthood. Battery power, both internal and external, can allow unrestricted portability in the home and the community. The equipment must also be impervious to electromagnetic interference and must be relatively easy to operate and troubleshoot.

Children who are chronically ventilated on positive pressure require a tracheostomy. The child's caregivers (parents, family members, and home nursing staff) are instructed in all aspects of tracheostomy care: stoma care, elective and emergency tracheostomy change, recognition of obstruction or decannulation, and appropriate suctioning techniques. The child's caregivers have to demonstrate competency prior to home discharge.

AIRWAY CLEARANCE

Thick, copious secretions may contribute to increased airway resistance and provide a substrate for bacterial and fungal growth. Respiratory infections in turn may also increase the amount of secretions and viscosity and thus contribute to airway clearance issues.

Patients with neuromuscular weakness often have discoordinated or even absent swallow and are at risk for aspiration of secretions and food. Reflux, resulting in aspiration, is also common. Many patients have poor or nonexistent cough and may have ciliary dysfunction.

Modalities that help with clearance of secretions include manual or mechanical percussion, postural drainage, vibration, and vest or wrap percussion therapy. Cough-assist devices and/or abdominal binders may enhance cough. Additionally, oropharyngeal or tracheal suction help clear secretions. Intermittent positive ventilation devices are useful adjuncts. Pharmacologic agents such as anticholinergics or botulinum toxin may help control secretions, or selective ligation of the salivary glands may be an option. In extreme cases laryngotracheal separation may be considered. In case of thick tenacious secretions, review of the patient's hydration and anticholinergic medications is indicated. Nebulized dornase alfa, N-acetylcysteine, hypertonic saline, or sodium bicarbonate may be helpful. In selected cases bronchoscopy may be indicated for removal of inspissated secretions and re-expansion of atelectatic lung.

PHYSICAL, OCCUPATIONAL, AND SPEECH THERAPY

Therapies are essential in the management of chronic respiratory failure. Some of the goals of physical therapy are strengthening of the muscles, with an emphasis on muscles essential to breathing such as truncal and abdominal. Occupational therapy goals are in support of child development. Child life therapy focuses on providing a developmentally appropriate environment and age-appropriate play. Speech therapy initially focuses on oromotor skills for feeding and communication. Evaluation of swallow is very important. Equally important is evaluation of hearing, as hearing loss is relatively common in ventilator-dependent patients. Sign language may be taught in order to ease communication.

INFECTIONS

Respiratory infections such as tracheitis, bronchitis, and pneumonia are common in patients with chronic respiratory failure. Community-acquired viral or bacterial pathogens are common. Bacterial infections must be distinguished from colonization in order to avoid overusage of antibiotics. Preventive measures such as immunizations and meticulous tracheostomy care are essential.

MONITORING

A patient who is ventilated in the home must be electronically and/or physically monitored at all times. Infants and young children, cognitively impaired patients, and patients who are tracheostomy dependent due to suprastomal obstruction must be under direct observation of the caregivers at all times. Caregivers should also closely monitor children whose pulmonary status is fragile or unstable. Continuous monitoring of heart rate and oxygen saturation is recommended during sleep and either continuous or intermittent monitoring during the daytime. Patients with pulmonary hypertension are prone to rapid drops in oxygen saturation. Patients with CCHS are particularly vulnerable to episodes of hypoxemia or hypercarbia.

Patients evaluated in the pulmonary clinic should be monitored at each visit for heart rate, oxygen saturation, and transcutaneous and end-tidal CO_2 levels. Pulmonary function tests should be considered for patients who are old enough (over 5 years) and able to cooperate. Patients with pulmonary hypertension should have serial echocardiograms. An increased level of monitoring is recommended for patients who have improved enough and are in the process of weaning off ventilator support. In addition to physiologic parameters, patients must be monitored for signs of stress, agitation, or fatigue.

WEANING OFF VENTILATOR SUPPORT

Patients recovering from chronic respiratory failure who are on stable ventilator settings, on low PEEP, and on minimal or no oxygen support should be evaluated periodically for readiness to wean off mechanical ventilation. Barriers to weaning may include residual lung disease, pulmonary hypertension, impaired central control of breathing, and muscle weakness. Muscle weakness may be due to underlying neuromuscular disease; use of sedatives, analgesics, or steroids; past use of muscle relaxants; prolonged immobility; and overuse of ventilator support. It is important to titrate ventilator needs in order to exercise respiratory muscles; however, caution must be taken to avoid fatigue.

Transitioning from full ventilation to spontaneous breathing requires conditioning of the respiratory muscles. This can be achieved by gradually decreasing the pressure or the rate, sprints of pressure support, retraining the respiratory muscles by breathing against resistance, or spontaneous sprints off the ventilator. The weaning program may be initiated prior to discharge from the hospital or during clinic visits. Typically one may start with sprints of 15 minutes two to three times a day under direct observation of a caregiver. The sprints are lengthened gradually with continuous monitoring in the home and frequent clinic visits. The patient is also monitored for respiratory distress, weight gain, energy levels, behavior, and sleep patterns. When the patient is weaned down to six hours/day of ventilator support, a polysomnogram is ordered prior to complete liberation off the ventilator.

SUGGESTED READINGS

Noah Z, Budek C. Severe chronic respiratory failure. In: Kliegman RM, Stanton BF, St. Geme JW, et al., eds. *Nelson Textbook of Pediatrics*. 20th ed. Philadelphia, PA: Elsevier; 2015.

Sobotka SA, Hird-McCorry LP, Goodman DM. Identification of fail points for discharging pediatric patients with new tracheostomy and ventilator. *Hosp Pediatr*. 2016;6:552-557.

Sterni LM, Collaco JM, Baker CD, et al. An official American Thoracic Society Clinical Practice Guideline: Pediatric chronic home invasive ventilation. *Am J Respir Crit Care Med*. 2016;193:e16-e35.

Cardiovascular

27 Cardiovascular Formulas and Parameters

Arterial oxygen content of the blood:

$$CaO_2 (mL\ O_2/dL) = (SaO_2 \times Hemoglobin \times 1.36) + 0.003*(PaO_2)$$

$0.003*PaO_2$ represents the fraction of dissolved oxygen in the blood

Venous oxygen content of the blood:

$$CvO_2 (mL\ O_2/dL) = (SvO_2 \times Hemoglobin \times 1.36) + 0.003*(PvO_2)$$

Arterial-mixed venous oxygen content difference:

$$avDO_2 = CaO_2 - CvO_2$$

CaO_2 ~20 mL/dL
CvO_2 ~15 mL/dL
Oxygen extraction is approximately 25%; it can also be estimated by:
$SaO_2 - SvO_2$

Cardiac Output: $CO = HR \times SV$ Units: L/min
Cardiac Index: $CI = CO/BSA$ in m^2 Nl 3.6 – 6 L/min/m^2

• CI more used for children as it normalizes for size

Oxygen Delivery: $DO_2 = CO \times CaO_2 \times 10$
Oxygen Consumption: $VO_2 = CO \times (CaO_2 - CvO_2) \times 10$
Oxygen Extraction Ratio: $O_2ER = VO_2/DO_2 = [(CaO_2 - CvO_2)/CaO_2]$
Pulmonary Vascular Resistance: $PVR = (PAP - PAOP)/CO \times 79.9$ dynes*sec/cm^5
Systemic Vascular Resistance: $SVR = (MAP - RAP)/CO \times 79.9$ dynes*sec/cm^5

If you don't multiply by 79.9, then use Woods units OR mmHg/L/min
PAP – Pulmonary artery pressure
PAOP – Pulmonary artery occlusion pressure
MAP – Mean arterial pressure
RAP – Right atrial pressure

SVR Index: $SVRI = SVR/BSA$ Nl: 800 to 1600 dyne-s/cm^5/m^2
PVR Index: $PVRI = PVR/BSA$ Nl: 80 to 240 dyne-s/cm^5/m^2
Normal Pediatric Hemodynamic Variables - See Table 27-1

TABLE 27-1	Normal Pediatric Hemodynamic Parameters	
Parameter	**Calculation**	**Normal Values (Children)**
Mean Arterial Pressure	$MAP = (SBP/3) + [(2 \times DBP)/3]$	
Cardiac Index (CI)	$CI = CO/BSA$	3.5–5.5 L/min/m^2
Stroke Index	$SI = CI/HR$	30–60 mL/m^2
Oxygen Delivery	$DO_2 = CI \times CaO_2$	570–670 mL/min/m^2
Fick Principle	$CI = VO_2/(CaO_2 - CvO_2)$	Infant 160–180 mL/min/m^2
		Child 100–130 mL/min/m^2
Mixed Venous O_2 Saturation		65%–75%
Oxygen Extraction Ratio*	$OER = (SaO_2 - SvO_2)/SaO_2$	0.24–0.28

(continued)

TABLE 27-1 (continued)		
Parameter	**Calculation**	**Normal Values (Children)**
Oxygen Excess Factor*	$W = SaO_2/(SaO_2 - SvO_2)$	3.6–4.2
Systemic Vascular Resistance Index (SVRI)	$[(MAP - CVP)/CI] \times 79.9$	800–1600 dyne*s*m²/cm⁵
Pulmonary Vascular Resistance Index (PVRI)	$[(MPAP - PCWP)/CI] \times 79.9$	80–240 dyne*s*m²/cm⁵
LV Stroke Work Index (LVSWI)	$(MAP) \times SI \times 0.0136$	50–62 gram*m/m² (adult values)

*Only valid if contribution of dissolved O_2 is negligible. Otherwise, utilize oxygen content values.
Used with permission from Wheeler DS, et al, eds. *Pediatric Critical Care Medicine: Basic Science and Clinical Evidence.* Springer-Verlag, London, 2014.

Using the Fick Principle to Calculate Cardiac Output

Fick principle: oxygen consumption can be measured by subtracting exhaled oxygen concentration from inhaled oxygen concentration
This value will be equal to the difference of oxygen content leaving the lungs ($CO \times CaO_2$) and the content returning to the lungs ($CO \times CvO_2$)
The Fick equation is:

$$VO_2 = CO \times (CaO_2 - CvO_2) \rightarrow CO = VO_2/(CaO_2 - CvO_2)$$

VO_2 = consumption of oxygen in mL/min
CO = L/min, sometimes noted by the variable Q
CaO_2 and CvO_2 = arterial and venous O_2 content

The Fick equation can be simplified to estimate CO
Bedside calculation: $CO = VO_2/(1.36 \times Hbg \times (SaO_2 - SvO_2) \times 10)$

VO_2 from reference for age (usually 100–200 mL/min/m²)
SaO2 = systemic arterial saturation
SvO2 = mixed venous saturation

Shunt Fraction

$$Qp/Qs = Qshunt/Qtotal = (CcO_2 - CaO_2)/(CcO_2 - CvO_2)$$

Qp:Qs = Systemic AVO₂ difference/pulmonary AVO₂ difference
Systemic AVO₂ difference = Aortic saturation – Mixed venous saturation
Pulmonary AVO₂ difference = Pulmonary venous saturation – Pulmonary artery saturation
CcO_2 = Capillary oxygen content of the blood
Nl shunt fraction is 3% to 7% (bronchial, thesbian circulations)

Bedside shunt calculation for patients with systemic to pulmonary shunts:

$$Qp:Qs = (SaO_2 - SmvO_2)/(SpvO_2 - SpaO_2)$$
$$= (SaO_2 - SmvO_2)/(1 - SaO_2)$$

SaO_2 = saturation in aorta, from arterial blood gases (ABG) or pulse oximetry
$SmvO_2$ = Mixed venous saturation (single ventricles—this is IVC saturation)
$SpvO_2$ ~ assume pulmonary venous saturation is 100%
$SpaO_2$ = same as in the aorta because systemic shunt goes to pulmonary artery

Right Atrial (or Central Venous) Waveform See Figure 27-1

A Wave	Atrial Contraction
C Wave	Tricuspid Valve Closure
V Wave	Passive Atrial Filling
X Descent	Atrial Relaxation
Y Descent	Atrial Emptying/Early Ventricular Filling

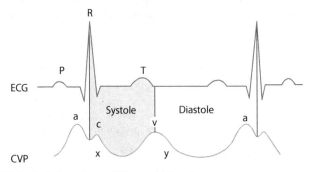

FIGURE 27-1 Right Atrial or (Central Venous) Waveform.

SUGGESTED READINGS

Atchabahian A, Gupta R. *The Anesthesia Guide*. www.accessanesthesiology.com, The McGraw Hill Companies, Inc.

West JB, Luks AM. *West's Respiratory Physiology: The Essentials*. 10th ed. 2015.Wolters Kluwer, Baltimore.

Wheeler DS, Wong HR, Shanley TP, eds. *Pediatric Critical Care Medicine: Basic Science and Clinical Evidence*. Springer, New York, 2007.

Shock

INTRODUCTION

Shock is a state of circulatory dysfunction that results in insufficient oxygen delivery and other substrate to meet tissue metabolic demands.[1] Inadequate oxygen delivery leads to a shift to anaerobic metabolism, eventually resulting in lactate production and metabolic acidosis.[2] If this state persists, it can lead to multiple organ dysfunction and death.

PHASES OF SHOCK

If unrecognized and untreated, shock progresses through three phases due to inadequate oxygen delivery.

- **Compensated:** Homeostasis is maintained by the body's compensatory mechanisms.
  - Increases in systemic vascular resistance and cardiac output through sympathetic nervous system activation and neurohormonal mechanisms lead to maintenance of blood pressure.
    - In younger children, cardiac output is maintained by increases in heart rate, leading to tachycardia.
  - Oxygen delivery is optimized by increasing oxygen extraction at the tissue level and maintaining blood flow to vital organs (e.g., heart, brain, and kidneys).
    - Blood flow to the gastrointestinal tract may be compromised.
    - Increased oxygen consumption leads to increased carbon dioxide (CO_2) production, often resulting in an increased respiratory rate for CO_2 elimination.
  - Early stages of all types of shock may be difficult to differentiate from the patient's normal status.
    - Tachycardia may be the only sign of shock.
- **Uncompensated:** Despite the body's compensatory mechanisms, cardiovascular compromise occurs, leading to inadequate microvascular perfusion.
  - This state is characterized by an imbalance of oxygen delivery (DO_2) and oxygen consumption (VO_2).
    - Decreasing mixed venous oxygen saturation (SVO_2) reflects a decrease in oxygen delivery relative to oxygen consumption.
    - Cellular metabolism and function deteriorate, leading to organ system dysfunction and metabolic acidosis from lactic acid production.
      - Increased lactate production can be seen in all forms of uncompensated shock.
  - As this phase evolves, the body loses the ability to maintain blood pressure due to cardiovascular compromise.
    - In children, hypotension is a late and ominous sign that may reflect up to a 25% to 40% loss of circulating blood volume.
- **Irreversible:** Terminal or irreversible shock results from damage to key organs of such magnitude that death occurs. This occurs even if therapy returns cardiovascular parameters to normal.

CLASSIFICATION OF SHOCK (SEE TABLE 28-1)

TABLE 28-1	Classification of Shock	
Type of Shock	**Primary Derangement**	**Common Causes**
Hypovolemic	Decreased circulating blood volume due to internal or external losses	Hemorrhage
		Fluid losses: gastrointestinal, renal
		Capillary leak
Distributive	Vasodilation, venous pooling, decreased preload Maldistribution of regional blood flow	Anaphylaxis
		Neurogenic
		Drug toxicity
		Sepsis
Cardiogenic	Decreased myocardial contractility and cardiac pump failure	Congenital heart disease
		Ischemic heart disease; Kawasaki disease
		Trauma
		Congestive heart failure
		Infections; Cardiomyopathies
		Drug toxicity
Obstructive	Mechanical obstruction to ventricular outflow	Massive pulmonary embolus
		Cardiac tamponade
		Tension pneumothorax
Dissociative	Oxygen not released from hemoglobin	Carbon monoxide poisoning
		Methemoglobinemia

RECOGNITION OF SHOCK AND ORGAN FAILURE

Early detection of shock states is crucial to treatment and outcome because delayed recognition can lead to organ failure and death. A thorough history and physical are essential. Frequent repeat examinations are necessary with careful attention paid to each organ system (Table 28-2). Early signs of shock may be subtle.

Organ failure is common in shock, and abnormalities should be treated quickly. Dysfunction of two or more organ systems that require medical intervention is defined as multiple organ dysfunction syndrome (MODS). MODS severity has been associated with increased mortality in PICU patients.[3,4]

TREATMENT OF SHOCK: GENERAL PRINCIPLES

Therapeutic efforts are directed toward increasing oxygen supply, decreasing oxygen demands, and correcting metabolic abnormalities.

TABLE 28-2	Organ System Dysfunction in Shock	
System	**Symptoms in Compensated Shock**	**Symptoms in Uncompensated Shock**
Central nervous system	Restless, lethargic, anxious	Agitated/confused, coma
Respiratory	↑ Ventilation	↑↑ Ventilation
Cardiovascular	Tachycardia	Tachycardia or bradycardia,
	Normotension or hypertension	Hypotension
	Delayed (cold shock) or bounding (warm shock) pulses	Diminished to absent peripheral pulses
Metabolism	Compensated metabolic acidemia	Uncompensated metabolic acidemia
Gastrointestinal tract	Impaired motility	Ileus
Kidney	Oliguria (<0.5 mL/kg/hour)	Oliguria/anuria
Skin	Cool extremities, delayed capillary refill	Mottled, cyanotic, cold extremities

$$\text{Oxygen Delivery (DO}_2) = CO \times CaO_2 \times 10$$
$$\text{Cardiac Output (CO)} = HR \times SV$$
$$\text{Arterial Oxygen Content (CaO}_2) = (1.34 \times sat \times Hemoglobin) + (0.003) \times PaO_2$$
$$\text{Oxygen Consumption (VO}_2) = CO \times (CaO_2\text{-}CvO_2) \times 10$$

1. **Decrease oxygen demands = decrease metabolic demands:**
- Assist ventilation
  - Can be accomplished by noninvasive positive pressure ventilation in some cases, though intubation may be required
  - Intubation and mechanical ventilation may also improve oxygen delivery
  - In cases of cardiogenic shock with left ventricular failure, intubation and mechanical ventilation result in decreased wall stress, thus leading to decreased myocardial oxygen consumption
- Decrease anxiety through calming measures or by sedation in intubated patients
- Restore neutral temperature
- Neuromuscular blockade
2. **Increase oxygen delivery:**
- Maintain arterial saturation
  - Can be accomplished by noninvasive positive pressure ventilation in some cases, though intubation may be required
- Correct anemia or relative anemia
- Increase cardiac output
  - Accomplished by using inotropes in most cases (see Chapter 30)
3. **Correct metabolic abnormalities:**
- Metabolic acidosis is common in shock states. It is usually the result of inadequate tissue perfusion and the resultant accumulation of acidic products of anaerobic metabolism.
  - Metabolic acidosis generally improves as oxygenation of tissues and renal function improve.

- pH correction occasionally is necessary before tissue perfusion can be restored.
  - Correction with sodium bicarbonate is indicated in serious metabolic acidosis (arterial blood pH <7.2) but has not been shown to improve outcomes.

TREATMENT OF SPECIFIC SHOCK STATES

HYPOVOLEMIC SHOCK

- This shock state is classified by decreased circulating blood volume due to internal or external losses.
- Treatment centers on replacement of volume with either crystalloid or colloid depending on the specific etiology.
- Hemorrhagic shock should be treated with replacement of total blood volume (including packed red blood cells [PRBCs], fresh frozen plasma [FFP], and platelets).
- In other cases of hypovolemic shock, resuscitation with colloid (e.g., albumin) has not been shown to be superior to resuscitation with crystalloid.

DISTRIBUTIVE SHOCK

- Distributive shock is caused by endothelial damage that leads to derangements in vascular tone.
- Treatment should address the etiology of shock (e.g., neurogenic shock, anaphylaxis, or sepsis).

NEUROGENIC SHOCK

- In neurogenic shock due to spinal cord injury, an α_1-adrenergic receptor agonist such as phenylephrine is preferred. This allows reversal of the shock state by improving vascular tone without unwanted β effects.

ANAPHYLAXIS

- Anaphylaxis is caused by an IgE-mediated response to an antigen in a sensitized patient.
- Common etiologies include latex, drugs, foods, or blood products.
- The mainstay of treatment for anaphylaxis is the administration of intramuscular epinephrine and withdrawal of the offending antigen if possible. Intravenous epinephrine may be administered in patients who already have IV access.
- If patients do not have IV access or have a single access point, clinicians should obtain additional vascular access and administer a bolus of crystalloid fluid (20 mL/kg).
- Additional doses of epinephrine and boluses of fluid may be necessary.
- Corticosteroids and histamine receptor antagonists (e.g., diphenhydramine and/or ranitidine) may also be administered to decrease the occurrence of late-phase reactions.

SEPTIC SHOCK

- Aggressive resuscitation of pediatric septic shock has led to improved outcomes.
- In general, the treatment of septic shock follows the guidelines outlined earlier in this chapter.
- In addition, rapid volume resuscitation with crystalloid fluid is recommended (at least 60 mL/kg in most cases).
- In cases of septic shock with myocardial dysfunction, use of inotropes may be preferred over the administration of additional fluid in order to decrease further cardiac dysfunction.
- Additional information regarding the treatment of septic shock can be found in Chapter 29.

CARDIOGENIC SHOCK

- Cardiogenic shock results from decreased myocardial contractility and cardiac pump failure.
- The most common manifestation of cardiogenic shock is left ventricular systolic failure; however, pediatric cardiogenic shock may involve both ventricles and both phases of the cardiac cycle.
- In all cases of cardiogenic shock, the primary goal of treatment is to restore cardiac output and provide oxygen delivery (DO_2) to the tissues.
- This may be accomplished by following the guidelines outlined earlier in this chapter and through the management strategies outlined in Chapter 32.

OBSTRUCTIVE SHOCK

- Obstructive shock results from mechanical obstruction to ventricular outflow of blood.
- This may result either from physical obstruction of blood within the vessel (e.g., pulmonary embolus) or external compression of vasculature (e.g., cardiac tamponade or tension pneumothorax).

Physical Obstruction

- Cases of massive pulmonary embolus that lead to obstructive shock and cardiac arrest are generally treated by thrombectomy at the discretion of the cardiac surgical team.
- Thrombolysis may also be attempted in specific cases.

External Compression

- In cases of external compression, the treatment of shock is aimed at removing the obstruction.
- To treat a tension pneumothorax, rapid needle decompression of the chest followed by thoracostomy tube placement is preferred.
- Cardiac tamponade may be treated by pericardiocentesis or surgical intervention, depending on the etiology (e.g., hemorrhage vs. effusion).

DISSOCIATIVE SHOCK

- Dissociative shock occurs when oxygen is not released from hemoglobin, leading to tissue hypoxia and lactic acidosis.
- Specific etiologies include carbon monoxide poisoning and methemoglobinemia.

Carbon Monoxide Poisoning

- Carbon monoxide poisoning results from the binding of carbon monoxide to hemoglobin, which leads to inadequate oxygen delivery to the tissues.
- Symptoms can occur with carboxyhemoglobin (COHb) levels over 10%, with levels over 70% being fatal.
- Treatment consists of administration of 100% FiO_2 through a nonrebreather until the COHb level is 5%.
- The use of oxygen decreases the elimination half-life of COHb from 5 to 6 hours (on room air) to 1.5 hours.
- Hyperbaric oxygen treatment is recommended for patients with neurologic changes or if the COHb level is over 25% (even in the absence of neurologic symptoms).
- Use of hyperbaric oxygen can decrease the elimination half-life of COHb to 1 hour.

Methemoglobinemia

- Methemoglobinemia results from an overproduction of methemoglobin (MetHb) and can be acquired or hereditary.
- MetHb is formed by the oxidation of ferrous hemoglobin to ferric hemoglobin and is incapable of oxygen transport.
- Thus, as in carbon monoxide poisoning, it can lead to tissue hypoxia and acidosis.
- Symptoms of methemoglobinemia are related to MetHb levels and generally do not appear until the level is 10% or greater.
- MetHb levels over 30% result in saturation of 85% as measured by pulse oximetry.
- First-line treatment for symptomatic methemoglobinemia consists of IV methylene blue.
- Hyperbaric oxygen administration or exchange transfusion may be considered for cases that are refractory to methylene blue.

REFERENCES

1. Smith LS, Hernan L. Shock states. In: Fuhrman R, ed. *Pediatric Critical Care*. 4th ed. Philadelphia, PA: Mosby, Inc.; 364-378.
2. Turner D, Cheifetz I. Shock. In: Kliegman R, ed. *Nelson Textbook of Pediatrics*. 20th ed. Philadeliphia, PA: Elsevier; 2016:516-552.
3. Graciano AL, Balko JA, Rahn DS, et al. The Pediatric Multiple Organ Dysfunction Score (P-MODS): development and validation of an objective scale to measure the severity of mulitple organ dysfunction in critically ill children. *Crit Care Med*. 2005;33:1484-1491.
4. Proulx F, Gauthier M, Nadwau D, et al. Timing and predictors of death in pediatric patients with multiple organ system failure. *Crit Care Med*. 1994;22:1025-1031.

Sepsis

INTRODUCTION

- Sepsis is a life-threatening condition that is characterized by an inflammatory response caused by an infection. Identifying and treating sepsis early is key to saving lives. Following are the sepsis definitions and treatment guidelines to help frame your approach to critically ill patients who have a suspected or confirmed diagnosis of sepsis.

DEFINITION

- An international pediatric sepsis consensus conference published a definition for pediatric systemic inflammatory response syndrome (SIRS), sepsis, severe sepsis, septic shock and organ dysfunction in 2005.[1]
- Definitions in Table 29-1.[1]
- Examples of organ dysfunction[1]:
  - Cardiovascular: Despite 40 cc/kg intravenous fluid given over 1 hour, patient has either hypotension, need for vasoactive infusion to maintain blood pressure, or evidence of decreased perfusion (ex: capillary refill >5 seconds, arterial lactate greater than two times normal)
  - Respiratory: Need for invasive or noninvasive positive pressure support, $PaO_2:FiO_2$ <300, requirement of >50% FiO_2 to maintain saturations ≥92%, or $PaCO_2$ >65 torr
  - Renal: Serum creatinine more than two times upper limit of normal for age or twofold increase in baseline creatinine
  - Hepatic: Total bilirubin ≥4 mg/dL (except newborns), ALT two times upper limit of normal
  - Neurologic: Glasgow Coma Score ≤11 or acute change in mental status
  - Hematologic: Platelet count <80,000/mm³ or 50% drop in platelet count from highest value in previous 3 days (for chronic hematology/oncology patients) or INR >2

TABLE 29-1	Definition of Sepsis
Systemic Inflammatory Response Syndrome (SIRS)	Presence of two out of four: • Core temperature >38.5°C or <36°C • HR >2 SD above normal for age (in absence of external stimulus such as pain) OR HR (if < 1 year of age) <10th percentile for age in absence of vagal stimulus • Mean RR >2 SD above normal for age OR mechanical ventilation for acute process (not due to neuromuscular disease or anesthesia) • Leukocyte count elevated or depressed for age OR >10% immature neutrophils
Infection	Suspected or proven (as with positive culture, PCR test) OR high probability of infection (such as presence of white blood cells in a usually sterile site)
Sepsis	SIRS in the presence of or as a result of infection
Severe Sepsis	Sepsis plus either cardiovascular organ dysfunction, acute respiratory distress syndrome, OR two or more organ dysfunctions
Septic Shock	Sepsis plus cardiovascular organ dysfunction

PATHOPHYSIOLOGY OF SEPSIS – THE BASICS

- The host response to infection triggers both an inflammatory and compensatory anti-inflammatory response (CARS) mediated by the immune system. The balance between these two determines the extent of organ injury and patient recovery.
- The **innate immune response** is nonspecific and triggered by the body's recognition of antigen resulting in an effector response. Components of the innate immune system include physical barriers like skin and phagycytic cells, such as macrophages, that recognize pathogens.
  - **Pattern-recognition receptors (PRRs)** are molecules in the host that recognize **pathogen-associated molecular patterns (PAMPs)** on pathogens.[2]
  - Specific types of PRR called **toll-like receptors (TLRs)** recognize several types of PAMPs implicated in sepsis. For example:
    - **TLR4** recognizes lipopolysaacharide present on gram-negative bacteria
    - **TLR2** recognizes lipotechoic acid on gram-positive bacteria
  - Once PRR recognizes PAMP, activation of signal transduction pathways occurs, leading to downstream production of inflammatory cytokines (such as IL-1β and TNF-α) and other mediators such as nitric oxide.
- The **adaptive immune response** involves a specific response to a pathogen and T- and B- cell proliferation with antibody response, as well as enhanced immunity (memory) upon re-exposure to that antigen.
- For additional information see chapter 73.

TREATMENT OF SEPSIS, SEVERE SEPSIS, AND SEPTIC SHOCK – EARLY GOAL-DIRECTED THERAPY:

- **Access and oxygen:** Within the first 5 minutes of recognition of sepsis, establish IV/IO access and start oxygen therapy.[3]
  - The goal of oxygen therapy is to maximize oxygen delivery (DO_2) by maximizing the oxygen content (CaO_2) in arterial blood because DO_2 = Cardiac Output $\times$ CaO_2 $\times$ 10 (unit conversion factor).
    - CaO_2 is dependent on hemoglobin, oxygen saturation (O_2 Sat %/100%), and arterial oxygen concentration (PaO_2) and is determined by the following equation:

$$CaO_2 = (1.39\,mL/g \times hemoglobin\,g/dL \times O_2\,saturation)$$
$$+ (PaO_2\,in\,mm\,Hg \times 0.003\,mL/dL/mmHg)$$

    - In order to achieve adequate ATP production and cellular function, oxygen delivery must meet or exceed demand. It is difficult to directly measure oxygen demand, though surrogates such as decreased mixed venous saturation provide evidence that delivery is not enough to meet demands. Lactic acid production is another sign of insufficient delivery (whether from low cardiac output, hypoxia, or other causes). Therefore, monitoring these indicators as interventions are made (such as fluid resuscitation to improve cardiac output, oxygen to increase CaO_2) can provide useful information about response to therapy and overall patient status.
- **Antibiotics:** Broad-spectrum antibiotics should be administered within the first 15 minutes of recognition of sepsis.
- **Fluid**: Initial resuscitation is fluids, fluids, and more fluids, as pediatric septic shock is often associated with significant volume depletion, low cardiac output, high systemic vascular resistance (SVR), and subsequently reduced oxygen delivery.[3] Reversal of the low cardiac output state with fluid resuscitation and continuous reassessment are essential in preventing death.[4]

- The constellation of signs of delayed capillary refill, difficult-to-palpate pulses, and cool peripheries is secondary to a high SVR, low cardiac output state called *cold shock*. *Warm shock* is characterized by bounding pulses, flash capillary refill, and reduced SVR (likely still with low cardiac output). Pediatric patients often quickly change between warm and cold shock.
  - Goal is to administer 60 cc/kg of crystalloid fluid or colloid (in 20 cc/kg aliquots in patients without known heart disease) within the **first hour** of resuscitation (whether in the emergency department, pediatrics ward, ICU, or elsewhere).[3]
  - If hepatomegaly, rales (in a patient without evidence of pneumonia), or other signs of right heart dysfunction develop, consider earlier addition of vasoactive support.
- **Fluid refractory hypotension:** When hypotension persists despite fluid resuscitation, initiate vasoactive support (see chapter 30). Goal is to achieve mixed venous saturation >70% and normal mean arterial blood pressure for age along with adequate end organ perfusion (i.e., improvement of organ dysfunction described earlier).
  - Norepinephrine or vasopressin for warm shock.
  - Epinephrine for cold shock.
  - Some argue that epinephrine should be used over dopamine in cold shock, as one study found an increased risk of mortality associated with dopamine vs. epinephrine use in children with septic shock.[5]
  - Consider adding vasodilator in order to reduce SVR if continued state of cold shock despite use of epinephrine. However, exercise extreme caution to avoid hypotension.
- **Catecholamine-resistant hypotension**: When hypotension persists despite initiation of vasoactive infusions, consider adding or changing vasoactive medications. Consider whether the patient might benefit from corticosteroids for adrenal insufficiency.
- **Additional factors:** Reverse hypoglycemia, hypocalcemia. Consider evaluation for pericardial effusion or other factors that could prevent improvement in cardiac output if the patient is unresponsive to therapy. Consider renal replacement therapy in patients with refractory shock and volume overload. Extracorporeal membrane oxygenation (ECMO) may also be an option where available in patients with refractory shock.

Remember, the overall goal is to improve cardiac output and end organ perfusion *quickly*! Frequent reassessment of the patient, titration of therapies, and monitoring of laboratory markers of shock will help you in this process.

REFERENCES

1. Goldstein B, Giroir B, Randolph A, International Consensus Conference on Pediatric S. International pediatric sepsis consensus conference: definitions for sepsis and organ dysfunction in pediatrics. *Pediatr Crit Care Med.* 2005;6(1):2-8.
2. Mogensen TH. Pathogen recognition and inflammatory signaling in innate immune defenses. *Clin Microbiol Rev.* 2009;22(2):240-273.
3. Brierley J, Carcillo JA, Choong K, et al. Clinical practice parameters for hemodynamic support of pediatric and neonatal septic shock: 2007 update from the American College of Critical Care Medicine. *Crit Care Med.* 2009;37(2):666-688.
4. de Oliveira CF, de Oliveira DS, Gottschald AF, et al. ACCM/PALS haemodynamic support guidelines for paediatric septic shock: an outcomes comparison with and without monitoring central venous oxygen saturation. *Intensive Care Med.* 2008;34(6):1065-1075.
5. Ventura AM, Shieh HH, Bousso A, et al. Double-blind prospective randomized controlled trial of dopamine versus epinephrine as first-line vasoactive drugs in pediatric septic shock. *Crit Care Med.* 2015;43(11):2292-2302.

30 Vasoactive Agents

INTRODUCTION

Vasoactive medications and inotropic agents are utilized frequently in the pediatric intensive care unit for patients in various states of shock. Selecting the proper pharmacologic therapy requires knowledge of the mechanism of action of each medication, as well as the etiology of the patient's physiologic derangement.

RECEPTOR CLASSES (SEE TABLE 30-1)

TABLE 30-1	Receptor Classes		
Receptor	**Cardiac Effects**	**Arterioles**	**Venules**
Alpha	None	Coronary, skeletal muscle, pulmonary, abdominal viscera, and renal vasoconstriction	Systemic vein vasoconstriction
Beta$_1$	Increase heart rate (S-A node), increase contractility and conduction velocity (atria and A-V node)	None	None
Beta$_2$	Increase in ventricle contractility and conduction velocity	Coronary, skeletal muscle, pulmonary, abdominal viscera, and renal vasodilatation	Systemic vein vasodilatation
Dopamine	None	Coronary, renal, cerebral, mesenteric vasodilation	Regional vasodilation

TERMINOLOGY

SYMPATHOMIMETIC AGENTS

- Dopamine
  - Dopamine is the precursor to epinephrine and norepinephrine. It has cardiac and vascular effects that are dose dependent.[1]
    - At moderate doses (4–10 mcg/kg/min), it acts as a weak partial agonist at myocardial β_1-receptors, resulting in positive inotropy.
      - Additionally, it causes the release of norepinephrine from sympathetic nerve terminals in the myocardium and vasculature, which may lead to vasoconstriction.
    - At high doses (10–20 mcg/kg/min), it stimulates α receptors, resulting in vasoconstriction.
- Epinephrine
  - Epinephrine is an endogenous catecholamine. It has potent cardiac and vascular effects.
    - It stimulates β_1- and β_2-receptors in the myocardium, resulting in positive chronotropic and inotropic responses.

- Higher doses of epinephrine may lead to tachycardia, increased risk of arrhythmia, and increased myocardial oxygen consumption.
  - It also has effects on α receptors, resulting in increased arterial and venous constriction.
- Norepinephrine
  - Norepinephrine is an endogenous catecholamine. It has potent vascular and some cardiac effects.
    - It primarily stimulates α receptors, resulting in vasoconstriction.
    - It has a weak effect on β_1-receptors in the myocardium.
- Isoproterenol
  - Isoproterenol is a synthetic sympathomimetic with a molecular structure that is similar to epinephrine.
    - It acts as a nonselective β-receptor agonist with limited to no alpha effects.
      - Stimulation of β_1- and β_2-receptors in the myocardium results in positive chronotropic and inotropic responses.
      - Stimulation of β_2-receptors in the vasculature results in pulmonary and skeletal muscle vasodilation, which may result in hypotension.
- Phenylephrine
  - Phenylephrine is a synthetic sympathomimetic
    - It is a selective alpha-1-adrenergic receptor agonist, resulting in vasoconstriction
    - Reflex bradycardia may occur

NONSYMPATHOMIMETIC AGENTS

- Milrinone:
  - Milrinone is a phosphodiesterase-3 inhibitor.
    - Inhibition results in improved Ca^{2+} release and increased myocardial contraction.[2]
    - It is a positive inotrope, lusitrope, and vasodilator.
    - Vasodilation results in decreased afterload.
  - *Does not* increase intrinsic myocardial oxygen consumption.
  - Dosing adjustment is required in renal failure.
    - Drug accumulation in cases of renal failure may occur, resulting in hypotension.
- Vasopressin:
  - Vasopressin is an endogenous hormone released by the posterior pituitary.
  - It acts on smooth muscle receptors (V_2) in the capillaries and small arterioles, causing them to vasoconstrict.
  - It may be used in catecholamine-resistant shock.
  - It has no effect on heart contractility or heart rate due to lack of β-receptor effects.

SUGGESTED READINGS

Biolo A, Colucci WS, Givertz MM. Inotropic and vasoactive agents in the cardiac intensive care unit. In: Jeremias A, ed. *Cardiac Intensive Care*. 2nd ed. Philadelphia, PA: Saunders; 2010;470-478.

Goldberg LI. Dopamine: clinical uses of an endogenous catecholamine. *N Engl J Med*. 1974;291:707.

Sturgill MG, Kelly M, Notterman DA. Pharmacology of the cardiovascular system. In: Fuhrman and Zimmerman eds. *Pediatr Crit Care*. Philadelphia, PA: Elsevier; 2011;277-305.

31 Hypertension

DEFINITIONS

Prehypertension is defined as blood pressures between the 90th and 95th percentiles for age, gender, and height.[1]

• Note that these definitions are based on blood pressures across a population of nonstressed children in outpatient settings. As such, some discretion should be used in strictly applying these standards to patients under stresses of a pediatric intensive care unit.

Hypertension is defined as systolic blood pressure (SBP) and/or diastolic blood pressure (DBP) greater than 95th percentile for age, gender, and height on at least three occasions.[1,2]

Hypertensive urgency implies profound hypertension, as in hypertensive emergency, but *without* evidence of end-organ dysfunction.

Hypertensive emergency is a syndrome of profound hypertension (generally greater than 95th percentile for age) with accompanying end-organ dysfunction. Common systems involved include central nervous system (CNS) (encephalopathy, infarction, hemorrhage), cardiovascular (heart failure, ischemia, aortic dissection), and renal (acute kidney injury, hematuria, proteinuria).

ETIOLOGY

Hypertension can be **primary (essential)** or **secondary.** Primary hypertension is rare in children, but is becoming more common as pediatric obesity becomes more prevalent.[1] Secondary hypertension is due to an inciting cause, which can be transient or sustained.

• Transient causes common in the pediatric intensive care unit include *pain, agitation,* and *delirium.* A thorough physical exam—including assessment of other vital signs (tachypnea, tachycardia), pupils, tearing, and movements—is essential to identifying and treating these causes. This can be especially difficult to assess in patients with neurologic injury or patients treated with neuromuscular blockade.

• Sustained causes are vast, but important considerations in the ICU are listed in Table 31-1. Hypertension, like any change in vital signs, warrants a thorough assessment of the patient, including examination, review of other vital signs (including four-limb blood pressures), input/output, past history, and medication list for clues as to the cause.

  ○ Accompanying bradycardia and irregular respirations could indicate elevated intracranial pressure. Intake in excess of output could indicate volume overload or renal injury. Cardiac exam, including assessment for hepatomegaly, auscultation of lungs for rales, and examining neck for jugular venous distension (or elevated central venous pressure if a central line is present), should be performed to assess for heart failure. All patients should have a thorough neurologic exam for the various causes listed in Table 31-1.

  ○ Initial diagnostic workup will depend on clinical assessment, but likely should include assessment of renal function via electrolytes, including blood urea nitrogen (BUN) and creatinine and a urinalysis. Consideration should be given to renal/bladder ultrasound as well. If there is reason to suspect coarctation of the aorta or other cardiac anomalies, an echocardiogram can be performed. Similarly, head imaging can be considered depending on clinical context.

TABLE 31-1	Causes of Hypertension
Iatrogenic	Inaccurate blood pressure measurements (inappropriate size cuff)
	Volume overload
	Drug induced (see separate section)
Neurologic	Elevated intracranial pressure
	Dysautonomia
	Guillain-Barre syndrome
	Seizures
	Spinal cord injury
Renal	Acute glomerulonephritis
	Acute kidney injury
	Chronic renal insufficiency/failure
	Congenital renal anomalies
	Obstructive uropathy
	Autoimmune/antibody mediated (Henoch-Schonlein purpura, lupus, hemolytic uremic syndrome, vasculitis)
	Tumor
Vascular	Renovascular (renal artery stenosis, renal artery compression, thrombosis)
	Coarctation of the aorta
Endocrine	Adrenal disease (congenital adrenal hyperplasia, Cushing's disease, Conn's syndrome)
	Hyperthyroidism
Tumor	Pheochromocytoma
	Neuroblastoma
Drug-induced	Vasopressor/inotrope excess
	Withdrawal (benzodiazepines, alcohol, narcotics)
	Sympathomimetics (amphetamine, cocaine, ephedrine)
	Exogenous steroids
	Cyclosporine, tacrolimus
	Caffeine, theophylline

MONITORING

- Accurate measurement of blood pressures is essential for appropriate management. Initial screening is generally done by automatic (oscillometric) cuff measurements. In the event of hypertension, this should be confirmed by manual (auscultory) measurement. It is also important to ensure proper cuff sizing prior to treatment for hypertension.
- Generally speaking, if there is evidence of end-organ dysfunction, continuous, invasive blood pressure monitoring should be obtained via an arterial line.

MANAGEMENT

- Blood pressure management strategies depend on the etiology of the elevated blood pressure. Secondary causes such as pain, agitation, delirium, and volume overload should be treated aggressively prior to initiation of pharmacotherapies for hypertension.
- The rate at which blood pressure should be lowered should also be considered, as not every patient should be corrected to normotension immediately.
  - Patients with suspected elevated intracranial pressure may need to maintain elevated mean arterial pressures to ensure adequate cerebral perfusion. In these patients, consideration should be given to permissive hypertension.
  - Similarly, patients with long-standing hypertension may have organ hypoperfusion if blood pressure is lowered too quickly. This is due to constriction of the patients' end-organ capillary beds to restrict flow in the setting of hypertension. This can result in diminished flow when blood pressure is lowered too quickly. Blood pressure should generally be reduced by no more than 25% in the first hour, with a goal of normotension in 24 to 48 hours.

PHARMACOTHERAPY - SEE TABLE 31-2

TABLE 31-2	Pharmacotherapy for Hypertension			
Agent	**Mechanism of Action**	**Dose**	**Route**	**Side Effects/ Precautions**
Enalapril	Angiotensin-converting enzyme (ACE) inhibitor	0.1–0.5 mg/kg/day divided q12 hr	Oral	May exacerbate renovascular hypertension Can cause hyperkalemia Can cause cough from bradykinin accumulation
Enalaprilat	ACE inhibitor	5–10 µg/kg/dose, repeated every 6–24 hr as needed	Intravenous bolus	Same as for enalapril
Captopril	ACE inhibitor	Infants: 0.1–0.5 mg/kg/dose every 6–12 hr Children: 0.3–0.5 mg/kg/dose every 6–12 hr	Oral	Same as for enalapril
Clonidine	Central alpha-2 agonist	3–10 µg/kg/d every 6–8 hr up to 25 µg/kg/day	Oral (also available in patch for chronic usage)	Can cause sedation Useful adjunct for pain or drug withdrawal
Hydralazine	Direct vasodilator	0.1–0.2 mg/kg/dose as starting dose. Can escalate to 20 mg total dose. Can be dosed every 4–6 hr. Max of 3.5 mg/kg/day	Intravenous bolus Intramuscular	Can cause reflex tachycardia, fluid retention

(continued)

TABLE 31-2	*(continued)*			
Agent	**Mechanism of Action**	**Dose**	**Route**	**Side Effects/ Precautions**
Labetalol	Alpha and beta receptor blocker (beta >> alpha)	0.2–1 mg/kg bolus, up to 40 mg total dose. Can repeat every 10 min.	Intravenous bolus	Relative contraindication in reactive airway diseases and decompensated heart failure
Esmolol	Beta$_1$ receptor blocker	500 µg/kg/minute bolus followed by 50–500 µg/kg/ minute infusion	Intravenous infusion	Can cause significant brady-cardia Relatively contraindicated in reactive airway diseases, decompensated heart failure
Nicardipine	Calcium channel blocker	0.5–5 µg/kg/min, increase in incre-ments of 0.5 µg/kg/ min every 15 min to desired effect	Intravenous infusion	Can cause peripheral phlebitis
Isradipine	Calcium channel blocker	0.05–0.1 mg/kg/dose every 6–8 hr (max 0.8 mg/kg/day to max 20 mg/day)	Oral	Can cause tachycardia, headache, dizziness, flushing
Nifedipine	Calcium channel blocker	0.1–0.25 mg/kg/dose every 4–6 hr	Oral	
Nitroprusside	Stimulation of nitric oxide and venous and arterial dilatation	0.3–4 µg/kg/minute Maximum rate: 10 µg/ kg/minute	IV infusion	Can cause cyanide toxicity; consider administration with sodium thiosulfate
Nitroglycerin	Nitric oxide stimulation and venous dilatation	0.25–20 µg/kg/minute	IV infusion (also available sublingual and as spray, but not approved in pediatric patients)	
Phentolamine	Alpha receptor blocker	0.05–0.1 mg/kg bolus dose, maximum of 5 mg	IV bolus	Indicated for pheochromocy-toma, generally 1–2 hr prior to surgery

REFERENCES

1. The fourth report on the diagnosis, evaluation, and treatment of high blood pressure in children and adolescents. *Pediatrics*. 2004;114:555-576.
2. National Heart, Lung, and Blood Institute. *Blood Pressure Tables for Children and Adolescents*. Bethesda, MD: National Heart Lung and Blood Institute; 2004.

32 Congestive Heart Failure

BACKGROUND

Heart failure is a syndrome of cardiac dysfunction that, left untreated, results in the myocardium's inability to maintain adequate cardiac output.[1] It may present as systolic and/or diastolic dysfunction. With progressive dysfunction, cardiac output is further diminished, resulting in impaired oxygen delivery to the body. As a result, many patients present to the pediatric intensive care unit or cardiac intensive care unit with signs and symptoms of cardiogenic shock (see Chapter 28).

ETIOLOGY

The heart failure syndrome may result from several etiologies, including states of altered preload, afterload, contractility, and abnormal heart rate or rhythm.[2] The most common etiology of heart failure in children is secondary to congenital malformations and cardiomyopathies.[3] Additional etiologies include arrhythmias, ischemia, toxins, or infections.[2]

NEUROHORMONAL MECHANISMS

In the setting of decreased cardiac output and decreased oxygen delivery to the kidney, the renin-angiotensin-aldosterone system is activated by the juxtaglomerular apparatus.[1] This adaptive response leads to increased sodium and water retention, thus increasing circulating blood volume. Initially, stroke volume is increased as a result of this increased volume by way of the Frank-Starling mechanism.[1] However, as volume overload develops, there is increased stretch of the ventricle, leading to decreased ejection fraction, increased wall stress, and increased myocardial oxygen consumption.[4]

THERAPEUTIC OPTIONS FOR ACUTE HEART FAILURE

The goal of acute heart failure treatment is to maintain or restore adequate oxygen delivery to end organs. This may be accomplished by improving oxygen delivery (DO_2) or decreasing oxygen consumption (VO_2) by decreasing the metabolic demands of the patient.

$$\textbf{Oxygen Delivery (DO}_2\textbf{)} = CO \times CaO_2 \times 10$$

$$\textbf{Cardiac Output (CO)} = HR \times SV$$

$$\textbf{Arterial Oxygen Content (CaO}_2\textbf{)} = (1.34 \times Sat \times Hemoglobin) + (0.003) \times PaO_2$$

$$\textbf{Oxygen Consumption (VO}_2\textbf{)} = CO \times (CaO_2 - CvO_2) \times 10$$

INCREASING OXYGEN DELIVERY

This strategy is aimed at improving oxygen delivery to the tissues. It may be accomplished by augmenting preload, decreasing afterload, or augmenting cardiac contractility to improve cardiac output.[2] Continuous infusions of catecholamines/catecholamine analogs (e.g., epinephrine, dopamine, or dobutamine) may be used for their beta-effects to increase cardiac contractility. However, these agents may increase myocardial oxygen consumption (VO_2), resulting in myocardial cell apoptosis.[2]

Milrinone, a phosphodiaesterase-3 inhibitor, is increasingly being used after cardiac surgery and in cases of heart failure.[5,6] It acts as an inodilator, resulting in improved myocardial contractility as well as pulmonary and systemic vasodilatory effects.[2] This vasodilation results in decreased afterload to the right and left sides of the heart, leading to increased cardiac output. Additionally, it improves diastolic relaxation (lusitropy) of the myocardium through its enhanced reuptake of calcium. Each of these effects occurs without increasing myocardial oxygen consumption. In many cases of acute decompensated heart failure, milrinone is used in combination with an inotrope (e.g., epinephrine).

DECREASING OXYGEN CONSUMPTION

This strategy is aimed at decreasing the metabolic demands of the patient. It is generally used in conjunction with strategies to increase oxygen delivery. Mechanisms to decrease oxygen consumption include:

• Temperature control
• Intubation and mechanical ventilation
• Sedation and analgesia
• Neuromuscular blockade

REFERENCES

1. Ralphe J. Pathophysiology of chronic myocardial dysfunction. *Pediatr Crit Care.* 230-234.
2. Graciano AL, Joashi U, Kocis K. Myocardial dysfunction, ventricular assist devices, and extracorporeal life support. In: Fuhrman and Zimmerman, eds. *Pediatr Crit Care.* 5th ed. Philadelphia, PA: Elsevier; 2017;302-324.e3.
3. Kantor PF, Lougheed J, Dancea A, et al. Presentation, diagnosis, and medical management of heart failure in children. Canadian Cardiovascular Society Guidelines. *Can J Cardiol.* 2013;29:1535-1552.
4. Schwinger RH, Bohm M, Koch A, et al. The failing human heart is unable to use the Frank-Starling mechanism. *Circ Res.* 1994;74:959-969.
5. Chang AC, Atz AM, Wernovsky G, et al. Milrinone: Systemic and pulmonary hemodynamic effects in neonates after cardiac surgery. *Crit Care Med.* 1995;23:1907-1914.
6. Hoffman TM, Wernovsky G, Atz AM, et al. Efficacy and safety of milrinone in preventing low cardiac output syndrome in infants and children after corrective surgery for congenital heart disease. *Circulation.* 2003;107:996-1002.

33 Arrhythmias

BASIC RHYTHM INTERPRETATION

Electrocardiograms (ECGs) of normal infants and children are different from those of normal adults. Neonates and infants will demonstrate right ventricular (RV) dominance related to the relative hypertrophy of the RV caused by the fetal circulation. Left ventricular (LV) dominance develops over the course of childhood.

- Sequence of Interpretation: Specific order is less important than having your own systematic approach to rhythm interpretation (Figure 33-1). Here is one example:
  - *Rate:* Heart rate
    - **Clinical Tip:** Estimated HR = 300 / # of big boxes
  - *Rhythm:* Sinus or nonsinus
    - **Clinical Tip:** Normal sinus rhythm requires the presence of:
      - P before every QRS
      - Regular PR interval
      - NL P wave axis (0–90 degrees) – P wave upright in I and aVF
  - *Axes:* QRS axis, T wave axis. An upright wave in any given lead means the vector forces travel towards that lead.
  - *Intervals:* Measure the PR, QRS, QTc intervals
  - *Morphology:* P wave amplitude and duration, QRS amplitude and duration, presence of abnormal Q waves, ST and T wave morphology

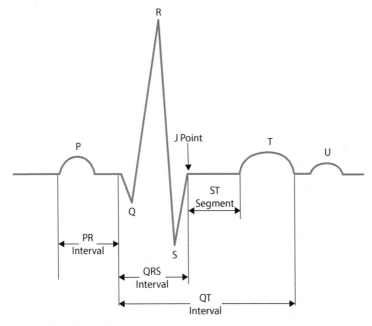

FIGURE 33-1 **Basic ECG tracing.**

- Telemetry: Continuous monitoring of the cardiac rhythm is standard of care in the cardiac intensive care unit (CICU)
  - Cardiac monitoring is used to identify pathologic rhythms in patients at risk for arrhythmia.
  - Real-time cardiac monitoring is *not* an ECG. Full interpretation of axis and morphology cannot be performed due to differences in electrode positioning compared to standard 12-lead ECG.
  - Continuous cardiac monitoring is indicated in patients who have undergone cardiac surgery; have a history of heart failure or arrhythmias; or have been admitted to the ICU for major trauma, acute respiratory failure, shock, pulmonary embolus, renal failure with electrolyte abnormalities, or toxic ingestion. Also used for monitoring in patients receiving proarrhythmic medications.

RHYTHM ABNORMALITIES

PATHOLOGIC TACHYCARDIA

- Sinus Tachycardia: An elevated heart rate for age with the rhythm still originating from the sinus node. May be caused by cardiac pathology or systemic disease. Treat underlying cause.
- Premature Beats: Premature beats are common in patients admitted to the PICU (figure 33-2).
  - *Premature atrial contractions (PACs)*
    - **Description:** An early heartbeat caused by premature activation of atrial tissue outside of the sinus node.
    - **Appearance:** P wave with an abnormal morphology will occur sooner than the anticipated sinus beat. This may be obscured by the preceding T wave. The PR interval may be prolonged. If the beat is very early, the QRS complex may be abnormally wide (PAC with aberrancy) or even absent (nonconducted PAC).
    - **Treatment:** Usually no treatment necessary for isolated PACs.
  - *Premature ventricular contractions (PVCs)*
    - **Description:** An early heartbeat caused by premature activation of ventricular tissue.
    - **Appearance:** Wide QRS complex will occur sooner than the anticipated sinus beat. T wave typically points in the opposite direction. Multiple PVCs can occur at regular intervals (bigeminy, trigeminy) or in a row (couplets, triplets) and can be uniform (monomorphic) or variable in morphology (polymorphic or multifocal).
    - **Treatment:** Treat underlying cause. In children with otherwise normal hearts, isolated monomorphic PVCs often do not require treatment. Symptomatic, frequent, or sustained ventricular ectopy may require intervention (see "Ventricular Tachycardia" later).
  - **Clinical Tip:** Both PACs and PVCs can have a wide QRS. With PACs there is typically an incomplete compensatory pause (the length from the beat preceding the PAC to the beat following is less than the length of two normal cycles). With PVCs a complete compensatory pause frequently occurs (the length from the beat preceding the PVC to the beat following is the same as that of two normal cycles). In other words, a PAC will typically "reset" the sinus cycle length, whereas a PVC usually does not.
- Narrow Complex:
  - *Atrioventricular reentrant tachycardia (AVRT):*
    - **Description:** Most common type of SVT in children. Reentrant circuit formed using the AV node and an anatomically separate accessory pathway. If the accessory pathway has anterograde conduction properties, the patient will demonstrate ventricular preexcitation (Wolff-Parkinson-White [WPW] pattern) in sinus rhythm (Figure 33-3B).

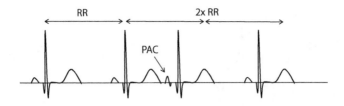

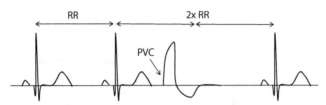

FIGURE 33-2 **PACs and PVCs.** PACs often demonstrate incomplete compensatory pause (the length from the beat preceding the PAC to the beat following is less than the length of two normal cycles). With PVCs a complete compensatory pause frequently occurs (the length from the beat preceding the PVC to the beat following is the same as that of two normal cycles).

- **Appearance:** Paroxysmal onset and termination with fast, regular heart rate. If a P wave is visible, it will be retrograde (just after the QRS complex).
- **Clinical Tip:** QRS is usually narrow. If the reentrant circuit conducts down the atrioventricular (AV) node and up the accessory pathway (orthodromic, most common), the QRS will be narrow (Figure 33-3D). If the reentrant circuit conducts down the accessory pathway and up the AV node (antidromic, less common), the QRS will be wide (Figure 33-3E). The QRS may also be wide if there is aberrant conduction.
- **Treatment:**
  - Acute Termination: Vagal maneuvers, adenosine, rapid atrial pacing (temporary pacing wires or transesophageal pacing leads).
  - Unstable SVT: Synchronized cardioversion.
  - Incessant or recurrent SVT: Beta blockers, sodium channel blockers (procainamide acutely, flecainide for chronic/refractory), or amiodarone. Avoid digoxin if pre-excitation present.
  - *AV nodal reentrant tachycardia (AVNRT):*
    - **Description:** Rare in infants. More common in older children. Reentrant circuit formed within the AV node due to the presence of dual AV nodal pathways: one with fast and the other with slow conduction properties (Figure 33-3F). Most often, the reentrant circuit conducts down the slow pathway and up the fast pathway (typical).
    - **Appearance:** Heart rate is usually rapid and regular. Rapid onset and termination (paroxysmal). In typical AVNRT, the P wave may be invisible because the retrograde P will be hidden in the QRS complex.
    - **Treatment:**
      - Acute Termination: Vagal maneuvers, adenosine, rapid atrial pacing (temporary pacing wires or transesophageal pacing leads)
      - Unstable SVT: Synchronized cardioversion
      - Incessant or recurrent SVT: Beta blockers, sodium channel blockers, amiodarone, or digoxin

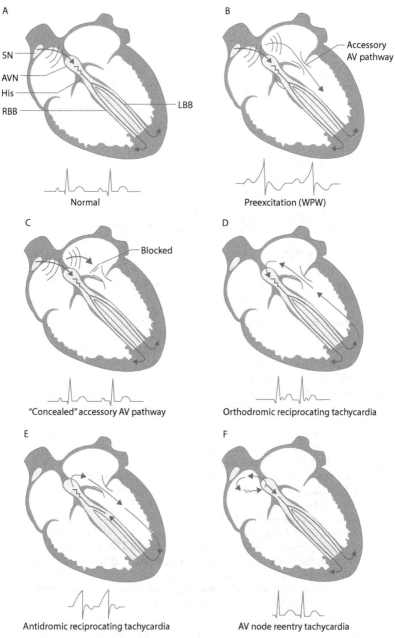

FIGURE 33-3 **Reentrant circuits.** Creation of a reentrant circuit that is capable of sustained SVT requires dual conduction pathways either within the AV node or utilizing the AV node with an accessory pathway. In the most common scenario, the signal will encounter a refractory fast pathway and instead conduct down the slow pathway. By the time the signal comes back around, the fast pathway will no longer be refractory and the signal will conduct retrograde setting up the circuit.

○ *Junctional ectopic tachycardia (JET)*
- **Description:** Most frequently seen in the early postoperative period after surgery for congenital heart disease. Occurs due to activation of an automatic focus in or near the AV node. May result in hemodynamic instability due to loss of AV synchrony in patients with poor cardiac reserve.
- **Appearance:** Narrow QRS complex at a rate of 180 to 240 bpm. There may be ventriculoatrial (VA) dissociation (with ventricular rate faster than atrial rate) or retrograde VA conduction.
  - **Clinical Tip:** If temporary atrial pacing wires are present, an atrial electrogram may help make the diagnosis.
  - **Clinical Tip:** In patients with a bundle branch block at baseline, the QRS may be wide, making it difficult to distinguish from ventricular tachycardia.
- **Treatment:**
  - Decrease sympathetic stimulation: Wean inotropes if possible, antipyretics, therapeutic cooling, avoid acidosis, initiate sedation/paralysis.
  - Drugs that decrease automaticity: Procainamide or amiodarone.
  - Pace the atrium at a rate faster than the junctional tachycardia to restore AV synchrony. Unlike reentrant SVT, this will *not* break the tachycardia.

○ *Ectopic Atrial Tachycardia (EAT)*
- **Description:** Tachycardia triggered by an abnormal focus within the atrium. Because it is often incessant and relatively slow tachyarrhthmia, it may lead to associated cardiac dysfunction.
- **Appearance:** Often gradual onset and resolution (warm-up and cool-down). Although it may appear similar to sinus tachycardia, P wave morphology will differ from normal sinus appearance. PR interval may be prolonged.
  - **Clinical Tip:** Like sinus rhythms, the heart rate (HR) in EAT will increase in response to catecholamines.
- **Treatment:**
  - Decrease sympathetic stimulation: Wean inotropes if possible, antipyretics, therapeutic cooling, avoid acidosis, increase sedation/paralysis.
  - Optimize electrolytes.
  - Drugs that slow conduction: Digoxin, beta blockers, amiodarone.
  - Drugs that decrease automaticity: Sodium channel blockers.

○ *Atrial Flutter*
- **Description:** Reentrant circuit formed within the atrium itself that triggers ventricular activation at intervals that are multiples of the atrial circuit. The atrial rate is fast enough that not every P wave will be able to be transmitted through the AV node.
- **Appearance:** Classic sawtooth pattern may be visible beneath the QRS complexes. Atrial rate typically approaches 300 bpm. AV nodal block results in ventricular activation in a 2:1, 3:1, 4:1, etc., pattern. QRS will be narrow and may be regular (if consistently conducting at a particular ratio) or irregular (if variably conducting).
  - **Clinical Tip:** Although adenosine will not break the tachycardia, it may unmask difficult-to-see flutter waves.
  - **Clinical Tip:** Intra-atrial reentrant tachycardia (IART) is a reentrant atrial rhythm that may be seen in patients who have undergone prior congenital heart surgery. Atrial rate is often slower, and sawtooth pattern may be absent.
- **Treatment:** Must first assess duration of arrhythmia. Prolonged (>24–48 hr) atrial flutter is associated with formation of intracardiac thrombi. May need transesophageal echo prior to therapy to assess risk of clot embolization.

- Cardioversion: Synchronized cardioversion or rapid atrial pacing; drugs that decrease automaticity: class I and class III antiarrhythmics (ex: procainamide, ibutilide).
  - **Clinical Tip:** Procainamide's anticholinergic properties may enhance AV nodal conduction and lead to a 1:1 ventricular response and severe tachycardia, especially as the flutter circuit slows. Consider pre-administration of a beta blocker or digoxin to avoid this effect.
- Rate Control: Drugs that slow AV conduction: beta blocker, calcium channel blocker, digoxin, amiodarone.
- Anticoagulation: IV anticoagulation if concern for intracardiac thrombus.

- *Atrial Fibrillation*
  - **Description:** Chaotic atrial activation resulting in irregular activation of the ventricle. Relatively rare in young, healthy patients.
  - **Appearance:** Irregularly irregular rhythm without clear P waves.
    - **Clinical Tip:** QRS may be wide in the presence of an accessory pathway (WPW) that can conduct antegrade to the ventricle. Risk of deterioration to ventricular fibrillation and sudden death in these patients.
  - **Treatment:** Must first assess duration of arrhythmia. Prolonged (>24–48 hr) atrial fibrillation is associated with formation of intracardiac thrombi. May need transesophageal echo prior to therapy to assess risk of clot embolization.
    - Cardioversion: Synchronized cardioversion; drugs that decrease automaticity: Class I (procainamide, flecainide) and class III antiarrhythmics (ex: sotalol, ibutilide).
      - **Clinical Tip:** Avoid digoxin and calcium channel blockers in patients with atrial fibrillation and WPW, as this may enhance conduction down the accessory pathway.
    - Rate Control: Drugs that slow AV conduction: Beta blocker, calcium channel blocker, digoxin, amiodarone.
    - Anticoagulation: IV anticoagulation if concern for intracardiac thrombus.

- *Multifocal Atrial Tachycardia (MAT)*
  - **Description:** Tachycardia results from multiple ectopic foci within the atrium. Most commonly seen in patients with underlying systemic critical illness (respiratory failure, pulmonary embolism, sepsis, etc.).
  - **Appearance:** Irregular rhythm with three or more separate non-sinus P wave morphologies. Variable PR, PP, and RR intervals.
  - **Treatment:**
    - Treat underlying systemic illness.
    - Beta blockers, drugs that decrease automaticity (class Ia, Ic, or III), amiodarone.

- Wide Complex:
  - *Ventricular tachycardia (VT)* (Figure 33-4):
    - **Description:** Series of three or more PVCs. VT that lasts >30 seconds is labeled "sustained." Although VT can be benign, it is often associated with ventricular dysfunction/cardiomyopathy, metabolic/electrolyte abnormalities, or toxic exposures.
    - **Appearance:** Usually complete VA dissociation. P waves may be absent or buried in QRS. HR typically 120 to 200 bpm. Wide QRS complex will have a distinct morphology compared to sinus QRS. Uniform QRS morphology in VT is monomorphic. Variable QRS morphology is polymorphic.
      - **Clinical Tip:** Torsades de pointes is a form of polymorphic VT caused by a prolonged QT interval. The QRS complex repetitively twists around the baseline. If sustained, will deteriorate into ventricular fibrillation.
    - **Treatment:**
      - Correct reversible causes (acidosis, electrolyte abnormalities, etc.).

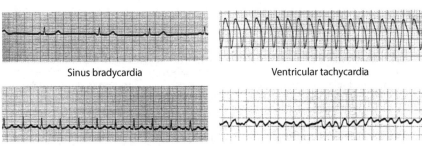

Sinus bradycardia	Ventricular tachycardia
Sinus tachycardia	Ventricular fibrillation

FIGURE 33-4 **ECGs.**

- Pulseless VT: Defibrillation and PALS algorithm (see Chapter 7).
- Unstable VT: Synchronized cardioversion.
- Stable VT: Amiodarone, beta blockers, sodium channel blockers.
- Torsades de pointes: IV magnesium, remove QT-prolonging agents, correct electrolytes, PALS algorithm.
  - *SVT with aberrancy:*
    - **Description:** Rate-dependent bundle branch block that results in a wide QRS complex. Can be seen in particularly rapid SVT or in patients with conduction abnormalities.
    - **Appearance:** See "Narrow Complex" earlier.
    - **Clinical Tip:** SVT with aberrancy can be extremely difficult to distinguish from VT. VA dissociation (i.e., more QRS complexes than P waves) is diagnostic of VT. Generally, a wide complex rhythm should be treated like VT until proven otherwise.

PATHOLOGIC BRADYCARDIA

- Sinus Bradycardia: A decreased heart rate for age with the rhythm still originating from the sinus node. May be caused by cardiac pathology or systemic disease. Treat underlying cause.
- Sinus Node Dysfunction: Frequently observed in congenital heart disease patients, especially after corrective or palliative surgery. May result in a symptomatic junctional rhythm. Treatment may require atrial pacing or chronotropic infusions.
- AV Nodal Dysfunction:
  - *First-Degree AV Block:*
    - **Description:** Delayed conduction through the AV node. Can be associated with underlying cardiac pathology (myocarditis, intrinsic disease of the conduction system), medications, or infections (Lyme disease, endocarditis, rheumatic fever, etc.).
    - **Appearance:** Prolonged PR interval, but conduction is still 1:1.
    - **Treatment:** No treatment usually necessary. Treat underlying cause. Watch for progression to more advanced block.
  - *Mobitz Type I Second-Degree AV Block (Wenckebach)*
    - **Description:** Second-degree heart block characterized by normal conduction through the AV node usually related to increased vagal tone.
    - **Appearance:** Gradual increase in each subsequent PR interval with eventual dropped QRS.
    - **Treatment:** No treatment usually necessary, but isoproterenol may be considered if symptomatic. Treat underlying cause.

- ○ *Mobitz Type II Second-Degree AV Block*
  - **Description:** Second-degree heart block characterized by intermittent failure of AV conduction due to pathology in the bundle of His. May progress to higher-grade block.
  - **Appearance:** Repeated pattern of conducted beats alternating with dropped beats. May occur in a regular (2:1, 3:1, 4:1, etc.) or irregularly recurring pattern. With higher-grade block, multiple P waves can be seen in a row without conduction to the ventricle.
  - **Treatment:** Treat reversible causes (medications, underlying cardiac pathology). Watch for progression to more advanced block. If symptomatic, may require atropine or isoproterenol until pacing can be initiated.
- ○ *Third-Degree AV Block (Complete Heart Block)*
  - **Description:** Complete failure of conduction of atrial impulses to ventricles. Can be congenital (maternal lupus, complex congenital heart disease) or acquired (myocarditis, postsurgical, etc.).
  - **Appearance:** Complete loss of AV synchrony. PP interval will be regular at an age-appropriate rate. The RR interval will be regular. The width of the QRS complex depends on the location within the conduction system that is generating the escape rhythm.
  - **Treatment:** Some asymptomatic congenital patients will not need treatment. Symptomatic patients require atropine or isoproterenol until pacing can be initiated.
    - **Clinical Tip:** A permanent pacemaker is indicated in postoperative cardiac surgical patients who develop persistent high-grade heart block that persists ≥7 to 10 days after surgery.

ANTIARRHYTHMIC MEDICATIONS

See Table 33-1 and Figure 33-5

PACEMAKERS

Pacemakers stimulate the heart with extrinsic electrical rhythms to restore a normal rhythm. The most common indications for a permanent pacemaker are heart block and symptomatic bradycardia. Many postoperative cardiac surgical patients will return to the ICU with temporary pacemaker wires. Unlike a permanent pacemaker, the pulse generator of a temporary pacemaker is located outside the body, and the temporary pacemaker box is available for real-time manipulation of the rhythm at the bedside (Table 33-2).

- Pacemaker Properties:
  - ○ *Pacing:*
    - The pacemaker will deliver an electrical pulse to the atrium and/or ventricle at the set voltage or current for a set duration in order to trigger depolarization of the cardiac tissue.
    - The stimulation threshold is the minimum amount of energy required to produce consistent depolarization of the heart tissue. Failure of a pacemaker impulse to depolarize the cardiac tissue is called loss of capture.
      - **Clinical Tip:** Can test the ventricular thresholds at the bedside by forcing the pacemaker to pace and systematically lowering the threshold until loss of capture. The last voltage/pulse width at which capture consistently occurs is the threshold. Set the pacemaker to two to three times the threshold ("safety margin"). In patients with temporary pacing wires (epicardial or transvenous), this should be done daily.

TABLE 33-1	Vaughan Williams Classification of Antiarrhythmic Medications			
Class	Mechanism of Action	Examples	Clinical Uses	Side Effects
Class I: Sodium channel blockade				
• Ia	Decreases atrial and ventricular automaticity, vagolytic effect	• Procainamide • Quinidine • Disopyramide	• Block reentrant SVT circuit in the accessory pathway • Treatment of JET (procainamide) • Treatment of PVCs, VT • Chemical cardioversion of a-fib/flutter	• Proarrhythmic • QTc prolongation • Negative inotropic effect (especially disopyramide) • Hypotension • Improved conduction through AV node may precipitate rapid ventricular response in a-fib/flutter (procainamide)
• Ib	Affects ventricular tissue	• Lidocaine • Mexiletine • Phenytoin	• Treatment of ventricular arrhythmias • Treatment of digoxin toxicity (phenytoin)	• Proarrhythmic but does not usually affect QT or QRS duration
• Ic	Slows conduction velocities throughout the myocardium	• Flecainide • Propafenone	• Affects both accessory pathway and AV node to break reentrant SVT Good for refractory cases • Treatment of PVCs, VT	• Proarrhythmic (especially in children with impaired LV function or prior surgery) • QRS prolongation • Negative inotropic effect

(continued)

TABLE 33-1 *(continued)*

Class	Mechanism of Action	Examples	Clinical Uses	Side Effects
Class II: Beta blockers	Lowers HR, decreases automaticity, slows AV nodal conduction	• Esmolol • Propranolol • Metoprolol	• Rate control of a-fib/flutter, EAT • Block AV node to break reentrant SVT • Treatment of PVCs, VT • Treatment of long QT syndrome	• Negative inotropic effect • Hypotension, bradycardia • May precipitate complete heart block • Bronchospasm (nonselective agents)
Class III: Potassium channel blockers	Prolong repolarization and refractoriness of atrial, nodal, and ventricular tissue	• Ibutilide • Dofetilide • Sotalol (also class II) • Amiodarone (also class I, II, IV)	• Affects both accessory pathway and AV node to break reentrant SVT (amiodarone, sotalol) • Treatment of JET • Treatment of EAT (amiodarone, sotalol) • Chemical cardioversion of a-fib/flutter (ibutilide, amiodarone) • Treatment of VT/VF (amiodarone)	• Proarrhythmic • QTc prolongation • Hypotension, bradycardia • May precipitate sinus arrest or heart block (amiodarone, sotalol)
Class IV: Calcium channel blockers	Slow conduction in sinus and AV nodes	• Verapamil • Diltiazem	• Block AV node to break reentrant SVT • Rate control of a-fib/flutter	• Negative inotropic effect • Hypotension, bradycardia • May precipitate sinus arrest or heart block • Can cause cardiac arrest in infants • Can precipitate VF in patients with WPW and a-fib/flutter

TABLE 33-1 (continued)

Class	Mechanism of Action	Examples	Clinical Uses	Side Effects
Other				
• Digoxin	Causes AV conduction delay and enhanced vagal tone		• Block AV node to break reentrant SVT • Rate control in a-fib/flutter	• Proarrhythmic (especially in the setting of electrolyte abnormalities) • Can precipitate VF in patients with WPW and a-fib/flutter • Digoxin toxicity (bradycardia, heart block, nausea/vomiting, altered mental status, hyperkalemia)
• Adenosine	Produces sinus bradycardia and transient block of AV node		• Block AV node to break reentrant SVT	• Dyspnea, flushing, chest discomfort, bronchospasm • Use with caution in patients with asthma or status post heart transplant
• Magnesium	Unknown mechanism		• Treatment of torsades de pointes	
• Atropine	Vagolytic that increases sinus rate and AV conduction		• Improve AV node conduction in heart block (very short acting)	
• Isoproterenol	Nonselective beta agonist		• Increases heart rate in setting of pathologic bradycardia	• Hypotension due to vasodilatory effects • Increases myocardial oxygen demand

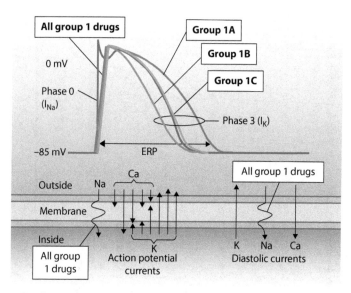

FIGURE 33-5 **Cardiac action potential and antiarrhythmic action.**

TABLE 33-2	National Association of Pacing and Electrophysiology Pacemaker Code		
Chamber Paced	**Chamber Sensed**	**Response to Sensing**	**Rate Modulation**
O = None	O = None	O = None	R = Rate responsive
A = Atrium	A = Atrium	T = Trigger	
V = Ventricle	V = Ventricle	I = Inhibited	
D = Dual (A + V)	D = Dual (A + V)	D = Dual (T + I)	

- ○ *Sensing:*
  - ▪ Sensing is the pacemaker's ability to detect the heart's intrinsic electrical signal (what the pacemaker "sees").
  - ▪ The programmed sensitivity is the minimum cardiac signal that will be sensed by the pacemaker. The programmed sensitivity is like a fence. A signal that rises above the fence will be seen by the pacemaker lead and initiate the appropriate pacemaker response (trigger or inhibit depending on the settings). The higher the programmed sensitivity, the less the pacemaker will see.
    - • **Clinical Tip:** Setting the programmed sensitivity too high will result in overpacing/undersensing. Setting the programmed sensitivity too low may result in underpacing/oversensing.
- ○ *Timing:*
  - ▪ **Lower Rate Limit:** The maximum time allowed between beats (paced or sensed).
  - ▪ **Refractory Period:** A programmed period of time during which the pacemaker will not respond to sensed events. This keeps the pacemaker from oversensing (for example, keeps the ventricular lead mistaking a T wave for a ventricular signal ("T wave over-sensing") or the atrial lead sensing an R wave as a P wave ("far field sensing"), but it

can also lead to dropped beats ("upper rate behavior" such that the next electrical signal falls into the refractory period and therefore does not trigger an appropriate pacemaker response).

- Typical Pacemaker Settings in the ICU
  - VVI-Ventricular backup pacing
    - Lead paces and senses the ventricle
    - If an impulse is sensed prior to the next timed impulse, the pacemaker will inhibit pacing
    - Useful for intermittent heart block or symptomatic pauses
  - AAI
    - Lead paces and senses the atrium
    - Useful only if there is good AV nodal function
    - Advantages over VVI include AV synchrony and coordinated ventricular contraction due to use of the conduction bundles
  - DDD-AV synchronous pacing
    - Provides synchronized pacing, particularly good for heart block.
    - Allows ventricular rate to track sinus rate for more physiologic cardiac output.
    - Allows for atrial pacing as well in case of sinus node dysfunction.
    - Provides a lower rate and an upper tracking rate. Note that a patient may have a rate above the upper limit if there is normal AV nodal function and the sinus rate goes above the upper rates.

SUGGESTED READINGS

Brugada J, Blom N, Sarquella-Brugada G, et al. Pharmacological and non-pharmacological therapy for arrhythmias in the pediatric population: EHRA and AEPC-Arrhythmia Working Group joint consensus statement. *Europace*. 2013;15:1337-1382.

Hebbar AK, Hueston WJ. Management of common arrhythmias. *Am Fam Physician*. 2002;65(12):2479-2487.

Jaeggi E, Ohman A. Fetal and neonatal arrhythmias. *Clin Perinatol*. 2016;43(1):99-112.

Saleh F, Greene EA, Mathison D. Evaluation and management of atrioventricular block in children. *Curr Opin Pediatr*. 2014;26(3):279-285.

Traditi DJ, Hollenberg SM. Cardiac arrhythmias in the intensive care unit. *Semin Respir Crit Care Med*. 2006;27(3):221-229.

Cardiac Defects and Surgical Repairs

34

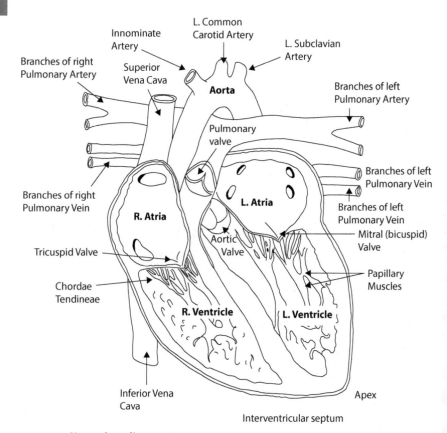

FIGURE 34-1 **Normal cardiac anatomy.**

ACYANOTIC LESIONS

PATENT DUCTUS ARTERIOSUS (PDA) (SEE FIGURE 34-2)

Occurrence: The ductus arteriosus is a normal part of fetal circulation. It is a vessel that connects the aorta to the pulmonary artery. Closure of the ductus usually occurs within the first 12 to 24 hours of life as a result of the increase in arterial oxygen tension and decrease in pulmonary vascular resistance. When the ductus closes, it becomes fibrous, forming the ligamentum arteriosus.

In neonates with ductal-dependent cyanotic heart lesions, prostaglandin will be administered to maintain the patent ductus arteriosus (PDA) until palliation or corrective surgery can be accomplished. In utero, the placenta was a major source of prostaglandin. In neonates

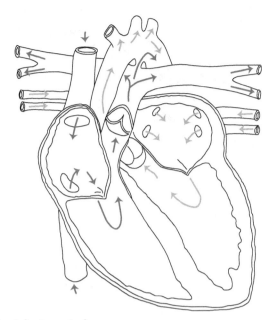

FIGURE 34-2 **Patent ductus arteriosus.**

with cyanotic lesions or premature infants with lung immaturity or disease, the ductus may remain patent due to the lack of a rise or delayed rise in arterial oxygen tension or due to scarring of the duct from rubella during fetal life.

Preoperative symptoms: If the ductus remains patent after birth, blood will flow from the aorta to the pulmonary artery due to decreased pulmonary vascular resistance. This left-to-right shunting will cause pulmonary overcirculation. Patients may present with congestive heart failure due to pulmonary overcirculation and left heart enlargement. Pulses will be noted to be bounding in older infants and demonstrate a widened pulse pressure as a result of a decrease in diastolic blood pressure and ventricular hypertrophy. Patients may present with tachypnea, poor feeding, and diaphoresis. Symptoms are directly proportional to the hemodynamics of the PDA.

Operative repair: If the PDA remains open and detected in the first two weeks of life, treatment options may include a prostaglandin synthetase inhibitor. After the first two weeks it may be surgically corrected by ligation or division and oversewing. It may also be closed with coil occlusion in the cardiac catheterization lab if the PDA is of the right size and configuration.

Postoperative considerations: Complications of coil occlusions in small patients include increased risk of embolization and pulmonary artery occlusion with the device, so surgical closure is preferred. Postoperative complications for surgical repair include chylous effusion and recurrent laryngeal nerve damage.

ATRIAL SEPTAL DEFECTS (SEE FIGURE 34-3)

Occurrence: An atrial septal defect (ASD) is an abnormal opening in the atrial septum. In the fourth to sixth week of gestation the common atrium is divided into two chambers. The first septum starts in the dorsal wall of the atrium and grows toward the endocardial cushions. The space between these two structures is called the ostium primum (first hole).

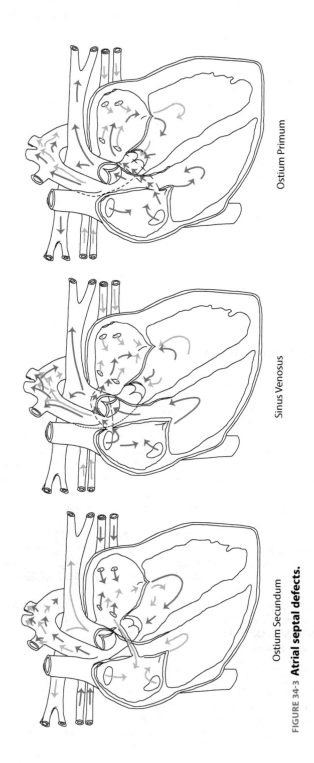

Ostium Secundum   Sinus Venosus   Ostium Primum

FIGURE 34-3 **Atrial septal defects.**

As the first septum grows the ostium secundum (second hole) appears in its center. A second septum, the septum secundum, begins to grow, and eventually the two septa form the foramen ovale. The foramen ovale allows blood to bypass the lungs. Defective development of the septum secundum or the septum primum leads to the development of an ASD.

Normally the left atrial pressure is greater than the right atrial pressure after birth, which helps to close the foramen ovale. Incomplete closure of the foramen ovale results in an ASD. When an ASD is present there is left-to-right shunting, but in the early postnatal period shunting is minimized because the wall thickness of the ventricles is similar. As the pulmonary bed matures, the right ventricular wall thickens, pulmonary vascular resistance diminishes, and the significance of the left-to-right shunting increases. This will lead to increasing right ventricular output and workload and increased pulmonary blood flow. The chronic volume overload increases the work of the right side and right atrium and may cause enlargement of these chambers. The three most common ASDs are ostium secundum, sinus venosus, and ostium primum.

Preoperative symptoms: Patients may be asymptomatic until school age, especially with secundum ASDs and sinus venosus ASDs. Prolonged dilatation of the right atria may cause arrhythmias. Long-standing pulmonary overcirculation can lead to pulmonary vascular obstructive disease. ASDs are the most commonly missed cause of congestive heart disease. With ostium primum, symptoms include a murmur (pulmonic ejection murmur at the left upper sternal border). If there is significant mitral valve insufficiency, the patient may exhibit heart failure in infancy. Symptoms include dyspnea, fatigue, and recurrent respiratory infections. Preoperative chest x-ray will show pulmonary congestion secondary to pulmonary overcirculation.

OSTIUM SECUNDUM

Occurrence: Most common, accounting for 80% to 85% of ASDs. Three times more likely in females, shows significant family inheritance. Patient will show normal growth and development. The secundum ASD is located in the center of the septum.

Operative procedure: Ostium secundum ASDs may be closed during cardiac catheterization with the placement of a septal occlude, or they may be surgically repaired in combination with other defects. This is the only type of ASD that may be able to be closed with a surgical device in a cardiac catheterization lab.

SINUS VENOSUS

Occurrence: The sinus venosus is located high in the septum near the junction of the right atrium and superior vena cava. It is often associated with total anomalous pulmonary venous return (TAPVR), with the right upper pulmonary vein draining into the right atrium.

Operative procedure: Closure includes placement of a pericardial patch with baffling of anomalous pulmonary venous drainage and coronary sinus blood to the left atrium.

OSTIUM PRIMUM

Occurrence: The ostium primum defect is located in the lower end of the septum and frequently involves the atrioventricular valves, most commonly the mitral valve with a cleft on the mitral valve.

Operative repair: Surgical correction includes patch closure of the ostium primum defect, atrioventricular (AV) valve assessment, and valvuloplasty individualized to the specific patient.

Postoperative considerations: Postoperative complications include atrial dysrhythmias, heart block, residual defects, anemia, and AV valve regurgitation. If patient has arrhythmia in the operating room, patient will return from surgery with an AV sequential pacemaker, either temporary or permanent. Heart block may be due to injury to the conduction system during surgery. Mitral valve regurgitation will be demonstrated by increased left arterial pressures and low cardiac output. Chest x-ray will show pulmonary congestion.

VENTRICULAR SEPTAL DEFECT (SEE FIGURE 34-4)

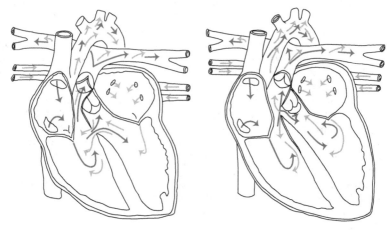

Peri-membranous VSD

Outlet, Infundibular, Subpulmonary,
Subarterial, Conal or Supracristal VSD

FIGURE 34-4 **Ventricular septal defects.**

Occurrence: A ventricular septal defect (VSD) is an abnormal opening between the right and left ventricles. The ventricular septum is established in the fourth to eighth week of gestation from the muscular membranous tissues that fuse with the endocardial cushions and bulbus cordis.

Preoperative symptoms: Generally a VSD shunts left to right. At birth, when pulmonary vascular resistance (PVR) is elevated, there may be minimal shunting. As the PVR and right heart pressures fall below systemic pressures, a left-to-right shunt will develop resulting in pulmonary overcirculation and detectable symptoms. VSDs are often not detected until 4 to 6 weeks of age unless they are very large. The size of the shunt will affect the patient's clinical presentation. The larger the VSD, the greater the shunting of blood from the left to the right and the subsequent increase in signs and symptoms of congestive heart failure. Over time, the effect of excessive pulmonary blood flow will cause volume overload on the left ventricle, causing left heart enlargement. Long-standing pulmonary overcirculation will lead to the development of pulmonary hypertension.

Operative repair: Endocarditis prophylaxis is recommended for all patients with a VSD, regardless of the size. Closure of small VSDs is controversial, but arguments to close the VSD include prevention of future cardiomegaly and decreased risk of endocarditis, arrhythmias, and progressive aortic regurgitation.

Timing of the repair is critical in preventing long-term complications. Surgical closure is completed on bypass with hypothermia, and sutures or a patch are used to close the defect. Because the surgical correction is near the AV node and His bundle in many VSDs, care is taken to avoid the conduction system. Most VSDs are repaired through a right atriotomy and visualized through the tricuspid valve.

Postoperative considerations: Postoperative complications include a residual VSD, heart block, low cardiac output, and junctional ectopic tachycardia. Patients with preoperative elevated pulmonary pressures may develop right heart failure. Aortic insufficiency may develop after repair of subarterial defects and is identified by the presence of a widened pulse pressure and a diastolic murmur.

Types of VSDs are identified by the location on the septum.

COMMON ATRIOVENTRICULAR CANAL

Occurrence: Common atrioventricular canal is a defect resulting from the nonfusion of the endocardial cushions leading to abnormalities in the atrial and/or ventricular septum. The defect also presents with varying defects of the AV valve, including malformation or malposition of the AV valves, resulting in variable mixing. It generally involves a primum ASD, AV valve abnormalities, and a VSD. When the ventricles are of equal size, the defect is balanced. If one ventricle is larger than the other, it is an unbalanced defect.

An incomplete AV canal usually consists of a primum ASD and two AV valve orifices with a cleft mitral valve. A transitional AV canal consists of an ASD above and below the AV valves but has two distinct AV valves. Both valves, although separate from each other, are abnormal. A complete defect consists of a primum ASD, VSD in the upper ventricular septum, and a common AV valve with five leaflets. A complete AV canal (ASD, VSD, common AV valve) is prevalent in children with trisomy 21. The complete AV canal allows significant left-to-right shunting and pulmonary overcirculation.

Preoperative symptoms: Hemodynamic symptoms of an incomplete AV canal will vary by the size of the septal defect, the degree of mitral valve incompetence, and the patient's pulmonary vascular resistance. Symptoms will vary from asymptomatic to those of a primum ASD. Once the PVR is normal, shunting from left to right will occur. If the mitral valve is insufficient, it will produce a left ventricular to right atrial shunt, increasing the load on the right heart.

The hemodynamic symptom of a complete AV canal is a significant left-to-right shunting with pulmonary overcirculation. Pulmonary resistance, systemic resistance, ventricular pressures, and myocardial compliance will affect the degree of shunting present. The patient will exhibit signs and symptoms of congestive heart failure (CHF). These children are also at increased risk for developing respiratory infections and pneumonia. Evidence of increasing pulmonary hypertension is the main indication for surgical repair.

INCOMPLETE (PARTIAL) AV CANAL (SEE FIGURE 34-5)

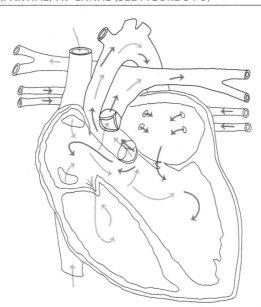

FIGURE 34-5 **Incomplete (partial) AV canal.**

COMPLETE AV CANAL (SEE FIGURE 34-6)

Operative repair: Surgical repair of an incomplete AV canal is similar to repair of a primum ASD. Surgery requires bypass, hypothermia, pericardial, or synthetic patch closure of the ASD and valvuloplasty of the mitral valve. Surgery is generally recommended before 1 year of age to prevent pulmonary complications. Earlier repair is recommended in Down's syndrome patients because of their likelihood to develop pulmonary vascular disease.

Surgical repair of a complete AV canal will require preoperative treatment for congestive heart disease (CHD) if present. Surgery is generally recommended before 1 year of age to prevent pulmonary complications. Surgery includes ASD and VSD closure and a surgical separation of the common AV valve. As in repair of the incomplete AV canal, surgery requires bypass and hypothermia. The AV valves are repaired using tissue from the common AV valve leaflets. Occasionally, mitral valve replacement may be needed. The AV valve is partially anchored to the patch and repair of the mitral or tricuspid valves. Care is taken during suturing to prevent heart block.

Postoperative considerations: In surgical repair of an incomplete AV canal, left atrium (LA) and pulmonary artery (PA) pressures will be watched for early diagnosis of pulmonary hypertension. Elevated LA pressures could indicate left heart failure. Aggressive volume resuscitation should be avoided because it may increase left AV regurgitation, decrease cardiac output, and cause hypotension.

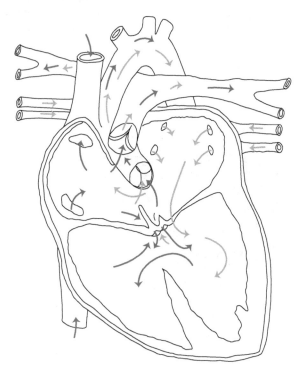

FIGURE 34-6 **Complete AV canal.**

Postoperative complications for a complete AV canal repair include heart block, arrhythmias, residual shunt, and AV valve insufficiency. Pulmonary hypertension may be treated with oxygen, sedation, alkalosis, and possibly nitric oxide. Like the incomplete AV canal repair, aggressive volume resuscitation should be avoided because it may increase left AV regurgitation, decrease cardiac output, and cause hypotension. Inotropes and afterload reduction may be used.

ACYANOTIC DEFECTS: OBSTRUCTIVE LESIONS

COARCTATION OF THE AORTA (SEE FIGURE 34-7)

Occurrence: Coarctation of the aorta is a constriction or narrowing of the aorta that may vary from slight to severe. Coarctation is often associated with other cardiac defects. In neonates, a PDA is often present, which provides distal aortic blood flow.

Preoperative symptoms: With severe coarctation, when the PDA closes, neonates have acute cardiovascular collapse, metabolic acidosis, and end-organ ischemia. If the development of the coarctation is slow or the ductal closure delayed, these infants present with CHF and differential blood pressures between their upper and lower extremities. Lower body perfusion may be entirely dependent on ductal patency. In older children, the coarctation may be detected with a routine physical because of hypertension. The hypertension may need to be treated preoperatively.

Operative repair: Balloon dilation of a coarctation may be possible in some cases. Surgical management techniques include resection of the narrowed aorta and end-to-end or end-to-side anastomosis, subclavian flap aortoplasty, and synthetic patch aortoplasty.

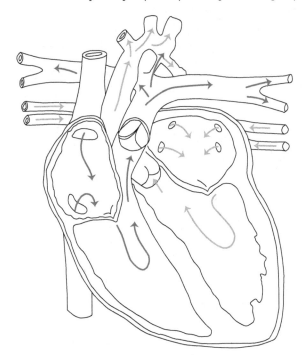

FIGURE 34-7 **Coarctation of the aorta.**

End-to-end anastomosis requires a greater degree of technical difficulty and has a potential for tension on the suture line. Subclavian flap aortoplasty ligates the subclavian artery and uses it to patch the aorta. With synthetic patch aortoplasty, the area of coarctation is incised and a pericardial or synthetic patch is placed to widen the area of hypoplasia. The advantage of the patch aortoplasty is that the patch may be much larger than a subclavian-flap patch without affecting perfusion to the left arm. However, the patch aortoplasty has increased risk of aneurysm opposite the patch. A rare complication of coarctation repair is paraplegia. Because of this, aortic cross-clamp time is limited and a test clamp is performed prior to the aortic cross-clamp.

Postoperative considerations: Complications of the subclavian flap repair include disruption of blood flow to the left arm with a potential to affect right arm growth, retention of abnormal ductal tissue in the aorta, and potential for development of an aneurysm.

Postoperative complications of the end-to-end anastomosis and the subclavian flap aortoplasty may include uncontrolled rebound hypertension causing an ileus and abdominal pain. These are medically treated with beta blockers and bowel rest. Other postoperative complications include chylous effusion and recurrent laryngeal nerve damage.

PULMONARY ATRESIA WITH INTACT VENTRICULAR SEPTUM (SEE FIGURE 34-8)

Occurrence: Pulmonary atresia is the complete absence of a pulmonary valve with hypoplasia of the right ventricle (RV) and tricuspid valve. Systemic venous blood enters into the

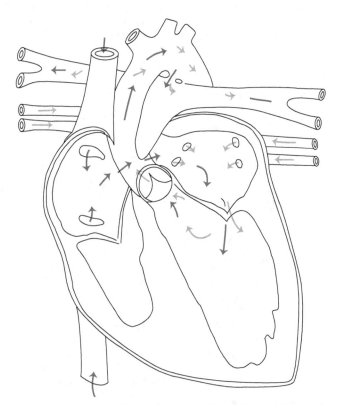

FIGURE 34-8 **Pulmonary atresia with intact ventricular septum.**

RA but cannot be ejected into the RV, so it is shunted through the patent foramen ovale into the LA. In the LA, the blood is mixed with oxygenated blood entering by way of the pulmonary veins. The LA functions as a single atrium and passes blood through the mitral valve to the LV. The blood is then ejected through the aorta with the lungs supplied by a PDA. If the tricuspid valve is competent, the blood that enters the RV has no method of escape. A small amount may enter the coronary circulation as a result of dilation of sinusoidal channels and hypertension of the RV. If the tricuspid valve is incompetent, blood may exit through the tricuspid valve during ventricular systole and hypertrophy of the RV is minimized.

Preoperative symptoms: The lack of a RV outflow tract causes a constant high RV afterload resulting in severe RV hypertrophy and RV hypertension. Prostaglandin is started as soon as the diagnosis is suspected.

A balloon atrial septostomy may be indicated to improve right-to-left shunting so that arterial circulation will improve. Surgical correction in the neonatal period will include a modified Blalock-Tausig (B-T) shunt with ligation of the PDA.

Postoperative complications of the modified B-T shunt include progressive RV dysfunction, low cardiac output, malignant ventricular arrhythmias, and CHF due to venous congestion.

Operative repair: Final corrective surgery with RV and right and left pulmonary arteries of adequate size involves a transannular patch or conduit inserted between the RV and pulmonary artery and closure of the ASD and ligation of the PDA.

Postoperative considerations: In 80% of patients with pulmonary atresia with intact ventricular septum, the RV is too hypoplastic to completely support pulmonary circulation, so the final repair is a Fontan or modified Fontan.

MIXING LESIONS

TRANSPOSITION OF THE GREAT ARTERIES (TGA)

Occurrence: There are two types of transposition of the great arteries defects: L-TGA or congenitally corrected TGA and D-TGA.

LEFT TRANSPOSITION OF THE GREAT ARTERIES (SEE FIGURE 34-9)

Occurrence: In L-TGA the right and left ventricles and AV valves are transposed. The pulmonary artery arises from the left ventricle on the right side, and the aorta arises from the right ventricle on the left side. Venous blood flows to the pulmonary artery, and the arterial blood flows to the aorta. The patient is not cyanotic.

Preoperative symptoms: Heart failure can occur in young adulthood because the RV is not functionally structured to be the systemic pump. It is frequently accompanied by pulmonary valve obstruction relieving pulmonary overcirculation until surgical repair can be performed.

Operative repair: Surgical repair is similar to repair of a single ventricle with a bidirectional Glenn shunt followed by a Fontan repair.

DEXTROTRANSPOSITION OF THE GREAT ARTERIES (SEE FIGURE 34-10)

Occurrence: In D-TGA the aorta arises from the anatomic right ventricle carrying desaturated blood to the body, and the pulmonary artery arises from the anatomic left ventricle carrying oxygenated blood to the lungs. Patients must have a PDA or septal defect to be compatible with life. The most common form (D-TGA) occurs when the ventricles are normally positioned and the aorta is anterior and to the right of the pulmonary artery.

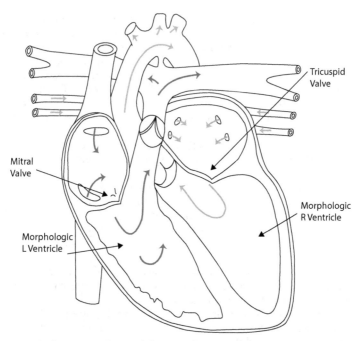

FIGURE 34-9 **Left transposition of the great arteries (L-TGA).**

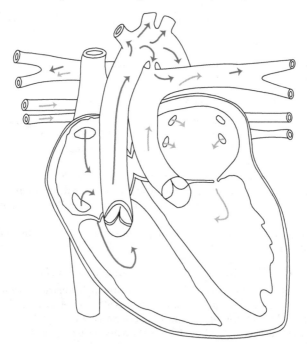

FIGURE 34-10 **Dextrotransposition of the great arteries (D-TGA).**

Preoperative symptoms: Survival of D-TGA patients is dependent on shunting, allowing adequate mixing of oxygen-saturated blood until surgical repair may be made. Immediate intervention with prostaglandins is necessary to maintain patency of the PDA. Pulmonary artery banding is performed in the neonatal period to increase mixing of oxygen-saturated blood. Patients are cyanotic at birth. Infants demonstrate signs and symptoms of CHF, dyspnea, and poor feeding. They have severe arterial hypoxemia that does not respond to oxygen inhalation.

Operative repair: In the arterial switch procedure the aorta and pulmonary artery are transected and reanastomosed above the valves to the correct ventricle positions. The pulmonary artery is now correctly positioned on the right side of the heart. The aorta is correctly positioned on the left side of the heart. Coronary arteries are removed from the aortic root on the right side of the heart and anastomosed onto the pulmonary root on the left side of the heart. If pulmonary stenosis is present and significant, the patient may require a RV-to-PA conduit because the pulmonary stenosis will become aortic stenosis.

Surgery is done in the neonatal period so that the LV, which is supporting low-resistance pulmonary circulation, does not become too weak to support systemic resistance. In children who present later, surgical repair is two-staged, first banding the pulmonary artery to increase LV pressure followed by the arterial switch and take-down of the PA band.

Postoperative considerations: Potential postoperative complications include (1) arrhythmias related to ischemic changes related to transfer of coronary arteries, (2) LV dysfunction related to myocardial ischemia or acute dysfunction due to an unprepared LV, or (3) acute increase in preload causing increased left arterial pressure and pulmonary congestion resulting in low cardiac output.

ARTERIAL SWITCH (SEE FIGURE 34-11)

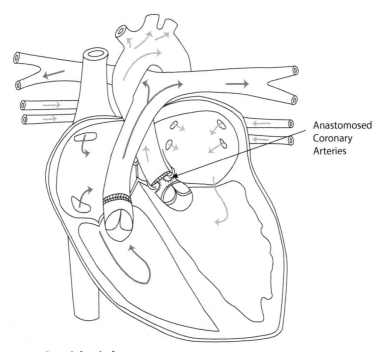

Anastomosed
Coronary
Arteries

FIGURE 34-11 **Arterial switch.**

CYANOTIC LESIONS

TETRALOGY OF FALLOT (SEE FIGURE 34-12)

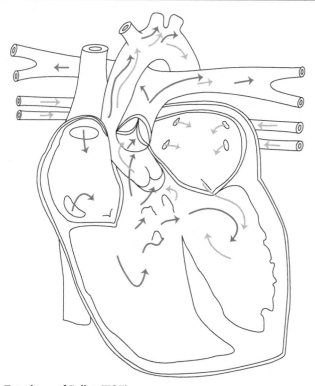

FIGURE 34-12 **Tetralogy of Fallot (TOF).**

Occurrence: Tetralogy of Fallot (TOF) consists of four defects: ventricular septal defect, pulmonary stenosis, right ventricular outflow tract obstruction (right ventricular hypertrophy), and dextraposition of the aorta (i.e., overriding aorta displaced to the right). The severity of the defect is determined by the severity of the pulmonary stenosis and obstruction to the pulmonary blood flow. In mild stenosis, right ventricle pressure will be only mildly increased and minimal right-to-left shunting will occur. In severe stenosis, right-sided pressure may exceed left and a large amount of shunting may occur.

Preoperative symptoms: Characteristic of TOF patients are "tet spells" in which the infant becomes acutely cyanotic, tachypneic, irritable, and diaphoretic after an episode of crying, defecation, or feeding in which increased right-to-left shunting occurs. The infant may even lose consciousness. Tet spells may be periods of agitation. If severe or untreated, severe hypoxemia may result in brain injury or even patient death. Treatment of hypoxic spells is to position the infant or child in a knee-to-chest position (so long as it does not increase the patient's agitation), give oxygen, and treat with morphine. Infants may be started on propranolol drip to decrease infundibular spasms and decrease right-to-left shunting.

Toddlers with unrepaired TOF may learn to squat or assume a knee-to-chest position to decrease systemic arterial blood flow, decrease the right-to-left shunt, and increase pulmonary blood flow. Prolonged cyanosis stimulates bone marrow production of red blood cells leading to increased hemoglobin levels and hyperviscosity. Patients are at risk for cerebral abscesses, cerebrovascular accidents, or death from the hypercyanotic spells. TOF patients have a systolic ejection murmur due to blood flowing through the stenotic RV pulmonary outflow tract.

Operative repair: Surgical correction is electively done in infancy at most institutions to normalize the cardiopulmonary physiology and avoid complications of palliative surgery as well as complications of prolonged cyanosis. Palliative surgical repair involves placement of a systemic-to-pulmonary artery shunt to improve pulmonary blood flow. If the patient has severe cyanosis, a modified B-T shunt will be placed to increase pulmonary blood flow.

Complete surgical repair is done between 3 and 9 months. The repair depends on the degree and location of the right ventricular outflow tract (RVOT) obstruction. Efforts to avoid a right ventriculotomy are made. A right atriotomy is made, and the right ventricular tract obstruction is relieved first with a resection of the obstructive muscle, the VSD is closed, the infundibular stenosis is resected, and a pulmonary arterioplasty or pulmonary valvotomy is performed. The pulmonary valve annulus is spared whenever possible. However, when a pulmonary valve annulus hypoplasia exists, a transannular patch may be placed to correct the RVOT obstruction.

A patent foramen ovale (PFO) may be left in place or incised to allow right-to-left atrial shunting if there is right ventricular dysfunction. This allows maintenance of systemic cardiac output despite RV dysfunction.

Postoperative considerations: If the PFO is left intact or incised to allow shunting, the patient will exhibit cyanosis. The PFO spontaneously closes when RV dysfunction resolves. Postoperative complications for palliation include shunt occlusion and for complete repair include heart block, junctional ectopic tachycardia (JET), low cardiac output due to RV dysfunction, residual RVOT obstruction, and pulmonary regurgitation.

HYPOPLASTIC LEFT HEART SYNDROME (SEE FIGURE 34-13)

Occurrence: Hypoplastic left heart syndrome (HLHS) includes a wide variation of disease involving varying degrees of the left side of the heart, including mitral valve atresia, a small left ventricle, aortic valve atresia, and aortic atresia. Hypoplasia of the left ventricle is always present, making the heart incapable of supporting systemic circulation. Survival at birth is dependent on a patent PDA to maintain systemic circulation. With no outflow from the left atrium to the left ventricle, blood completely shunts across the ASD or PFO. Mixing of blood occurs at the atrial level and flows across the tricuspid valve into the right ventricle and out the pulmonary artery. Some blood flows to the lungs and some shunts across the PDA to the aorta. At birth prostaglandin is started to retain a patent PDA. HLHS may be diagnosed by echocardiogram.

Preoperative symptoms: Preoperative complications may be pulmonary overcirculation or pulmonary undercirculation. Pulmonary overcirculation creates increased pulmonary blood flow (PBF) and decreased systemic output. Symptoms of pulmonary overcirculation include high systemic saturations (90%), poor peripheral perfusion, and low diastolic blood pressure. It is the result of a drop in pulmonary vascular resistance (PVR) after birth. Management is focused on increasing PVR by inducing respiratory acidosis. Some institutions utilize a hypoxic gas mixture (17%–20%). Respiratory acidosis or hypoxic gas stimulate pulmonary vasoconstriction and decrease PBF. The goal is to achieve an oxygen saturation of 75% to 80%.

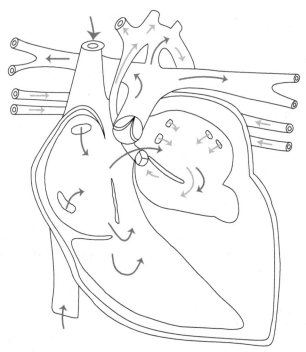

FIGURE 34-13 **Hypoplastic left heart syndrome (HLHS).**

Pulmonary undercirculation occurs when the PVR is too high. Medical management focuses on decreasing the PVR by ventilating with 100% oxygen and inducing alkalosis by hyperventilation and bicarbonate administration. Nitric oxide may also be used. Typically pulmonary overcirculation occurs. A systemic saturation of 75% to 80% indicates an appropriate PBF.

Operative plan: Treatment includes cardiac transplant or reconstructive surgery. Reconstructive surgery consists of three stages:

1) The Norwood procedure to establish unobstructed flow from the right ventricle to the aorta and regulate PBF.
2) The bidirectional Glenn shunt, which directs venous blood from the head and upper body into the superior vena cava to the pulmonary artery, improving PBF and decreasing the workload of the right side of the heart. Decreasing the volume load of the single ventricle preserves myocardial function, tricuspid valve function, and myocardial perfusion.
3) The Fontan procedure allowing systemic venous blood from the head and neck to directly enter the pulmonary circulation via the superior vena cava and from the lower body via the inferior vena cava.

Refer to the specific surgical procedures for postoperative complications. Patients who undergo a Glenn and Fontan procedure are dependent on a low PVR to maintain adequate pulmonary blood flow.

CARDIOVASCULAR SURGICAL INTERVENTIONS: MULTIPLE-STAGED SURGICAL PROCEDURES

STAGED REPAIR OF A HYPOPLASTIC LEFT HEART SYNDROME

These procedures are used for surgical repairs of multiple congenital cardiac defects, but are demonstrated with the repair of an HLHS heart.

STAGE I

NORWOOD PROCEDURE (SEE FIGURE 34-14)

There are three goals for this procedure:

1. To establish arterial mixing and avoid pulmonary venous hypertension.
2. To establish pulmonary blood flow, allowing adequate pulmonary vascular development and minimizing load on one ventricle.
3. To provide unobstructed outflow to the systemic circulation.

The first stage of repair is done on cardiopulmonary bypass. The ductus arteriosus is ligated on the PA side. The atrial septum is completely divided. The main pulmonary artery is divided close to the branch pulmonary arteries, and the divided end of the main

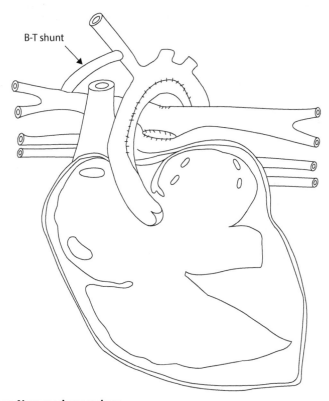

FIGURE 34-14 **Norwood procedure.**

pulmonary artery is surgically closed with sutures or a patch. The atretic aortic arch is incised along the underside of the transverse arch and a pulmonary homograft placed to augment the aorta. A distal Blalock-Taussig shunt is placed. As the heart is recirculated, coronary artery perfusion is watched closely.

Interoperatively, inotropic support is used to wean off bypass. The goal is to have oxygen saturations between 75% and 85%, indicating balanced pulmonary and systemic circulation.

Postoperative considerations: Acidosis should be avoided postoperatively. Postoperatively, the patient's chest will be closed with a Silastic patch for 48 to 72 hours. Low-dose epinephrine may be started for hypotension. Patients are sedated and paralyzed. Aspirin will be administered after the first 24 hours to prevent shunt thrombosis.

HYBRID PROCEDURE (SEE FIGURE 34-15)

Procedure: The hybrid procedure is an alternative method to the Norwood procedure that avoids cardiopulmonary bypass and circulatory arrest in the neonatal period.

The hybrid procedure involves pulmonary artery banding and placement of a stent in the PDA. One week later, a balloon atrial septectomy (BAS) is performed in the cardiac catheterization lab to increase blood flow on the right side of the heart.

Postoperative considerations: The patient will be intubated and treated with sedation as needed. The patient's saturations will be between 75% and 85%. The patient will be extubated as soon as tolerated. Cardiovascular Surgery should be notified if saturations are higher, because it may indicate higher pulmonary blood flow and decreased systemic blood flow.

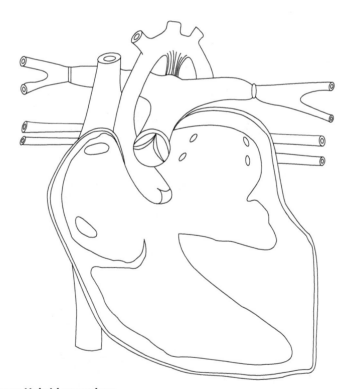

FIGURE 34-15 **Hybrid procedure.**

Small changes in patient status can precipitate cardiac failure, so fluid and electrolyte balance or changes in assessment must be watched and closely treated.

The patient must be closely monitored for signs and symptoms of necrotizing enterocolitis (NEC). Early signs include temperature instability, lethargy, apnea, bradycardia, increased gastric residuals, poor feeding, emesis (bilious or Hemoccult positive), abdominal distension, and occult blood in stool. Advanced signs include abdominal radiographs with significant intestinal distension with ileus, small bowel separation, and pneumatosis intestinalis.

The patient will go home with daily monitoring, which includes daily saturation measurements and daily weights.

The patient will need a bidirectional Glenn and aortic arch reconstruction around 4 to 6 months of age and a Fontan at about age 3.

STAGE II

BIDIRECTIONAL GLENN SHUNT AND BIDIRECTIONAL CAVOPULMONARY SHUNT (SEE FIGURE 34-16)

Occurrence: The bidirectional Glenn procedure is used in single-ventricle patients to decrease the workload on the right side of the heart in preparation for a Fontan procedure. This is generally performed at approximately 4 to 6 months of age once the patient

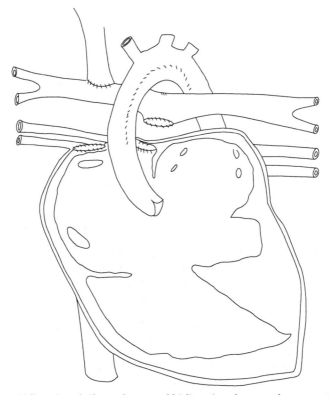

FIGURE 34-16 **Bidirectional Glenn shunt and bidirectional cavopulmonary shunt.**

demonstrates decreased pulmonary vascular resistance. It increases effective pulmonary blood flow by directing unoxygenated blood directly to the lungs while reducing overall pulmonary blood flow. Most importantly, it also reduces volume load on the single ventricle and the tricuspid valve, preserving the ventricle for a Fontan-type procedure.

Operative repair: The superior vena cava is divided from the right atria and anastomosed to the right branch of the pulmonary artery. The B-T shunt is removed and the cardiac end of the superior vena cava is closed. Any valve reconstruction necessary in preparation for a Fontan procedure is usually done at this time. All blood from the superior vena cava directly enters the pulmonary artery; all blood from the inferior vena cava enters the common atria, mixes with the pulmonary venous blood, and exits the aorta. Systemic arterial oxygen saturation is 75% to 85%.

Postoperative considerations: Inotropic support is used to improve cardiac output and minimize atrial pressures. Minimal maintenance fluids and blood products are used to prevent pulmonary edema and effusion. Early extubation is planned for.

The head and upper body are elevated and kept midline to prevent superior vena cava syndrome (obstruction at the anastomosis site or pulmonary artery distortion or elevation in PVR, demonstrated by upper body edema and flushing) and to improve blood return to the right atria. Frequent evaluation for SVC syndrome is required as well as neurologic assessment because SVC syndrome may preclude cerebral perfusion.

Troubleshooting postoperative Glenn desaturations:
Pulmonary venous desaturation
  1. Pulmonary cause
    a. Pneumonia, effusion, chylothorax, hemothorax, V/Q mismatch, etc.
Systemic venous desaturation
  1. Extrapulmonary causes
    a. Decreased cardiac output, anemia, fever (increased oxygen utilization), etc.
Decreased pulmonary blood flow
  1. Obstruction of flow through the Glenn circuit or decreased amount of blood through the circuit
    a. Narrowing/obstruction of Glenn or clot.
    b. Cerebral vasoconstriction can cause decreased perfusion and decreased Glenn flow. Do not overventilate Glenn patients (low CO_2 causes vasoconstriction, causing decreased cerebral blood flow and consequently decreased pulmonary blood flow).

STAGE III

EXTRACARDIAC FONTAN (SEE FIGURE 34-17)

Operative repair: The inferior vena cava (IVC) is separated from the right atria and a Gore-Tex conduit sewn to the IVC and connected to the right pulmonary artery. This technique avoids the risk of elevated RA pressures, decreasing the risks of arrhythmias and effusions. All systemic venous blood is directly diverted to the pulmonary circulation, but coronary sinus blood enters the atria, mixes with the saturated venous blood, and is returned to the systemic circulation, leaving a systemic arterial oxygen saturation of about 95%.

Postoperative considerations: Postoperative pulmonary blood flow is dependent on systemic blood pressure and pulmonary vascular resistance. Cardiac output must be monitored closely for changes in pulses, blood pressure, urine output, and capillary refill time. Low cardiac output may be caused by inadequate preload or myocardial dysfunction. Systemic vasoconstriction is treated with vasodilators. If changes in cardiac output cannot be treated pharmacologically, surgical intervention may be required. These patients are at risk for pleural effusions.

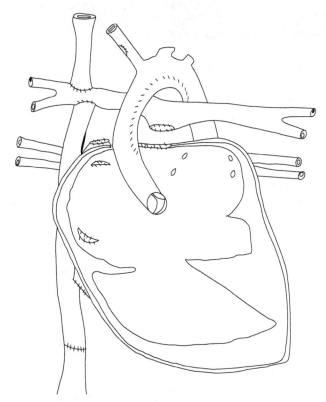

FIGURE 34-17 **Extracardiac Fontan procedure.**

SUGGESTED READINGS

Amin Z, Cao Q, Hijazi Z, et al. Closure of muscular ventricular septal defects: Transcatheter and hybrid techniques. *Catheter Cardiovasc Interv*. 2008;72:102-111.

Curley M. *Critical Care Nursing of Infants and Children*. 2nd ed. Philadelphia, PA: Lippincott Williams & Wilkens; 2007.

Mavroudis C, Backer C. *Pediatric Cardiac Surgery*. 2nd ed. St Louis, MO: Mosby; 1994.

Sabiston DCJr, Spencer FC. *Surgery of the Chest*. 6th ed. Phildadelphia, PA: W.B. Saunders; 1995.

ANESTHESIA/SURGICAL HANDOFF

A thorough understanding of what occurred intraoperatively is critical to postoperative management after cardiac surgery.

- Cardiac Anesthesia:
  - Induction technique and maintenance of anesthesia depend on the underlying anatomic defect, cardiac function, and degree/duration of sedation required. The goal is to minimize hemodynamic instability, particularly in patients with low cardiac reserve.
  - *Premedication*: Often utilizes a benzodiazepine or barbiturate orally.
  - *Airway management*: Skillful manipulation of the airway and management of ventilation are critical to minimize unfavorable cardiopulmonary interactions.
  - *Induction and maintenance of anesthesia*: Wide variety of agents administered alone or in combination. Neuromuscular blockade typically utilizes a nondepolarizing muscle relaxant.
- Cardiopulmonary Bypass (CPB): Cardiothoracic surgery may be performed with or without cardiopulmonary bypass.
  - Considerations include pump prime strategy and dilutional effect on blood volume, use of hypothermia, use of regional low-flow perfusion or circulatory arrest, use of modified ultrafiltration (MUF), acid–base strategy, use of intraoperative steroids.
  - Sequelae of CPB include renal dysfunction, capillary leak, systemic inflammation, abnormal glucose regulation, hemodilution, and neurologic injury.
- Hemostasis: Bleeding is often a problem after CPB due to a combination of systemic anticoagulation, platelet dysfunction, and systemic inflammation. Intraoperative concern about bleeding, last activated clotting time (ACT), and blood product administration should be quantified. Assess need and timing for postoperative anticoagulation (ex: aspirin for shunt).
- Hemodynamics: Mean arterial pressure maintained with combination of CPB and vasoactive medications. Any intraoperative hemodynamic instability should be discussed at handoff. Invasive monitoring devices (arterial lines, intracardiac lines, central venous access, Foley catheter, chest tubes, pacing wires, etc.) placed during surgery should be identified.
- Anatomic Considerations: Technical aspects of the surgical repair and postoperative cardiac function often assessed by transesophageal echocardiography intraoperatively.

POSTOPERATIVE MONITORING

Postoperative status should be monitored both invasively and noninvasively.

- Noninvasive Monitoring:
  - *Vital signs:* Heart rate, blood pressure, respiratory rate, near-infrared spectroscopy (NIRS), end-tidal CO_2, chest radiograph, electrocardiogram, echocardiogram
  - *Physical exam:* Pulses, perfusion, capillary refill, mental status (if applicable), urine output, chest tube output
- Invasive Monitoring: Peripheral or central arterial line, central venous pressure, intracardiac lines, Swan-Ganz pulmonary artery catheter
- Laboratory Monitoring: Blood counts, coagulation profile, electrolytes, renal and hepatic function, blood gas analysis (including mixed venous saturation), lactate

POSTOPERATIVE MANAGEMENT

- **Pain Control/Sedation:** Depends on degree of postoperative clinical instability. Awake, extubated patients can be managed with an intermittent opioid regimen. Patients moving towards extubation may benefit from adjunctive dexmedetomidine to minimize respiratory depression. Ketorolac and other nonsteroidal anti-inflammatory drugs (NSAIDs) may reduce narcotic burden, but should be used cautiously in setting of renal dysfunction and/or bleeding concerns.
- **Fluid and Nutrition Management:**
  - CPB results in release of circulating hormones that promote sodium and fluid accumulation. At the same time, capillary leak may result in intravascular volume depletion. Frequent clinical reassessments are required to manage dynamic changes in volume status.
  - Diuretics are typically started 12 to 24 hours post-CPB, once hemodynamics have stabilized.
  - Enteral nutrition should be withheld until acidosis is improved and postoperative hemodynamics have stabilized.
  - For patients requiring nutritional support, a restrictive fluid strategy should be used initially with careful monitoring of electrolytes (K > 3.5–4 mmol/L, Mg > 2 mg/dL, iCa > 1mmol/L). Total parenteral nutrition (TPN) is usually deferred for the first 24 hours.
  - Existing data does not support a strategy of tight glycemic control in the postoperative pediatric cardiac surgery population. Dextrose composition is 10% in neonates, 5% for infants and children.
- **Inotropic Support:** See Chapter 14 and Chapter 30.
  - Milrinone (phosphodiesterase inhibitor) is commonly used in the postoperative period to provide inotropy, lusitropy, and afterload reduction. It can be associated with excessive vasodilation and hypotension, particularly in patients with abnormal renal clearance.
  - Catecholaminergic agents (epinephrine, dopamine) are commonly used in the postoperative setting to provide inotropy. They can also increase vascular tone and augment blood pressure at higher doses. They can both be associated with arrhythmias.
  - Vasoconstrictive agents (vasopressin, norepinephrine) may be required to augment vascular tone in hypotensive patients, but should be used cautiously in patients with depressed ventricular function, as they will increase afterload on the systemic ventricle.
- **Mechanical Circulatory Support:** In some circumstances, particularly in the setting of complex congenital lesions, patients may be unable to separate from mechanical circulatory support and may require transition to extracorporeal membrane oxygenation (ECMO) postoperatively (see Chapter 25).
  - **Clinical Tip:** Postoperative ECMO is required in approximately 10% of patients undergoing stage 1 Norwood palliation for hypoplastic left heart syndrome.
- **Mechanical Ventilation:** Early postoperative extubation has been utilized in appropriate patients at many centers and decreases resource utilization and length of stay.
  - Positive pressure ventilation will decrease left ventricular afterload, but may increase pulmonary vascular resistance (PVR) and decrease preload, particularly after Glenn/Fontan procedure.
  - *Extubation readiness:* Appropriate mental status, stable hemodynamics, adequate oxygenation and ventilation on minimal support, control of bleeding, sternum closed, appropriate volume status, adequate pain control.

COMMON POSTOPERATIVE COMPLICATIONS

- Bleeding: Occurs due to surgical site bleeding and abnormal coagulation cascade post-CPB.
  - Coagulation studies and platelet count may be abnormal in the immediate postoperative period. Treatment of abnormal coagulation studies is reserved for marked derangement or excessive clinical bleeding (protamine, recombinant factor 7).
  - Replace ongoing losses using the 4:1:1 Rule (4 units packed red blood cells [PRBCs]: 1 unit platelets: 1 unit fresh frozen plasma [FFP]).
    - **Clinical Tip:** Bloody chest tube output >5 to 10 mL/kg/hr suggests acute postoperative hemorrhage. Lack of chest tube output does not rule out hemorrhage (may be accumulating in chest but not draining).
    - **Clinical Tip:** Watch for drop in iCa related to citrate preservatives and rise in K+ related to cell breakdown if administering large volume of blood products.
- Cardiac Dysfunction
  - *Low cardiac output syndrome (LCOS):* Transient slump in cardiac output that typically occurs between 6 and 18 hours after cardiac surgery.
    - Treat by decreasing oxygen consumption (sedation, avoid fever, support respiration, paralysis if necessary), optimizing preload (volume resuscitation, monitor for bleeding), decreasing afterload (milrinone, nitroprusside), augmenting contractility (milrinone, dopamine, epinephrine, ECMO in extreme cases), and managing rhythm abnormalities (avoid arrhythmia, maintain atrioventricular synchrony). May require transient pacing.
    - **Clinical Tip:** The multicenter, randomized, controlled PRIMACORP study demonstrated a 50% reduction in the relative risk of LCOS in postoperative pediatric cardiac surgical patients treated prophylactically with high-dose milrinone.
  - *Tamponade:* Accumulation of blood, fluid, or clots in the thoracic cavity may cause tamponade physiology and cardiovascular collapse. Treat with volume resuscitation, manipulation of chest tubes, and drains to restore drainage. May require urgent drainage.
    - **Clinical Tip:** Acute decrease in chest tube output in a patient with previously significant drainage may suggest evolving tamponade.
  - *Residual anatomic lesions:* Hemodynamically significant residual lesions may affect cardiac output (ex: residual ventricular septal defect [VSD], outflow tract obstruction, valvular abnormalities) and should be ruled out with imaging if concerns.
  - *Pulmonary hypertension (PH):* Patients with congenital heart disease (CHD) may be at risk for underlying PH (defects with excessive pulmonary blood flow, transposition of the great arteries, left-sided obstructive lesions). This may be exacerbated after surgery due to vasoreactivity, thrombus formation, inflammation, and acute lung injury. Acute increase in pulmonary artery (PA) pressure can result in acute right heart failure. Presence of a right-to-left shunt may result in acute hypoxia but relative preservation of cardiac output.
    - Treat with deep sedation, optimizing cardiopulmonary interactions (ventilate at functional residual capacity, maintain normal PaO_2/saturation, avoid acidosis), pulmonary vasodilators (inhaled nitric oxide [iNO], milrinone, nitroprusside, isoproterenol, sildenafil, prostacyclin), support right ventricle (dopamine, epinephrine, milrinone).
- *Hypoxemia*
  - May occur due to respiratory abnormalities or to residual intracardiac mixing/shunting. Treat the underlying cause.
    - **Clinical Tip:** Causes of excessive hypoxemia in patients with complete mixing lesions (ex: postop stage 1 Norwood or systemic-to-PA shunt)

- Pulmonary venous desaturation (lung disease, pulmonary edema, atelectasis, intrapulmonary shunting)
- Decreased pulmonary blood flow (shunt obstruction, pulmonary hypertension, pulmonary stenosis, pulmonary venous obstruction)
- Mixed venous desaturation
  - Increased systemic oxygen consumption (seizures, agitation, fever, sepsis)
  - Decreased cardiac output
  - Anemia
  - **Clinical Tip:** Acute worsening of hypoxemia in a patient with shunt-dependent pulmonary blood flow is a life-threatening shunt obstruction until proven otherwise. Shunt obstruction cannot be definitively ruled out with noninvasive imaging and may require an urgent diagnostic catheterization. In the interim, temporize shunt obstruction with heparin and pharmacologic manipulation of systemic vascular resistance (SVR) (bolus fluids, vasopressors) to force an increase in pulmonary blood flow.
- Arrhythmias
  - See Chapter 33.
  - An abnormal postoperative rhythm may cause hemodynamic instability. Sinus tachycardia, inappropriate sinus bradycardia, and AV dyssynchrony may result in inefficient cardiac filling and pumping and lead to low cardiac output. Some surgeons may place temporary atrial and/or ventricular pacing wires intraoperatively.
- Respiratory Failure
  - Positive pressure ventilation reduces left ventricular (LV) afterload and increases right ventricular (RV) afterload. Patients with passive pulmonary blood flow or RV dysfunction may benefit from early extubation where possible.
  - Postoperative respiratory failure can occur related to central nervous system (CNS) depression, diaphragmatic paresis, fluid overload, or cardiac output state.
- Acute Kidney Injury (AKI)
  - Neonates and patients with low cardiac output postoperatively are at higher risk for AKI. Risk is higher in patients with longer CPB times.
  - Postoperative AKI is associated with increased ICU length of stay, morbidity, and mortality.
  - Treat by optimizing renal perfusion and minimizing fluid overload (diuretics, peritoneal dialysis, continuous renal replacement therapy).
- Neurologic Dysfunction
  - Cardiac surgery and CPB can lead to periods of relative cerebral hypoxia-ischemia, release of excitatory neurotransmitters, and/or thromboembolic events. A careful postoperative neurologic examination must be done to identify abnormalities.
  - Neonates are at particularly high risk of neurologic injury following cardiac surgery, especially if utilizing deep hypothermic circulatory arrest.
    - **Clinical Tip:** Nearly 10% of neonates will have subclinical seizures in the immediate postoperative period. Postoperative seizures are associated with increased mortality and worse neurodevelopmental outcomes.
    - **Clinical Tip:** Approximately 50% of neonates will demonstrate postoperative white matter injury on magnetic resonance imaging (MRI), which may correlate with neurocognitive and functional deficits in the long term.
    - There is not currently an expert consensus on the utility of routine postoperative electroencephalogram (EEG) monitoring or MRI imaging.
  - Strong evidence that children who have undergone cardiac surgery are at risk for a spectrum of neurodevelopmental abnormalities at long-term follow-up.

SUGGESTED READINGS

Bastero P, DiNardo JA, Pratap JN, et al. Early perioperative management after pediatric cardiac surgery: Review at PCICS 2014. *World J Pediatr Congenit Heart Surg.* 2015;6(4):565-574.

Beca J, Gunn JK, Coleman L, et al. New white matter brain injury after infant heart surgery is associated with diagnostic group and the use of circulatory arrest Circulation. 2014;127(9):971-979.

Bronicki RA, Chang AC. Management of the postoperative pediatric cardiac surgical patient. *Crit Care Med.* 2011;39(8);1974-1984.

Greeley WJ. Anesthesia for pediatric cardiac surgery. In: Nichols DG, ed. *Critical Heart Disease in Infants and Children.* 2nd ed. Philadelphia, PA: Mosby Elsevier; 2006.

Hoffman TM, Wernovsky G, Atz AM, et al. Efficacy and safety of milrinone in preventing low cardiac output syndrome in infants and children after corrective surgery for congenital heart disease. *Circulation.* 2003;107(7):996-1002.

Naim MY, Gaynor JW, Chen J, et al. Subclinical seizures identified by postoperative electroencephalographic monitoring are common after cardiac surgery. *JTCVS.* 2015;150(1):169-180.

Ofori-Amanfo G, Cheifetz IM. Pediatric postoperative cardiac care. *Crit Care Clin.* 2013;29(2):185-202.

Sherwin ED, Gauvreau K, Scheurer MA, et al. Extracorporeal membrane oxygenation after stage 1 palliation for hypoplastic left heart syndrome. *JTCVS.* 2012;144:1337-1343.

36 Mechanical Circulatory Support

INDICATIONS FOR MECHANICAL CIRCULATORY SUPPORT

Children with severe cardiac or respiratory failure that is refractory to medical management may require mechanical cardiorespiratory support. Transient respiratory and/or circulatory support can be accomplished using extracorporeal membrane oxygenation (ECMO) (see Chapter 25), but prolonged use of ECMO is associated with increased morbidity and mortality due to the inflammation, thromboembolic complications, and issues with durability related to the oxygenator. Longer-term circulatory support without an oxygenator can be accomplished using a ventricular assist device (VAD) in patients with adequate pulmonary status. Currently, only the Berlin EXCOR is approved by the Food and Drug Administration (FDA) for pediatric use, but a number of adult VADs are being used in older children and adolescents.

CHOOSING A DEVICE

The type of device used depends on expected duration of therapy, patient size, and hemodynamic considerations (see Table 36-1 and Figure 36-1).

- Duration of Therapy: The anticipated duration of therapy is an important component of device selection.
  - *Short-Term Therapy (CentriMag/PediMag, RotaFlow, Impella, TandemHeart):*
    - Patients experiencing an acute process (classically myocarditis) with hope of possible recovery may benefit from a short-term device that is easier to explant.
    - These devices typically last 2 to 4 weeks (similar duration to ECMO without the sequelae of the oxygenator).
    - These devices can be used while the medical team weighs options ("bridge to decision") or as a pathway to eventual device explant ("bridge to recovery") or conversion to a long-term VAD ("bridge to bridge"). On some occasions a donor heart may become available fast enough for the device to serve as a "bridge to transplant."
  - *Long-Term or Destination Therapy:*
    - Patients requiring long-term support as a bridge to transplant will be candidates for a different set of devices.
    - Currently, the devices routinely available for pediatric long-term use are the Berlin EXCOR, HeartWare VAD, HeartMate II, and the SynCardia Total Artificial Heart (TAH).
    - Some centers are also beginning to offer VAD placement as destination therapy in those who are not candidates for transplant (ex: Duchenne's muscular dystrophy).
- Type of Flow: There are two types of flow patterns: pulsatile and centrifugal. Whereas pulsatile flow more closely mimics the normal heart function, continuous-flow devices are smaller and more durable.
  - *Pulsatile Pumps*
    - Berlin EXCOR: Only available device for infants and young children
      - Pump system sits outside the body (paracorporeal).
      - The pump is composed of a blood chamber and an air chamber, which are separated by a diaphragm. A driving unit forces air into and out of the chamber, which moves the diaphragm. The diaphragm's movement draws blood into the chamber via the inflow cannula and then pushes it out to the body via the outflow cannula.

TABLE 36-1 Types of Ventricular Assist Devices

Device	Duration of Therapy	Implantation Approach	Flow Characteristics	Patient Size	Special Considerations
Percutaneous TandemHeart	Temporary	• Percutaneous • Extracorporeal	• Centrifugal continuous flow pump	• BSA >1.3 m²	• Cannula is placed transseptally into the left atrium via percutaneous femoral venous access in the catheterization lab • FDA approved for 6 hr of use
CentriMag/ PediMag	Temporary	• Surgical sternotomy	• Centrifugal continuous flow pump	• PediMag <20 kg, CentriMag >20 kg	• Can be used with an oxygenator as an ECMO circuit • PediMag is only FDA approved for 6 hr of use
RotaFlow	Temporary	• Surgical sternotomy • Extracorporeal	• Centrifugal continuous-flow pump	• All sizes	• Can be used with an oxygenator as an ECMO circuit • Only FDA approved for 6 hr of use • Hand crank available if device malfunctions • Very short-term use only
Impella	Temporary	• Percutaneous	• Axial continuous-flow pump	• BSA >1.3 m²	• In-hospital therapy only
Surgical TandemHeart	Longer-term	• Surgical sternotomy • Paracorporeal	• Centrifugal continuous-flow pump	• Has been used in BSA as small as 0.4 m²	• Recirculation circuit added to enable use in smaller patients (similar concept to ECMO bridge) • Can be used with an oxygenator

Device	Duration of Therapy	Implantation Approach	Flow Characteristics	Patient Size	Special Considerations
TABLE 36-1 (continued)					
Berlin EXCOR	Longerterm	• Surgical sternotomy • Paracorporeal	• Pulsatile pump	• Generally >3 kg (better outcomes in patients > 5 kg)	• Only FDA-approved pediatric device • Transparent pump housing allows for early thrombus detection • In-hospital therapy only • Can be used as an LVAD, RVAD, or bi-VAD • Manual pump available if device malfunctions
HeartMate II	Longerterm	• Surgical sternotomy • Intracorporeal	• Axial continuous-flow rotary pump	• BSA >1.3 m² (but has been used in patients as small as 1.0 m² and as young as 10 yr)	• Can be used as destination therapy or bridge to transplant • Outpatient management is possible
HeartWare HVAD	Longerterm	• Surgical sternotomy • Intracorporeal	• Centrifugal continuous-flow rotary pump	• BSA >1.0 m² (but has been used in patients as small as 0.7 m² and as young as 4 yr)	• Can be used as destination therapy or bridge to transplant • Outpatient management is possible
SynCardia Total Artificial Heart	Longerterm	• Surgical sternotomy and explantation of native heart • Intracorporeal	• Pulsatile pump	• Large device requires BSA >1.7 m² and appropriate thoracic dimensions (but currently investigating use in patients with BSA as small as 1.2 m² with adequate thoracic dimensions)	• May be useful in patients with biventricular failure, refractory arrhythmias, or restrictive physiology • Native heart is removed so can *only* be used as destination therapy or bridge to transplant • Outpatient management is possible • Manual pump available if device malfunctions

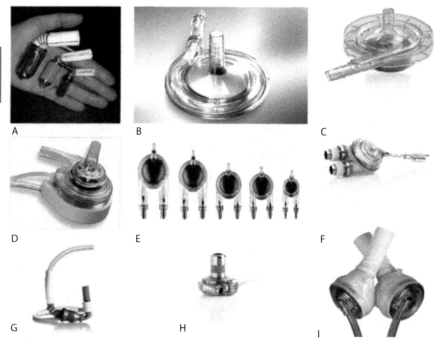

A B C

D E F

G H I

FIGURE 36-1 Ventricular assist devices commonly used in pediatrics. (A) The adult, child, and infant Jarvik devices (Used with permission from Dr. Robert Jarvik). (B) The RotaFlow assist device (Used with permission from Getinge). (C) The PediMag assist device (Reproduced with permission of St. Jude Medical, ©2018. All rights reserved). (D) The TandemHeart assist device (Used with permission from CardiacAssist Inc). (E) The Berlin Heart EXCOR 60, 50, 30, 25, and 10 mL devices (Used with permission from Berlin Heart Inc). (F) The Thoratec assist device (Reproduced with permission of St. Jude Medical, ©2018. All rights reserved). (G) The HeartMate II assist device (Reproduced with permission of St. Jude Medical, ©2018. All rights reserved). (H) The HeartWare assist device (Reproduced with permission of Medtronic, Inc). (I) The SynCardia Total Artificial Heart (Courtesy of syncardia.com).

- Each pump has valves to ensure that blood can only flow forward.
- The inflow cannula typically drains the patient's atrium. The outflow cannula pumps blood back into one of the great vessels (RA, PA for RVAD vs. LA, Ao for LVAD).
▪ Syncardia Total Artificial Heart
  - Native ventricles and heart valves are explanted so that artificial right and left ventricular pumps can be placed in situ.
  - Each half of the device consists of a chamber with a tilting-disk artificial valve in both the inflow and outflow position. Each pumping chamber is connected to the native atrium and to the corresponding great vessel.
○ *Continuous Flow-Rotary Pump Devices* (see Figure 36-2): Pump is made of a single rotating element that drives blood forward. Continuous-flow devices are smaller and more efficient than pulsatile pumps and are associated with improved mortality. Continuous-flow devices have largely replaced pulsatile pumps in adults. The long-term effects of decreased arterial pulsatility on various organ systems are not yet completely understood.

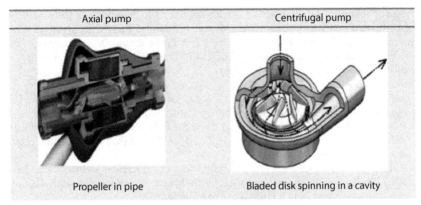

Axial pump	Centrifugal pump
Propeller in pipe	Bladed disk spinning in a cavity

FIGURE 36-2 **Continuous-flow rotary pumps.** Mechanism of flow generation in axial vs. centrifugal continuous-flow rotary pumps. Axial pumps function like a propeller in a pipe to spin blood forward. Centrifugal pumps act as a rotating bladed disk to accelerate blood around the outer edge of the chamber and subsequently out the outflow.

- Axial Flow (HeartMate II, DeBakey VAD, infant Jarvik):
  - Generates flow by rotating its internal impeller.
  - Because the impeller is very small, it has to be operated at a very high revolutions per minute (RPM) to generate adequate flow.
  - TandemHeart is placed percutaneously, which limits feasibility in smaller children. Some centers use an open surgical approach, which allows use in smaller patients.
- Centrifugal Flow (CentriMag, PediMag, Rotaflow, TandemHeart, HeartWare HVAD):
  - Generates flow by rotating a bladed disk that "throws" blood forward
  - Typically operates at a lower RPM than an axial flow device, which may lead to less red blood cell (RBC) shearing/hemolysis
  - Even the smallest long-term device is not recommended by the manufacturer for use in infants or very small children, although there are case reports of use after device modification in some centers
- Size considerations:
  - The Berlin EXCOR can be used successfully in infants as small as 3 kg
  - Continuous-flow devices are designed for adults, but have been adapted for use in smaller children
    - Some long-term continuous-flow devices have been used in children as small as ~0.7 m^2 in body surface area (BSA) (ex: HeartMate II) at centers with significant VAD expertise.
    - The infant Jarvik device can be used in even smaller children, but its use has been limited by associated significant intravascular hemolysis. The new infant Jarvik 2015 model is currently undergoing study in the "PumpKIN" clinical trial.
    - TandemHeart is placed percutaneously, which limits feasibility in smaller children. Some centers use an open surgical approach and placement of a recirculation bridge, which allows use in smaller patients who require lower flows and cannot accommodate large percutaneous cannulae.
  - The SynCardia Total Artificial Heart has specific size requirements (BSA and anteroposterior [AP] chest diameter), which currently limits its use to larger adolescents. A smaller SynCardia device is currently undergoing investigation.

- Single vs. biventricular support: VAD selection must take into account the functioning of both ventricles. Many times LVAD support will offload the RV such that an RVAD is unnecessary. The most bi-VAD experience is with the Berlin EXCOR, although other devices have also been attempted. In patients who are large enough, the SynCardia TAH may be the best option for bi-VAD support.
- Special populations:
  - Patients with restrictive physiology or refractory arrhythmias may benefit from explanting the native heart and placement of the SynCardia TAH.
  - Patients with complex congenital heart disease may be anatomically ill suited for traditional VAD and may benefit from SynCardia TAH. In these patients, complex atrial reconstructions may be necessary.
  - Although patients with single-ventricle physiology have increased mortality after Berlin EXCOR placement compared to patients with dilated cardiomyopathy, mortality while awaiting transplant is still improved compared to ECMO.
    - Many centers have extensive experience with Berlin VAD placement in single-ventricle patients.
    - Outcomes better after Glenn or Fontan procedure than after stage I Norwood.
    - Failing Fontan physiology is best supported if pathophysiology is ventricular pump failure rather than elevated central venous pressure (protein-losing enteropathy [PLE], plastic bronchitis, etc.)

VAD MANAGEMENT

Postoperative VAD management requires monitoring and manipulation of multiple organ systems in order to optimize performance and avoid complications.

- Cardiovascular concerns: A transesophageal echocardiogram is performed to guide a VAD titration ("ramp study") in the operating room at the time of placement. Hemodynamic goals include adequate blood pressure and cardiac output, sufficient unloading of the ventricle, evaluation of the right heart function, and occasional aortic valve opening. Refractory right heart failure after LVAD placement may require placement of a second device to support the right ventricle.
  - *Continuous-Flow Devices:* The optimal pump setting (in RPMs) is determined during a VAD titration study ("ramped study") under echocardiographic guidance. This is typically done at the time of placement in the operating room.
    - The device will typically report speed (RPMs), power, pulsatility index, and flow.
    - Hemodynamic goals include adequate blood pressure and cardiac output, sufficient unloading of the ventricle (flat septal position, LA pressure <20), evaluation of the right heart function, and occasional aortic valve opening.
    - Use a ramped study to set RPMs and then modify preload, afterload, and contractility as needed to alter cardiac output. Once RPMs are optimized, the patient's physiology is titrated to affect cardiac output—preload, afterload, and contractility—using fluid, vasodilators, and inotropes.
      - **Clinical Tip:** A change in cardiac output should trigger an investigation of the patient's physiologic status rather than a reflexive adjustment of the VAD RPMs. A sudden decrease in LVAD cardiac output at stable RPMs requires evaluation of preload (RV failure, pulmonary hypertension, tamponade, volume depletion), afterload (relative hypertension, device thrombus), or contractility (worsening LV function).

- *Berlin EXCOR Pulsatile Device:* The diaphragm inside the pump chamber is pulled downward by a vacuum to increase the space in the chamber and allow blood to enter. To eject blood, a puff of air pushes the diaphragm upward to expel blood from the chamber.
  - During the cardiac cycle, the pump should completely fill and empty without "crinkling" of the membrane. Because the device is paracorporeal, the membrane can be visualized by the clinician.
  - The device parameters include the systolic pressure, diastolic pressure, heart rate, and relative systolic duration (%). The diastolic pressure acts as a vacuum to fill the chamber. The systolic pressure drives blood out of the chamber to the body. The systolic driving pressure must be higher than the patient's systolic blood pressure for blood to move forward.
    - **Clinical Tip:** If the LVAD chamber is not filling or emptying fully, the actual cardiac output will be less than the calculated pump flow.
      - To improve filling, you may need to make the diastolic pressure more negative in order to increase suction, augment the preload, improve right heart function, shorten the relative systolic duration so there is more time for filling, or rule out a mechanical problem with the inflow cannula.
      - To improve emptying, you may need to raise the systolic pump pressure, lower the afterload, lengthen the relative systolic duration so there is more time for ejection, or rule out a mechanical problem with the outflow cannula.
- *SynCardia Total Artificial Heart:* The diaphragm inside the pump chamber is moved downward by passive venous flow (or pulled downward by applying a small amount of vacuum) to increase the space in the chamber and allow blood to enter. To eject blood, a puff of air pushes the diaphragm upward to expel blood from the chamber.
  - The device parameters include heart rate, percentage systole, left and right driving pressures, and vacuum. In contrast to the Berlin, this device is set for partial filling and complete ejection at the baseline settings. This allows for increases in cardiac ouput during exercise or volume loading without adjustment of the VAD settings. Because the chamber is intracorporeal, the degree of filling and emptying must be determined from the monitor (diaphragm is internal and cannot be visualized by the clinician). The right and left driving pressures must be higher than the patient's respective pulmonary artery and aortic pressures in order to drive blood forward.
- Hematologic Concerns:
  - All VADs require an anticoagulation regimen. Recommendations vary by center and by VAD type. Strategies may include unfractionated or low-molecular-weight heparin, warfarin, and/or antiplatelet agents.
  - Monitoring may include activated partial thromboplastin time (aPTT), international normalized ratio (INR), factor Xa level, activated clotting time (ACT), and/or thromboelastogram (TEG) monitoring, depending on agents used.
  - Patients are at high risk for thrombotic and hemorrhagic complications, and relative risks must be balanced.
    - Ischemic complications (pump thrombosis, stroke) are the primary cause of mortality in pediatric VAD patients.
    - Thirty to fifty percent of VAD patients will experience major bleeding requiring reoperation. This is most common during the early postoperative period.
    - Patients with long-term continuous-flow devices are at particulary high risk of gastrointestinal (GI) bleeding, which is thought to be due to development of acquired von Willebrand deficiency and vascular changes due to loss of pulsatile blood flow to the gut. Although this can be problematic, it is rarely life threatening.

- Neurologic Concerns:
  - High risk for both stroke and intracranial hemorrhage (see "Hematologic Concerns" earlier).
    - **Clinical Tip:** Original prospective Berlin EXCOR pediatric VAD trial reported an incidence of stroke of nearly 30%. Risk is less in adult continuous-flow devices, but true incidence in children is not yet known.
- Infectious/Inflammatory Concerns:
  - The risk of infectious complications is highest with paracorporeal devices due to the tract formed from the multiple cannulae to the intrathoracic space. Original prospective Berlin EXCOR trial reported major infection rate approaching 60%.
  - VAD patients are at increased risk for development of human leukocyte antigen (HLA) antibodies. Etiology is not well understood. This can complicate future transplantation.

SUGGESTED READINGS

Adachi I, Burki S, Zafar F, et al. Pediatric ventricular assist devices. *J Thorac Dis.* 2015;7(12):2194-2202.

Cooper DS, Pretre R. Clinical management of pediatric ventricular assist devices. *Pediatr Crit Care Med.* 2013;14:S27-S36.

Fraser CD, Jaquiss RDB, Rosenthal DN, et al. Prospective trial of a pediatric ventricular assist device. *NEJM.* 2012;367(6):532-541.

Mascio CE. The use of ventricular assist device support in children: The state of the art. *Artificial Organs.* 2015;39(1):14-20.

Monge MC, Kulat BT, Eltayeb O, et al. Novel modifications of a ventricular assist device for infants and children. *Ann Thorac Surg.* 2016;102(1):147-153.

37 Heart Transplantation

INDICATIONS FOR HEART TRANSPLANT

Heart transplantation can be utilized in patients with end-stage heart failure that is refractory to medical and surgical management.

- Common indications for transplant:
  - Cardiomyopathy requiring IV inotropes or mechanical respiratory or circulatory support
  - Palliated congenital heart disease with heart failure requiring IV inotropes or prostaglandin E (PGE) and/or mechanical support
  - Patients with heart failure due to cardiomyopathy or congenital heart disease that leads to severe limitation of exercise/activity or growth
  - Patients with life-threatening arrhythmias untreatable with medications or an implantable defibrillator
- Relative contraindications to transplant:
  - Severe multiorgan system disease
  - Severe pulmonary hypertension that is refractory to medical management
  - History of another medical condition that limits life expectancy in such a way that it would shorten graft survival
  - Severe psychosocial issues that may limit family's ability to care for the patient postoperatively

TRANSPLANT EVALUATION

In order to evaluate candidacy, a multidisciplinary team must assess the medical condition of the patient, but also the psychosocial functioning and resources of the entire family. Comorbidities must be taken into account.

- Cardiac evaluation
  - Fully evaluate past medical and surgical cardiac history.
  - Outline cardiac condition and degree of heart failure. In patients where there is concern for specific anatomic issues or pulmonary hypertension, a cardiac catheterization may be necessary.
  - Confirm that alternative medical and surgical treatment options have been exhausted.
- Immunologic evaluation
  - Vaccination history
  - Human leukocyte antigen (HLA) and blood typing for appropriate donor–recipient matching
- Infectious evaluation
  - Testing for human immunodeficiency virus (HIV), hepatitis C virus (HCV), cytomegalovirus (CMV), Epstein-Barr virus (EBV)
  - Evaluation of dental health
- General medical
  - Evaluation of brain, renal, intestinal, and hepatic systems, all of which can be affected by chronic heart failure or by underlying diagnosis
- Psychosocial
  - Psychological evaluation of patient and family

○ Social work evaluation of patient and family support systems, financial resources, insurance
○ Formal family meeting to complete informed consent after outlining specific details of transplant and necessary lifelong changes to lifestyle

UNOS LISTING

Once the team makes the decision to complete listing for transplant, the patient will be assigned a wait list category through the United Network for Organ Sharing (UNOS).

- UNOS Categories: Assigned based on clinical severity. Patients with severe disease that would otherwise be listed Status 2 can apply for an "exception" allowing them to be listed as Status 1A or 1B after review by a multicenter board.
  ○ *Status 1A* – Requiring mechanical ventilatory or circulatory (ECMO or VAD) support or congenital heart patients requiring inotropic support or with ductal dependent systemic or pulmonary blood flow who require a stent or PGE to maintain ductal patency. Patients remain hospitalized (VAD patients are exception).
  ○ *Status 1B* – Requiring inotropes but does not meet criteria for 1a or infants with restrictive or hypertrophic cardiomyopathy.
  ○ *Status 2* – Does not meet criteria for 1A or 1B.
  ○ *Status 7* – Temporary inactive status.
- Transplant Waiting List: Approximately 500 children are added to the heart transplant waiting list annually. Wait list mortality is nearly 20% per year waiting, but has improved over the past 2 decades.
  ○ In 2012, over 70% of patients were listed Status 1A (or assigned 1A via exception). This results in a waiting system that is largely based on time on the list.
  ○ Patients with weight <10 kg, congenital heart disease, blood type O, ECMO, mechanical ventilation, and renal dysfunction had increased waiting list mortality.
  ○ VAD implantation increases likelihood of survival to transplant.
  ○ Attempts made to decrease wait time by accepting hearts previously thought to be "marginal." According to UNOS, up to 40% of available pediatric donor hearts go unused. An evaluation of the Pediatric Heart Transplant Study Database failed to show an impact of traditional donor risk factors (high donor inotropes, donor CPR, mechanism of donor death) on recipient post-transplant survival. Ischemic time and older donor age may be risk factors for poor outcome in patients ≥10 years of age.

OPERATIVE TECHNIQUE

Surgical technique must take into account both recipient and donor anatomy, particularly in recipients with a history of complex congenital heart lesions. Extensive harvesting of the donor systemic veins and great vessels may be necessary.

- Systemic venous connection:
  ○ Biatrial anastomosis: donor heart is anastamosed to residual cuff of recipient left and right atrial tissue.
  ○ Bicaval anastomosis: donor superior vena cava (SVC) and inferior vena cava (IVC) are connected end to end to recipient SVC and IVC. Cuff of recipient left atrium is anastamosed to donor left atrium.
  ○ Patients with complex congenital systemic venous anatomy (ex: bidirectional Glenn) may require additional donor tissue (SVC +/− innominate vein).
- Great vessel connection:
  ○ Donor proximal main pulmonary artery (MPA) is anastamosed to recipient distal MPA. Patients with branch PA stenosis may require additional patch arterioplasty of branch PAs.

○ Donor proximal ascending aorta is anastamosed to recipient distal ascending aorta. Patients with a history of congenital arch anomalies/surgeries may require additional aortic reconstruction.
- Recipients with a history of multiple prior sternotomies and/or complex anatomy may also require extensive intrathoracic dissection and reconstruction, resulting in prolonged graft ischemic time and increased risk of bleeding.

POSTOPERATIVE CONSIDERATIONS

Perioperative complications after heart transplant are predominantly related to bleeding, myocardial dysfunction, rejection, arrhythmias, infection, and acute kidney injury.

- Bleeding
  ○ Particularly problematic in patients with multiple prior sternotomies or chronic hypoxemia with intrathoracic collaterals
- Myocardial dysfunction
  ○ Right ventricular (RV) dysfunction is common due to elevated pulmonary vascular resistance (PVR) in patients with chronic left atrial hypertension or congenital heart abnormalities. May require use of inhaled nitric oxide (iNO) or inotropes for RV support.
  ○ Prolonged donor ischemic time and resultant inflammatory response may result in biventricular graft dysfunction.
  ○ Diastolic dysfunction may result in need for relatively high central venous pressure (10–15 mmHg) to maintain adequate preload.
  ○ Often require inotropic support with dopamine and epinephrine. Milrinone should be used cautiously given risk of post-cardiopulmonary bypass (CPB) renal dysfunction and systemic inflammatory response syndrome (SIRS) response with low systemic vascular resistance.
  ○ Acute rejection may also contribute to early graft dysfunction (see next).
- Rejection
  ○ Some centers utilize induction therapy with a polyclonal anti-lymphocyte antibody in the immediate postoperative period.
  ○ Plasmapheresis may be necessary in patients with elevated panel reactive antibodies (PRA) or positive crossmatch.
  ○ Maintenance immunosuppression typically includes steroids and an antiproliferative agent (mycophenolate mofetil or azathioprine). A calcineurin inhibitor (tacrolimus or cyclosporine) is typically added once renal function has stabilized. Sirolimus (mTOR inhibitor) may be used as an adjunct or alternative to tacrolimus, particularly in retransplant patients with history of graft vasculopathy.
  ○ Rejection can be hyperacute (acute severe graft function due to preformed antibodies), acute cellular (T-cell–mediated immune response against allograft), or antibody-mediated (donor-specific antibodies against allograft).
- Arrhythmias
  ○ The donor sinus node will no longer receive autonomic innervation, which may contribute to sinus or junctional bradycardia in the early postoperative period requiring temporary atrial pacing to optimize heart rate and cardiac output
  ○ Maintain cardioprotective levels of magnesium, calcium, and potassium
- Infection
  ○ Aggressive induction regimen in the immediate postoperative period increases risk of infection with bacterial and opportunistic infections
  ○ Antibiotic prophylaxis is initiated in the immediate post-transplant period against *Pneumocystis jirovecii* pneumonia, candida, and CMV

- Acute kidney injury
  - Prolonged bypass time, SIRS response, low cardiac output, and nephrotoxic medications can all contribute to early postoperative acute kidney injury

SUGGESTED READINGS

Conway J, Chin C, Kemna M, et al. Donors' characteristics and impact on outcomes in pediatric heart transplant recipient. *Pediatr Transplantation*. 2013;17:774-781.

Dipchand AI, Kirk R, Mahle WT, et al. Ten years of pediatric heart transplantation: A report from the Pediatric Heart Transplant Study. *Pediatr Transplantation*. 2013;17:99-111.

Gazit AZ, Fehr J. Perioperative management of the pediatric cardiac transplantation patient. *Curr Treat Options Cardio Med*. 2011;13:425-443.

Mahle WT, Webber SA, Cherikh WS, et al. Less urgent (UNOS 1B and 2) listings in pediatric heart transplantation: A vanishing breed. *JHLT*. 2012;31(7);782-784.

Zafar F, Castleberry C, Khan MS, et al. Pediatric heart transplant waiting list mortality in the era of ventricular assist devices. *JHLT*. 2015;34(1):82-88.

Neurology

38 Neurologic Formulas and Parameters

INTRACRANIAL PRESSURE

• Normal 0 to 20 mmHg

CEREBRAL PERFUSION PRESSURE (CPP)

Formula: CPP = Mean Arterial Pressure (MAP) − Intracranial Pressure (ICP)

• Infants: 40 mmHg
• Adults: 65 mmHg
  ○ Changes throughout development: parallels changes in systemic blood pressure (BP); increases gradually throughout development to adult levels.
  ○ Consider patient's baseline BP: Baseline MAP should be considered when considering therapeutic target for CPP in setting of acute neurologic injury. A patient with baseline hypertension will need blood pressure supported to a level that approximates their baseline physiology.
  ○ In adults poor outcomes are associated with sustained CPP <40 mmHg.

CEREBRAL BLOOD FLOW (CBF)

• Infants: 40 mL/100 g/min
• Children (4 years): 100 mL/100 g/min
• Children (9 years): 50 to 70 mL/100 g/min
• Adults: 50 mL/100 g/min

CEREBRAL METABOLIC RATE FOR OXYGEN (CMRO$_2$)

• Normal: 3.0 to 3.8 mL O$_2$/100 g brain/min

CEREBROSPINAL FLUID (CSF)

Normal values:

• White blood cell count (WBC): 0 to 5
• Total protein: 22 to 38 mg/dL
• Glucose: 60% to 80% of serum glucose

GLASGOW COMA SCALE (GCS)

• See Table 38-1.

TABLE 38-1	Glasgow Coma Scale	
Eye Opening	**Verbal Response**	**Motor Response**
4 – Opens Spontaneously	5 – Normal Conversation	6 – Normal
3 – Opens to Voice	4 – Disoriented Conversation	5 – Localizes Pain
2 – Opens to Pain	3 – Words, Incoherent	4 – Withdraws from Pain
1 – None	2 – Incomprehensible Sounds	3 – Decorticate Posturing
	1 – None	2 – Decerebrate Posturing
		1 – None

SUGGESTED READINGS

Downard C, Hulka F, Mullins RJ, et al. Relationship of cerebral perfusion pressure and survival in pediatric brain injured patients. *J Trauma*. 2000;49(4):654-658.

Teasdale G, Jennett B. Assessment of coma and impaired consciousness. A practical scale. *Lancet*. 1974;304(7872):81-84.

39 Neurosurgical and Neurologic Emergencies

NEUROSURGICAL EMERGENCIES

MONRO KELLIE DOCTRINE

- Physiology: Most cases of neurosurgical emergencies are related to the volume-occupying relationship between the brain matter, cerebral blood volume, and cerebrospinal fluid volume sharing space in the fixed-volume compartment of the skull (See Figure 39-1)
  - ○ Changes in the relative volume of one of these components require compensatory change in the volume occupied by one or more of the other components
  - ○ In the event that a change in the volume of one component overwhelms compensatory mechanisms, brain matter may move along the path of least resistance as it is pushed by pathologically elevated pressure within the calvarium
    - ▪ Cerebellar herniation via the foramen magnum
    - ▪ Transtentorial herniation across the falx cerebri
    - ▪ Transcalvarial herniation via a surgical or traumatic defect in the skull
- Clinical presentation:
  - ○ *Cerebellar herniation (brainstem compression and hydrocephalus)*
    - ▪ Somnolence/coma
    - ▪ Pupillary dilatation
      - • Unilateral or bilateral
      - • Nonreactive or sluggishly reactive
      - • Due to compression of third cranial nerve
    - ▪ Respiratory pattern
      - • Hyperventilation
      - • Cheyne-Stokes
    - ▪ Decorticate or decerebrate posturing
  - ○ *Transtentorial herniation*
- Cushing's triad: Clinical presentation of acute intracranial hypertension
  - ○ Hypertension
  - ○ Reflex bradycardia

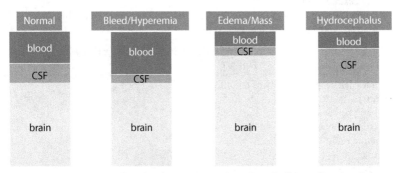

FIGURE 39-1 **The Monro Kellie doctrine states that the skull is a fixed-volume container and that an increase in the proportion of intracranial volume occupied by any of these tissues requires a compensatory decrease in the relative volume of the other tissues.**

○ Hypopnea
  ▪ May not be apparent in setting of intubated and mechanically ventilated patient
  ▪ May present as change in respiratory pattern
• Diagnostic approach: Aimed at determining underlying cause and developing definitive treatment plan
  ○ *Computerized tomography (CT) brain*
    ▪ Advantages
      • Rapid study
      • Readily available at most institutions
      • Can identify:
        ○ Blood collection
          ▪ Extraaxial
          ▪ Intraparenchymal
          ▪ Intraventricular
        ○ Hydrocephalus
        ○ Cerebral edema
        ○ Some masses
        ○ Skull defects
      • Contrast enhances ability to identify:
        ○ Vascular abnormalities (thromboses and anatomic variants)
        ○ Infectious processes (abscess)
      • CT angiography
    ▪ Disadvantages
      • Limited ability to image posterior fossa for mass (though this is often overcome with sagittal reconstructions)
      • Large ionizing radiation exposure
  ○ *Magnetic resonance imaging (MRI) brain*
    ▪ Advantages
      • Can reliably identify mass lesions in all parts of the central nervous system (CNS)
      • Can reliably identify acute ischemia, cerebral edema, and inflammatory parenchymal lesions
      • No ionizing radiation
    ▪ Disadvantages
      • Not readily available in all centers
      • Long duration study (the use of the fast-brain MRI has improved this greatly)
      • Material restrictions for magnet exposure

DISORDERS RESULTING IN INCREASE IN PARENCHYMAL VOLUME OF INTRACRANIAL COMPARTMENT

• Cerebral edema: Wide variety of conditions
  ○ Trauma
  ○ Diabetic ketoacidosis
  ○ Hepatic encephalopathy
  ○ Ischemic brain injury
    ▪ Stroke
    ▪ Hypoxic ischemic encephalopathy
    ▪ Encephalitis
  ○ Treatment
    ▪ Hyperosmolar therapy

- Hypertonic saline
  - 3 to 5 mEq/kg bolus
  - 1 mEq/kg can predictably increase serum sodium by 1
- Mannitol
  - 0.25 to 1 g/kg
  - Results in diuresis, which can cause hypotension and should be treated immediately
  - Decompressive surgery
  - Lesion
  - Skull
- Brain mass: Tumors
  - Discussion of specific tumor types is beyond the scope of this chapter
  - Surgical decompression as necessary
  - Surrounding edema may be treated with dexamethasone acutely or subacutely

DISORDERS RESULTING IN DECREASED INTRACRANIAL VOLUME

- Craniofacial disorders
  - Craniosynostosis
  - Trauma
  - Iatrogenic
- Neurosurgical postoperative
  - Epilepsy
  - Craniofacial repair

DISORDERS RESULTING IN INCREASE IN BLOOD VOLUME WITHIN THE INTRACRANIAL COMPARTMENT

- Hemorrhagic conditions
  - Frequently occur after trauma
  - Initial diagnosis via CT scan
  - Treatment involves surgical evacuation of blood collection and surgical repair of bleeding vessel
  - May occur in setting of coagulopathy or thrombocytopenia
    - Therapeutic anticoagulation
    - Pathologic coagulopathy
    - Liver failure
    - Multiple system organ failure
    - Sepsis
  - Intraparenchymal hemorrhage
    - Traumatic
    - Arteriovenous malformation rupture
      - May be definitively diagnosed and treated with interventional radiological procedures
  - Subdural hemorrhage
    - Traumatic injury
      - Accidental
      - Nonaccidental trauma
  - Subarachnoid hemorrhage (SAH)
    - Most common cause is post-traumatic
    - Can be aneurysmal SAH as a consequence of rupture of an aneurysm associated with cerebral vasculature
    - May be definitively diagnosed and treated with interventional radiological procedures

- Watch for clinical consequences of vasospasm
  - ○ Epidural hemorrhage
    - Often after trauma
    - Associated with skull fractures
  - ○ Tumor: hemorrhagic conversion

DISORDERS ASSOCIATED WITH INCREASE IN CEREBROSPINAL FLUID (CSF) COMPONENT OF INTRACRANIAL COMPARTMENT

- Hydrocephalus
  - ○ May develop as a result of anatomic changes resulting from a prior insult
  - ○ Ventriculoperitoneal shunt failure
  - ○ Treatment includes surgical diversion of CSF from the intracranial compartment to external ventricular drain, ventricular shunt, or removal of obstruction

INFECTIOUS DISORDERS

- Empyema from intracranial infections behaves in the same manner as the disorders listed earlier and can result in herniation syndrome.
- Require neurosurgical drainage, but must find primary cause. Most common in children is sinovenous infection. Concurrent treatment of cause (sinusitis) and consequence (intracranial infection) important.
- Require antibiotic therapy.
- Diagnosed via CT with or without contrast, but MRI is more sensitive and can see associated brain inflammation.
- Most require antiseizure therapy.

OTHER THERAPIES

- Normoxia
  - ○ Goal SaO_2 >95%
  - ○ Hypoxemia results in cerebral vasodilation, which can exacerbate a herniation event (See Figure 39-2)

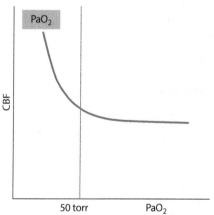

FIGURE 39-2 PaO_2 and cerebral blood flow. As PaO_2 decreases below 50 mmHg there is a reflexive vasodilation. This can increase cerebral blood volume and exacerbate intracranial hypertension—one of several reasons hypoxia should be avoided after brain injury. Hypoxemia is a cerebral vasodilator; hyperoxia does not have an effect on cerebral blood flow.

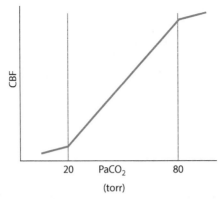

FIGURE 39-3 PaCO$_2$ and cerebral blood flow. As PaCO$_2$ decreases there is an associated decrease in cerebral blood flow (and therefore cerebral blood volume); as PaCO$_2$ increases there is an increase in cerebral blood flow/cerebral blood volume—approximately a 4% change in cerebral blood flow per 1 mmHg change in PaCO$_2$ across the range of PaCO$_2$ 20 to 80 mmHg.

○ Hypoxemia exacerbates cellular injury in the injured tissue and is associated with increased mortality and worsened functional outcome after a variety of cerebral injuries[1]
• Hyperventilation
  ○ Decrease in PaCO$_2$ results in cerebral vasoconstriction, which results in decrease in cerebral blood volume (See Figure 39-3)
  ○ This maneuver can be temporarily employed to prevent herniation while a definitive treatment plan is deployed
  ○ Prolonged hyperventilation cerebral vasoconstriction can result in ischemia—this maneuver should be considered a rescue maneuver
• Therapeutic temperature management
  ○ Normothermia (35.5–36.5°C) should be actively maintained
  ○ Hyperthermia results in cerebral vasodilation and may exacerbate a herniation event
  ○ No evidence to support therapeutic hypothermia to improve survival or improved functional outcome in setting of neurosurgical illness[2]
• Blood pressure: Should be maintained in the normal range for age[3] (See Figure 39-4)
  ○ Hypertension can exacerbate cerebral hemorrhage.
  ○ Hypotension can result in tissue ischemia and worsen survival/outcome.
  ○ IMPORTANT: Hypertension associated with Cushing's triad should not be directly treated; rather, the underlying cause should be identified and definitively treated before initiating antihypertensive therapy. These decisions should be made in consultation with neurosurgical partners.

SPINAL CORD INJURY

• Presentation: Acute change in sensation and motor function detected below a particular spinal dermatome. Frequently bilateral, may be unilateral.
• Causes
  ○ Mass
  ○ Hemorrhage
  ○ Trauma and cord compression

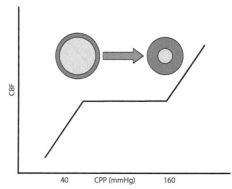

FIGURE 39-4 Cerebral autoregulation. Across a physiologic blood pressure range the cerebral vasculature can maintain steady blood flow and substrate delivery by vasodilating in the setting of lower mean arterial pressure (MAP) and vasoconstricting in the setting of higher MAP. At extremely low MAP, the dilatory mechanism is exhausted, and further decrease in MAP results in linear decrease in cerebral blood flow, resulting in tissue malperfusion/ischemia. At extremely high MAP, the constricting mechanism is exhausted, resulting in vascular injury, local edema, headache, and seizures (hypertensive encephalopathy).

- Diagnosis: MRI
- Requires urgent neurosurgical intervention to maximize neurologic recovery. Certain tumor syndromes respond to chemotherapy and will not need surgery.
- Postoperative care includes careful blood pressure management to ensure adequate cord perfusion.
  - ○ Phenylephrine frequently used to support blood pressure in physiologic range
  - ○ Spinal shock

NEUROLOGIC EMERGENCIES

HYPERTENSIVE ENCEPHALOPATHY

- Presentation: Headache, visual changes, somnolence/coma, seizure
- Pathophysiology: Unmitigated hypertension that exhausts the autoregulatory mechanism
  - ○ This causes increase in cerebral blood flow and injury to brain–blood barrier
  - ○ Causes tissue edema and injury to cerebral tissue
- Treatment:
  - ○ Correct hypertension
  - ○ Treat seizures (see Chapter 42)

SEIZURES – SEE CHAPTER 42

STROKE

- Presentation: Acute-onset focal neurologic deficit
  - ○ Motor weakness
  - ○ Sensory deficit
  - ○ Cranial nerve finding
  - ○ Alteration in consciousness

- <u>Diagnosis:</u> MRI with diffusion-weighted imaging and apparent diffusion coefficient sequences
- <u>Conversion:</u> Nascent strokes may undergo hemorrhagic conversion or develop diffuse edema, resulting in intracranial hypertension and herniation syndrome (Cushing's triad). Urgent neurosurgical evaluation along with therapeutic rescue maneuvers described earlier should be immediately employed.
- Please see Chapter 43 for a full discussion of stroke.

REFERENCES

1. Stochetti N, Furlan A, Volta F. Hypoxemia and arterial hypotension at the accident scene in head injury. *J Trauma*. 1996;40:764-776.
2. Hutchison JS, Ward RE, Lacroix J. Hypothermia therapy after traumatic brain injury in children. *NEJM*. 2008;358:2447-2456.
3. Pigula FA, Wald SL, Shackford SR. The effect of hypotension and hypoxia on children with severe head injuries. *J Pediatr Surg*. 1993;28:310-314.

Increased Intracranial Pressure 40

DEFINITION AND NORMAL INTRACRANIAL PRESSURE VALUES

Intracranial pressure (ICP) is the pressure of cerebrospinal fluid (CSF) within the cerebral ventricles. ICP is the product of the rate of cerebrospinal fluid (CSF) formation ($I_{formation}$), resistance to CSF drainage (R_{out}), and pressure in the dural venous sinuses (P_d), a formula proposed by Davson (ICP = $R_{out} \times I_{formation} + P_d$).[1] Thus, ICP is regulated by venous pressure, cerebral blood flow, and CSF circulation.

- Normal values for CSF production, sagittal sinus pressure, and resistance to CSF outflow are 0.2 to 0.7 mL/min, 5 to 8 mmHg, and 6 to 10 mm Hg/mL/min, respectively.
- ICP increases with age.
  - In the newborn, the normal value for ICP is approximately 82 mm H_2O, or 6 mmHg.[2]
  - Normal CSF pressure in healthy children obtained during lumbar puncture is a mean of 19.6 cm H_2O (10th to 90th percentile, 11.5 to 28.0 cm H_2O).
    - Sedation may increase opening CSF pressure by up to 3.5 cm H_2O.
- Volume status, blood pressure, and end-tidal CO_2 may also affect ICP and must be considered when deciding on interventions to treat intracranial hypertension.
- An opening pressure above 28 H_2O may not be "abnormal" if signs of increased ICP (papilledema, abducens nerve palsy, hydrocephalus, subdural fluid, other intracranial pathology) are absent.[3]

PATHOPHYSIOLOGY

- Monro-Kellie doctrine
  - The skull is a rigid cavity containing brain (1200–1600 mL), arterial and venous blood (100–150 mL), and CSF or other extracellular fluid (100–150 mL)
  - Expansion of one compartment is offset by a decrease in volume of the others. The pressure–volume relationship is expressed by the formula C ~ dV/dp, where C represents compliance and dV represents the change in volume that accompanies a change in pressure (dp) (Figure 40-1).
  - As ICP increases, compliance decreases. In cases of intracranial pathology, such as traumatic brain injury (TBI) or space-occupying lesions (tumors, arachnoid cysts, hemorrhage), compliance is decreased and small increases in the volume of one compartment result in large increases in ICP. Cranial causes of decreased compliance can include hyperostosis, craniosynostosis, and traumatic skull injury without brain injury such as a depressed skull fracture.
- Intracranial pressure, cerebral perfusion, and autoregulation
  - Under normal conditions, cerebral blood flow (CBF) is a constant of approximately 50 mL/100 gm brain/min.
  - CBF is determined by the vascular gradient across the cerebral beds and is a product of cerebral perfusion pressure (CPP) and cerebrovascular resistance (CVR), according to the formula CBF = CPP/CVR.[4]
  - The relationship between CPP and ICP is expressed by the formula CPP = MAP – ICP.
  - Autoregulation is the mechanism by which CBF is kept constant despite changes in CPP.

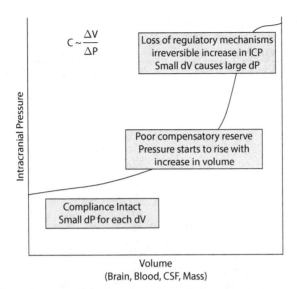

$$C \sim \frac{\Delta V}{\Delta P}$$

Loss of regulatory mechanisms irreversible increase in ICP Small dV causes large dP

Poor compensatory reserve Pressure starts to rise with increase in volume

Compliance Intact Small dP for each dV

Intracranial Pressure

Volume
(Brain, Blood, CSF, Mass)

FIGURE 40-1 **Compliance curve showing the relationship between intracranial pressure and volume.** As volume of one compartment increases, compliance within the cranial vault fails, and small increases in volume result in large increases in intracranial pressure.

- ○ When autoregulation is intact, increases in blood pressure lead to a decrease in cerebral artery caliber to maintain a constant CBF by increasing CVR.
- ○ When CPP falls below the lower limit of autoregulation (40–50 mmHg in the mature brain), CBF is dependent on MAP.
  - ▪ This is a "pressure-passive" circulation in which decreases in MAP result in corresponding decreases in cerebral perfusion and risk for ischemic injury.
- ○ Cumulative data from pediatric traumatic brain injury studies suggest ICP >20 mmHg or CPP <40 mmHg are associated with poor outcome.

CLINICAL SIGNS OF INTRACRANIAL HYPERTENSION

Diagnosis of intracranial hypertension requires a high index of clinical suspicion and cannot be excluded based on a normal computerized tomography (CT) or magnetic resonance imaging (MRI) scan. Imaging signs of intracranial hypertension include decrease in size or loss of cisterns, uncal and other herniation, midline shift, and loss of grey-white differentiation. Clinical signs range from subtle changes in mental status to cranial neuropathies, focal weakness, posturing, stupor, and coma.

DIAGNOSIS

The diagnosis may be made, and therapy initiated, based on the clinical exam (Table 40-1) and imaging findings (edema, midline shift, loss of grey-white differentiation) in the appropriate clinical context of a patient at risk for increased ICP.

TABLE 40-1	Clinical Signs of Herniation Syndromes	
Type	**Mechanism and Structures Affected**	**Clinical Findings**
Central	Swelling of both cerebral hemispheres	Early: Decline in consciousness, constricted pupils (sympathetic dysfunction), Cheyne-Stokes respiration
	Compression of diencephalon and midbrain	Late: Neurogenic hyperventilation, decerebrate posturing
		Loss of occulocephalic reflexes
Cingulate	Displacement of edematous cingulate gyrus under the falx cerebri	Variable symptoms
		Often occurs prior to other herniation syndromes
	Compression of ipsilateral or bilateral anterior cerebral arteries and internal cerebral vein	Associated with uncal herniation
Tonsillar	Cerebellar tonsils affected in the foramen magnum	Early: Abrupt loss of consciousness, opisthotonic posturing
	Compression of medulla and upper cervical spinal cord	Late: Irregular respiration, apnea
Transtentorial	Displacement of uncal portion of temporal lobe with entrapment in the tentorial notch	Ipsilateral dilated pupil (compression of pupilloconstrictor fibers)
		Progressive decline in consciousness Loss of occulocephalic reflexes Decorticate posturing
	Compression of the ipsilateral third cranial nerve, midbrain, cerebral peduncle, and posterior cerebral artery	Ipsilateral hemiparesis
Late stages	Later stages of uncal, central, and tonsillar herniation manifest as coma, flaccid limbs, midsize unresponsive pupils, loss of corneal and occulocephalic reflexes, and irreversible apnea	

- Papilledema is a late finding.
  - Visual acuity is typically preserved with intracranial hypertension.
  - The absence of papilledema does not rule out intracranial hypertension.
- Lumbar puncture (LP) may increase the risk for herniation and is contraindicated if there is a focal finding on the neurologic exam, concern for obstruction (noncommunicating hydrocephalus), or an intracranial mass lesion.

  - Neuroimaging (MRI or CT) should first be performed to confirm the absence of a mass lesion.
  - Under some circumstances, after consultation with Neurosurgery, the LP may be used as a diagnostic or therapeutic intervention to measure opening pressure or to allow drainage of CSF.

INTRACRANIAL PRESSURE MONITORING

Severe traumatic brain injury is the best-established indication for ICP monitoring, although this is a level III recommendation.[5] ICP-directed care in children with acute central nervous system (CNS) infections, acute liver failure, stroke, and diabetic ketoacidosis have been reported, but not linked to improved outcome.[6]

- ICP monitor types
  - ICP monitors are classified by mechanism (fluid or nonfluid coupled) and anatomy (extradural, subdural, ventricular, or parenchymal)
  - The gold standard for accurate ICP monitoring is the intraventricular drain, which both allows drainage of CSF and provides real-time measurement of ICP.[7]
  - Insertion may be difficult in certain clinical circumstances, including ventricular size and clinical status of the patient (location, coagulation/bleeding, other systemic abnormalities).
  - Noninvasive approaches to ICP monitoring include optic nerve sheath diameter measurement, tympanometry, and tonometry, none of which are in routine clinical use. MRI has been used to measure ICP, also without much adoption.
- Indications for ICP monitoring
  - Numerous pediatric studies report a relationship between intracranial hypertension (>20 mmHg) and poor outcome in severe TBI.[8]
    - Whether ICP monitoring improves outcome following severe TBI is controversial, with evidence for no benefit[9] or some survival advantage.[10]
  - ICP monitoring without complications has been reported in children with other acute neurologic insults, including diabetic ketoacidosis, CNS infections, stroke, and acute liver failure, and may be considered at the treating physician's discretion.

MANAGEMENT

First establish a neurologic exam and identify the primary cause of intracranial hypertension. Notify Neurosurgery, and determine whether emergent operative intervention or CSF diversion is needed. Decompressive craniectomy with duraplasty or continuous ventricular CSF drainage with ICP monitoring may improve outcome in children with intracranial hypertension following severe TBI. Start medical management of intracranial hypertension (Figure 40-2).[11]

- Key principles
  - Maintain ICP <20 to 25 mmHg; CPP > minimum of 40 mmHg
    - Use age-dependent goals for CPP thresholds
  - Limit interventions (suctioning, pain) that may cause increases in ICP
  - Prevent fever and use targeted temperature management if possible
  - Medical management may proceed without an ICP monitor
  - Be prepared to escalate the intensity of therapy based on serial neurologic examinations or imaging changes
  - If hypothermia is used to reduce ICP, rewarm slowly (0.5–1.0°C every 12–24 hours)
  - Ensure adequate access (arterial, venous, and central lines) if hyperosmolar and ICP-directed therapy are anticipated

1

1. Neurosurgery Consult
2. Stabilize patient (see below)
3. Correct volume status and optimize CPP
4. Treat **latrogenic causes** of increased ICP
5. Consider craniectomy, CSF diversion

2

Initial Stabilization

1. Head in midline to optimize jugular venous outflow
2. Keep temperature < 36.5°C
3. Head of bed at 0 or 30 degrees (depending on volume status and oligemic or hyperemic state), typically 30 degrees
4. O2 sat > 96%
5. PaCO2 35-40 mm Hg
6. Minimize stimulation. Start sedation as needed
7. Treat iatrogenic causes of ICP increases

3

Assess volume status and correct blood pressure to maintain adequate cerebral blood flow

1. For Low systolic BP or hypovolemia (CPP deficit), give normal saline bolus 10-20 ml/kg
2. Repeat and add pressors if needed to maintain CPP > **minimum of 40 mm Hg**

4

Consider placement of ICP monitor or external ventricular drain

1. Continue 'General Care and fluid support to maintain goal MAPs
2. For clinical or radiographic signs of increased ICP follow tiered therapy (Boxes 5-7)
3. If ICP monitor is in place, escalate therapy if ICP is > 20 - 25 mm Hg for > 5 minutes or is rising rapidly
4. Obtain stat CT and neurosurgical consult if clinical signs of herniation are present
5. Consider cEEG monitoring

5

First Tier Therapy for ICP > 20

1. CSF drainage (EVD)
2. Treat iatrogenic causes and check position of head
3. **Transient** hyperventilation to PaCO2 25-30 mm Hg

6

Second Tier Therapy

1. Sedation and neuromuscular blockage if needed
2. 3% hypertonic saline bolus (2-6 ml/kg) then infusion at 0.1-1 ml. kg-1 of body weight per hr). Hold if osmolarity > 360 or Na > 155. **OR** (may select based on volume status)
3. Mannitol 0.25 - 1.0 gm/kg IV every 4-6 hr. Hold if serum osmolarity > 320 mOsm/L
4. Check sodium and serum osmolarity q 6 hr

7

Third Tier Therapy

1. Barbiturate (pentobarbital, thiopental) titrated to ICP, BP and burst suppression
2. Stepwise hypothermia with first reduction to 35 ± 1°C then 32-33°C for up to 48 hr
3. Decompressive craniectomy

Physiologic Parameters

1. Goal ICP < 20 mm Hg
2. CPP (**minimum**) > 40 mm Hg
3. Age-dependent CPP recommendations:
   50 mm Hg (2-6 yr)
   55 mm Hg (7-10 yr)
   60 mm Hg (11-16 yr)
4. O2 sat > 96 %
5. PaCO2 35-40 mm Hg
6. Temperature < 36.5°C
7. Na > 140

General Principles

1. Escalate therapies quickly. If ICP is refractory or CT shows herniation, consider early decompression.
2. If hypothermia is used to decrease ICP, rewarm slowly (< 0.5-1.0°C per 12-24 hr)

Iatrogenic Causes of Increased ICP

1. Hypoxia or hypercarbia
2. Pain or insufficient sedation
3. Hyperthermia
4. Suctioning
5. ICP monitor malfunction
6. Consider EEG monitoring for seizures

REFERENCES

1. Davson H. Formation and drainage of the cerebrospinal fluid. *Sci Basis Med Annu Rev* 1966:238-259.
2. Welch K. The intracranial pressure in infants. *J Neurosurg.* 1980;52:693-699.
3. Avery RA. Reference range of cerebrospinal fluid opening pressure in children: Historical overview and current data. *Neuropediatrics.* 2014;45:206-211.
4. Harper A. Physiology of cerebral blood flow. *Br J Anaesth.* 1965;37:225-235.
5. Kochanek PM, Carney N, Adelson PD, et al. Guidelines for the acute medical management of severe traumatic brain injury in infants, children, and adolescents–second edition. *Pediatr Crit Care Med.* 2012;13(Suppl 1):S1-82.
6. O'Brien NF, Mella C. Brain tissue oxygenation-guided management of diabetic ketoacidosis induced cerebral edema. *Pediatr Crit Care Med.* 2012;13:e383-e388.
7. Padayachy L, Figaji A, Bullock M. Intracranial pressure monitoring for traumatic brain injury in the modern era. *Childs Nerv Syst.* 2010;26:441-452.
8. Adelson PD, Wisniewski SR, Beca J, et al. Comparison of hypothermia and normothermia after severe traumatic brain injury in children (Cool Kids): A phase 3, randomised controlled trial. *Lancet Neurol.* 2013;12:546-553.
9. Chesnut R, Temkin N, Carney N, et al. A trial of intracranial-pressure monitoring in traumatic brain injury. *N Engl J Med.* 2012;367:2471-2481.
10. Alkhoury F, Kyriakides TC. Intracranial pressure monitoring in children with severe traumatic brain injury: National Trauma Data Bank-Based Review of Outcomes. *JAMA Surg.* 2014;149:544-548.
11. Mhanna MJ, Mallah WE, Verrees M, et al. Outcome of children with severe traumatic brain injury who are treated with decompressive craniectomy. *J Neurosurg Pediatr.* 2015;16(5):508-514.

Traumatic Brain Injury 41

CHAPTER

MECHANISMS OF INJURY AND PATHOPHYSIOLOGY

INJURY PATTERNS

- Mechanism of Injury: It is important to know the cause of injury to determine severity of injury, triage the patient to the appropriate level of care, and anticipate possible complications.
- Primary Injury: Occurs on initial impact, either diffuse or focal. Often results in skull fractures. *Focal injuries* include contusions, lacerations, and hemorrhages. *Diffuse brain injuries* include concussions and diffuse axonal injury.
  - *Concussion:* Diffuse brain injury without associated head computerized tomography (CT) findings. Symptoms may include headache, disorientation, emesis, or brief loss of consciousness.[1]
  - *Diffuse axonal injury:* Shearing injury caused by acceleration and deceleration resulting in trauma between the gray and white matter.[1]
  - *Epidural hematoma:* Rapidly progressing arterial bleed occurring between the skull and dura.[2] Often secondary to middle meningeal artery and occasionally caused by a venous bleed.[1] Patients may have loss of consciousness followed by a lucid period prior to neurologic deterioration. Elliptical shape on head CT due to limitations of fluid spread by dural attachment at suture lines. See Figure 41-1.
  - *Subdural hematoma:* Venous bleed occurring between the dura and arachnoid. Caused by rupture of the bridging veins during rapid movement of the brain within the skull. Acute subdural hematomas progress rapidly and are associated with high morbidity and

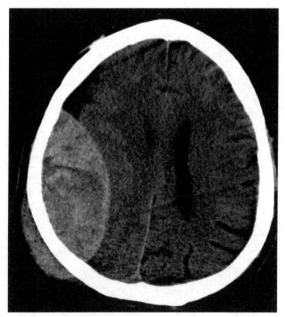

FIGURE 41-1 **Epidural hematoma.**

mortality.[2] Concave shape on neuroimaging, extending throughout the subdural space. See Figure 41-2.

- *Intracerebral hematomas*: Tearing of small vessels in any area of the brain. Symptoms vary depending on location of bleed, but often occur in the frontal and temporal lobes.[2]

- Secondary Injury: Occurs due to decreased perfusion of surviving tissue that causes reduction in oxygen delivery, metabolite delivery, and metabolic waste and toxin clearance. Additional injury results from cerebral herniation syndromes, which can cause focal ischemic injury and brainstem compression.[3]

  - *Vasogenic edema*: Swelling of interstitial space. Capillary leak from cerebral vasculature into interstitial space due to disruption of blood–brain barrier, occurring primarily in the white matter. Secondary to ischemia, hemorrhage, brain injury, infection, and tumors.[2]

  - *Cytotoxic edema*: Swelling of brain cells. Secondary to altered osmotic state caused by ischemia with associated extracellular acidosis secondary to anaerobic metabolism and cell membrane rupture.[2]

SEVERITY OF TRAUMATIC BRAIN INJURY

- Severity of traumatic brain injury (TBI) is determined by the Glasgow Coma Scale (GCS). See Tables 41-1 and 41-2.

MANAGEMENT OF SEVERE TRAUMATIC BRAIN INJURY

GUIDELINES FOR MANAGEMENT OF SEVERE TRAUMATIC BRAIN INJURY

- The second edition of the *Guidelines for the Acute Medical Management of Severe Traumatic Brain Injury in Infants, Children, and Adolescents* was published in 2012.[3] The extensive literature review is broken down into recommendations with supporting strength of evidence

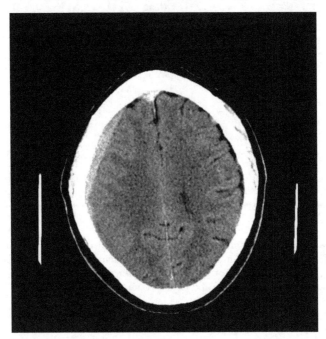

FIGURE 41-2 **Subdural hematoma.**

TABLE 41-1	Severities of Traumatic Brain Injury	
Classification of Traumatic Brain Injury by Severity		
	Glasgow Coma Scale	**Recommended Monitoring & Disposition**
Mild TBI	13–15	After initial evaluation, depending on neurologic status and history, may be monitored at home
Moderate TBI	9–12	Close monitoring in PICU
		Do not intubate unless clinically indicated by respiratory exam
Severe TBI	3–8	In presence of abnormal CT scan suggesting TBI
		Intubation and placement of ICP monitor as soon as possible

TABLE 41-2	Glasgow Coma Scale for Children and Infants. Total Score 3–15. Flexion is Decorticate Posturing. Extension is Decerebrate Posturing		
	Children	**Infants**	**Score**
Eye Opening	Spontaneously	Spontaneously	**4**
	To voice	To voice	**3**
	To pain	To pain	**2**
	None	None	**1**
Verbal	Oriented	Coos and babbles	**5**
	Confused	Irritable cries	**4**
	Inappropriate words	Cries to pain	**3**
	Incomprehensible sounds	Moans to pain	**2**
	None	None	**1**
Motor	Follows commands	Normal spontaneous movement	**6**
	Localizes pain	Withdraws to touch	**5**
	Withdraws to pain	Withdraws to pain	**4**
	Flexion to painful stimuli	Flexion to painful stimuli	**3**
	Extension to painful stimuli	Extension to painful stimuli	**2**
	None	None	**1**

and does not include recommendations made by expert opinion. These guidelines are endorsed by many important medical bodies, including the Society of Critical Care Medicine, Neurocritical Care Society, Pediatric Neurocritical Care Research Group, World Federation of Pediatric Intensive and Critical Care Societies, and American Academy of Pediatrics Section on Neurological Surgery.[3]

• Although the 2012 guidelines[3] include 40 years of TBI literature, due to a lack of high-quality pediatric TBI evidence, specific treatment plans cannot be made for infants and children with severe TBI.[4]

PREVENTION OF SECONDARY INJURY

- Goals of TBI Management:

Management of severe TBI
Maintain adequate cerebral perfusion pressure
Minimize intracranial hypertension and secondary injury

- *Intracranial hypertension (ICH) and systemic hypotension are associated with poor outcomes in severe TBI*[3]
- Neuroprotective Measures:
  - *Positioning*: **Improve cerebral venous drainage** by midline head positioning with head of bed elevated to 30 degrees.[5]
  - *Electrolyte monitoring*: **Avoid hypoglycemia and hyperglycemia.** Avoid rapid fluctuations in sodium and glucose levels. Hyponatremia can cause intracerebral swelling and seizures.[5]
  - *Temperature*: **Avoid hypothermia and maintain normothermia**[5] using antipyretics and hypothermia or hyperthermia blankets as necessary.
  - *Sedation*: **Provide adequate sedation and analgesia,** which can help lower intracranial pressure (ICP).[3,5]
    - Other benefits include preventing shivering, long-term psychological trauma, pain, stress, frequent coughing, and ventilator dyssynchrony.[3,5]
    - Pain and stress increase cerebral metabolic demand, cerebral blood volume, and ICP.[3]
  - *Normalize oxygenation and ventilation*:
    - **Maintain SpO_2 above 94%** and use caution, as increased intrathoracic pressure (due to increased positive end-expiratory pressure [PEEP]) can decrease cerebral venous return and thus cause ICH.[5]
    - **Goal pH is 7.35 to 7.45 with $PaCO_2$ 35 to 45mmHg** because hyperventilation lowers cerebral perfusion pressure (CPP) by vasoconstricting cerebral blood flow and should generally be avoided to prevent further ischemia.[3,5]
    - In severe, life-threatening periods of ICH, hyperventilation may be used briefly to a $PaCO_2$ of 20 mmHg while awaiting further treatment or surgical interventions.[5]
  - *Fluid management*: Avoid hypotonic fluids to avoid exacerbating cerebral edema; consider normal saline as fluid of choice
- Intracranial Pressure Monitoring: Placement of an ICP monitoring device is recommended in patients with severe TBI and may be considered in children with mild or moderate TBI with limited ability to undergo serial neurologic exams (i.e., sedation, anesthesia, or neuromuscular blockade).[3]
- Treatment Thresholds for Intracranial Hypertension: **Sustained intracranial hypertension above 20 mmHg for longer than 5 minutes should be treated.**[3]

Intracranial Hypertension (ICH) = ICP > 20 mmHg for > 5 minutes

  - Mortality and poor outcomes are associated with sustained increases in ICP.
  - ICP treatment thresholds should most likely be age dependent; however, the current literature does not provide enough evidence to determine ranges.[3]
- Cerebral Perfusion Pressure Thresholds: CPP is the pressure gradient providing cerebral blood flow and is calculated as the difference between the mean arterial pressure (MAP) and ICP.[3] *Survivors of severe TBI have higher CPP values than nonsurvivors.*[6]

$$CPP = MAP - ICP$$

Goal CPP[6] > 40 for infants to 5 year olds > 50 for 6 − 17 year olds
> 50 − 60 for > 17 year olds

  ○ **CPP should be maintained above a minimum level of 40 to 50 mmHg to prevent cerebral ischemia, with infants on the lower end and adolescents on the upper end.**[3]
  ○ In severe TBI, patients should have continuous MAP (arterial line) and ICP monitoring to provide accurate CPP monitoring.[3]
    ▪ Ideally, these pressure monitoring devices should be zeroed at the same level for accurate CPP monitoring.[3,5]
• Hyperosmolar Therapy: Used for medical management of ICH. Target euvolemic hyperosmolar state (may trend central venous pressure).[3]
  ○ *Hypertonic Saline*: Dose: 6.5 to 10 mL/kg for acute ICH[3] (dosing may range 2–10 mL/kg/dose[6])
    Continuous infusion: 0.1 to 1 mL/kg/hr[3] titrated for minimum effective dose.
    Maintain serum osmolarity less than 360 mOsm/L[3]

    ▪ Side effects of hypertonic saline: May include rebound ICP, central pontine myelinolysis (with rapid shifts in sodium levels), renal impairment, subarachnoid hemorrhage, dehydration, and hyperchloremic metabolic acidosis, masking symptoms of diabetes inspidius.[3]
  ○ *Foley catheter*: Should be used in patients on hyperosmolar therapy to monitor urine output and prevent bladder rupture.[3]
  ○ *Mannitol*: Dose: 0.25 to 1 gm/kg intermittent dosing for acute ICH.
    Maintain serum osmolarity less than 320 mOsm/L[3,5]

    ▪ Initial effects (<75 minutes) reduces blood viscosity, thereby increasing laminar flow.
    ▪ Osmotic effect (15–30 minutes) triggers diuresis of water from brain parenchyma into the systemic circulation, lasting about 6 hours.[3]
    ▪ Long-term effects of mannitol:
      • Accumulation in injured brain tissue may reverse osmotic shift, drawing water into parenchyma and increasing ICP.
      • Acute tubular necrosis, possibly due to renal excretion of mannitol, hyperosmolar state, or dehydration.[3]

  Note: Although used frequently in practice, there is no evidence to support or refute the efficacy of mannitol within the most recent guidelines.[3]

• Antiepileptic Prophylaxis:
  ○ Post-traumatic seizures: Occur early (within 7 days) or late (more than 8 days after injury) with increased risk depending on location and severity of injury, depressed skull fracture, and neurologic deficits.[3]
  ○ Electroencephalogram (EEG): In patients on sedation, barbiturates, or neuromuscular blockade, continuous EEG should be placed to monitor for subclinical seizure activity.
  ○ There is limited data to suggest the appropriate agent for use for antiepileptic prophylaxis in pediatric severe TBI. Current guidelines suggest phenytoin for consideration for prophylaxis of early post-traumatic seizure activity.[3] Antiepileptic medications may have sedating side effects, cause hypotension, or inhibit ability for recovery; thus, clinician assessment with neurology or neurocritical care–experienced physicians is useful.[5]

- Cerebrospinal Fluid Drainage: Cerebrospinal fluid (CSF) drainage may be considered in patients with ICH. Removal of CSF reduces the intracranial fluid volume and thus lowers ICP.[3]
  - External ventricular drain (EVD): Clinicians should consider intermittent vs. continuous fluid drainage.[3]
  - Lumbar drain: In patients with refractory ICH, open basal cisterns, EVD, and no mass lesions or shift on radiologic imaging.[3]
- Barbiturate Therapy: Barbiturates lower ICP by suppressing cerebral metabolic demand and altering vascular tone. High-dose barbiturates can be considered in refractory ICH after first-tier medical and surgical interventions, but are not supported for prophylactic use.[3]
  - Pentobarbital: Initial bolus dose range: 5 to 10 mg/kg; continuous infusion range: 1 to 4 mg/kg/hr[3,7]
  - EEG monitoring: To achieve burst suppression, titrate barbiturate infusion to effect.
  - Side effects: Hypoxia and lower CPP due to decreased cardiac output, hypotension, and increased intrapulmonary shunt. Patients should have close hemodynamic and respiratory monitoring with available vasoactive medications.[3]

NEUROIMAGING AND NEUROSURGICAL INTERVENTIONS

- Neuroimaging: Initial head CT should be used to determine severity of TBI.
  - *Repeat imaging*: May be necessary in patients with unchanged neurologic exam, persistent ICH, or inability to assess neurologic status.
  - *Risks of neuroimaging*: Medically unstable patients may not tolerate CT imaging. Radiation exposure increases risks of fatal cancer.
  - Routine use of follow-up imaging in the absence of neurologic deterioration is not recommended; risks and benefits should be weighed.[3]
- Decompressive Craniectomy (DC): Performed with unilateral or bilateral removal of skull bone flap to allow for cerebral edema. Location depends on underlying injury.[3]
  - *Primary DC*: For treatment of cerebral herniation or early refractory ICH.[3]
    - Consider in patients with early herniation or neurologic deterioration or refractory ICH resistant to early medical management.
    - Primary DC can decrease ICP; however, whether it improves functional and neurologic outcomes is unknown.[3]
  - *Secondary DC*: For removal of mass lesion or hematoma to treat associated cerebral edema.[3]

REFERENCES

1. Reuter-Rice K, Bolick BN. *Pediatric Acute Care: A Guide for Interprofessional Practice.* Burlington, MA: Jones & Bartlett Learning; 2012.
2. Grossman S, Porth CM. *Porth's Pathophysiology: Concepts of Altered Health States.* 9th ed. Philadelphia, PA: Wolters Kluwer Health, Lippincott Williams & Wilkins; 2014.
3. Kochanek PM, Carney N, Adelson PD, et al. Guidelines for the acute management of severe traumatic brain injury in infants, children, and adolescents- second edition. *Pediatr Crit Care Med.* 2012;13(1):S1-S82.
4. Bell MJ, Kochanek PM. Pediatric traumatic brain injury in 2012: The year with new guidelines and common data elements. *Crit Care Clin.* 2013;29:223-238.

5. Nichols DG, Shaffner DH. *Rogers' Textbook of Pediatric Intensive Care*. 5th ed. Philadelphia, PA: Wolters Kluwer; 2016.
6. Allen BB, Chiu YL, Gerber LM, et al. Age-specific cerebral perfusion pressure thresholds and survival in children and adolescents with severe traumatic brain injury. *Pediatr Crit Care Med*. 2014;15(1):62-70.
7. Lexicomp Online, Pediatric and neonatal Lexi-Drugs. Wolters Kluwer Clinical Drug Information, Inc.; Accessed August 8, 2016. http://online.lexi.com/lco/action/home.

42 Status Epilepticus

DEFINITION

Status epilepticus (SE) is defined as 5 minutes or more of (1) continuous clinical and/or electrographic seizure activity or (2) recurrent seizure activity without recovery (returning to baseline) between seizures.[1]

- May be convulsive (with motor features) or nonconvulsive (electrographic seizures only)
- SE progresses in phases
  - Early SE (5–30 minutes), established SE (>30 minutes), and refractory SE
  - Refractory status epilepticus
    - Clinical or electrographic seizures that persist after an adequate dose of an initial benzodiazepine and a second appropriate antiseizure medication
    - Associated with poor outcome, with mortality up to 30%, related to young age, etiology, and multifocal or generalized EEG abnormalities

BACKGROUND AND EPIDEMIOLOGY

- Epidemiology and morbidity of SE
  - Incidence of first-time SE is approximately 18 to 23 per 100,000 children per year[2]
  - Fifty percent of children with new-onset convulsive SE are neurologically healthy
  - One-year recurrence risk is 16% with 3% mortality, which is lower than adults
  - Risk for mortality and long-term morbidity related to primary cause of the seizure
- Factors associated with increased morbidity in SE
  - Time to the first dose of benzodiazepine in children with SE is often delayed or the drug not given until arrival at a hospital[3]
  - Delay in administration of the first anticonvulsant is associated with longer SE duration[4]

CAUSES OF SE

Prolonged febrile seizures and seizure due to remote neurologic injury account for 50% of SE cases in children.

- Other common causes in order of frequency include
  - Acute new neurologic injury
    - Central nervous system (CNS) infection; cardiac arrest, stroke; traumatic brain injury; drug or toxin
  - Acute exacerbation of underlying epilepsy
    - Missed anticonvulsant or subtherapeutic levels
    - Intercurrent illness
  - Progressive neurologic disorder

KEY PRINCIPLES OF SE MANAGEMENT

- After 5 to 10 minutes, most seizures will not stop unless treated with an anticonvulsant
- Early, sequential administration of adequate doses of anticonvulsants is essential[5]
- Treatment should be given in the field prior to arrival in the ICU
- Identify and treat precipitating cause

• Manage systemic complications
• All units should have a management pathway and agreed on time frame for treatment[6]

TREATMENT

Incipient SE 0 to 5 minutes of seizure onset

• Stabilize airway, breathing, and circulation
• Obtain fingerstick glucose in first-line labs
• Obtain IV access and administer IV benzodiazepine if seizure lasts 5 minutes
  ○ If IV access is not possible, administer benzodiazepine via intramuscular, intranasal, rectal, or buccal route (see Table 42-1)
  ○ Do not delay treatment in order to obtain IV access

Early (5–30 min) and established (>30 min) SE (Figure 42-1)
Refractory SE

• Continued seizures despite treatment with adequate doses of two to three anticonvulsants
• Load with midazolam 0.2 mg per kg
  ○ Continue with infusion at 0.05 to 0.2 mg per kg per hour *with EEG monitoring to suppress clinical or electrographic seizures*
  ○ No maximum rate established, but typical range is up to 1.0 to 1.5 mg per kg per hour
• If pharmacologic coma is required or insufficient response to midazolam, add pentobarbital 5 mg per kg bolus followed by infusion at 0.5 mg per kg per hour

TABLE 42-1	Anticonvulsant Medications	
Drug	**Route**	**Dose**
Midazolam	IV bolus	Loading dose: 0.15–0.2 mg/kg
	IV infusion	0.05–1.5 mg/kg/**hr**
	Intramuscular	0.2 mg/kg/dose, may repeat every 10–15 min; maximum dose 6 mg
	Buccal	0.2–0.5 mg/kg once; maximum dose 10 mg
	Intranasal	0.2 mg/kg once; maximum dose: 10 mg
Lorazepam	IV bolus	0.1 mg/kg maximum: 4 mg, slow IV over 2–5 minutes; may repeat in 5–15 min
Diazepam	IV bolus	0.1–0.3 mg/kg/dose given over 3–5 min, every 5–10 min; maximum dose 10 mg/dose
	Rectal	2–5 yr: 0.5 mg/kg
		6–11 yr: 0.3 mg/kg
		≥12 yr and adolescents: 0.2 mg/kg
Fosphenytoin	IV Bolus	15–20 mg PE/kg; maximum dose 1500 mg PE
Levetiracetam	IV Bolus	20–60 mg/kg; dose should not exceed adult initial range: 1000–3000 mg
Pentobarbital	IV bolus	Loading dose: 5 mg/kg
	IV infusion	Initial: 0.5–1 mg/kg/**hr**
Phenobarbital	IV bolus	15–20 mg/kg; maximum dose 1000 mg

- Optimal duration of treatment is not established, but guidelines suggest 24 to 48 hours of electrographic seizure control[1]
- For add-on drugs or other therapies, see Abend et al.[5]

Time 0 - 5 Minutes (Incipient Status Epilepticus)

1. Check ABCs
   Evaluate and maintain the airway - (reposition patient's head/suction)
   Provide 100% oxygen (non-rebreather). Place pulse oximeter. Maintain oxygen > 92%
   Assess and support ventilation
   Check and establish monitoring of vital signs (RR, BP, pulse, temperature, pulse oximetry)
2. Fingerstick Glucose (Glucose < 60 mg/dl, administer 2 ml/kg D25%W; children < 2 years: 4ml/kg D12.5W)
3. Attempt IV access. Obtain serum for Na, Mg, Ca levels
4. Order but do not administer:
   (i) **IV access present:**
       Lorazepam 0.1 mg per kg (maximum dose 4 mg) OR
       Diazepam 0.15 - 0.4 mg per kg (up to 10 mg)
   (ii) **No IV access;** Either
       (a) Intranasal Midazolam 0.2 mg per kg (maximum dose 10 mg; administer 1/2 dose in each nostril)
   Or (b) Rectal Diazepam (maximum dose 20 mg)
       Age 1month - 2 years: 0.2 mg per kg
       Age 2-5 years: 0.5 mg per kg
       Age 6-11 years: 0.3 mg per kg
       Age 12+:   0.2 mg per kg
   Or (c) Intramuscular Midazolam 5 mg (13-40 kg), 10 mg if > 40 kg
   Or (d) Buccal Midazolam 0.5 mg per kg
5. Determine if the patient has an individual specific status epilepticus plan (patients with known epilepsy)

Time 5 - 30 Minutes (Early Status Epilepticus)

1. **At 5 minutes** give the first dose of benzodiazepine.
2. If the seizure does not stop 5 minutes after the first dose, repeat x 1
3. Order, but do not administer one of;
       (a) Phenytoin or Fosphenytoin 20 mg per kg IV (maximum dose 1500 mg)
       (b) Levitiracetam 20-60 mg per kg IV   (maximum dose 1500 mg)
       (c) Phenobarbital 15-20 mg per kg IV
4. **If seizures continue after 2nd dose of benzodiazepine then at Time 15 minutes administer** one of either phenytoin, levitiracetam, or phenobarbital
5. Correct electrolyte abnormalities
6. Monitor for signs of respiratory depression or hypotension
7. See table for approach to diagnostic studies. Treat primary cause if known

---

Time > 30 Minutes (Established Status Epilepticus)

1. No proven definitive therapy
2. Consider continuous EEG monitoring and transfer to ICU. Confirm adequate IV access.
3. Repeat treatment with one of
       Fosphenytoin (max 30 mg per kg)
       Levitiracetam (max 60-80 mg per kg)
       Phenobarbital (max 60-80 mg per kg)
4. If seizures do not respond to one of these agents being Midazolam infusion with EEG monitoring
       Loading dose 0.1 - 0.2 mg per kg IV
       Initial Infusion rate 0.05 to 0.2 mg per kg per hour
       Increase rate by 0.05 mg per kg per hour every 15 minutes
       Titrate to cessation of clinical or electrographic seizures
       Maximum rate 1.0 - 1.5 mg per kg per hour
5. If no response at maximum rate, add pentobarbital
       Loading dose 6.0 - 8.0 mg per kg IV
       Maintenance rate 1.0 - 4.0 mg per kg per hour for 48 hours

---

FIGURE 42-1 **Summary of approach to management of pediatric status epilepticus and refractory status epilepticus.**

DIAGNOSTIC STUDIES

Zero to five minutes of seizure onset

- Goal is to identify rapidly reversible causes of SE within 5 minutes of seizure onset[1]
  - Fingerstick glucose
  - Electrolytes including magnesium and calcium
  - Anticonvulsant drug levels
  - Blood gas
  - Complete blood count

  Five to sixty minutes and beyond (Table 42-2)

TABLE 42-2	Approach to Diagnostic Testing in the Child with Status Epilepticus		
Fever or Suspected Inflammatory Disorder	**Normal MRI**	**Abnormal MRI**	**Developmental Regression or Abnormal Development**
Cerebrospinal fluid for:	New-onset epilepsy	Acute injury evaluation	Genetic testing
Infections	Toxin ingestion	Autoimmune epilepsy (may also be normal)	POLG1
			SCN1A
HSV, HHV6, HHV7	Toxicology screen		
Influenza A	Drug levels	Metabolic disorders	Cerebrospinal fluid
Adenovirus		Mitochondrial disorders (MELAS, POLG1, depletion syndromes)	Amino acids
			Lactate and pyruvate
			Neurotransmitters
West Nile	Metabolic disorders		
Epstein-Barr	Ammonia	Neuronal migration disorders	Neurodegenerative and storage disorder evaluation
RSV	Organic and amino acids		For example: Wilson's, Menkes', neuronal ceroid lipofuscinosis, Huntington's, sialidosis
Gram stain	Lactate and pyruvate		
Bacterial cultures			
	Autoimmune epilepsy		
Autoimmune epilepsy	Antibody studies		
Anti-NMDA receptor antibody	Screening for SLE		
Other antibodies	ACE (neurosarcoid)		
GAD, VGKC	Antithyroid antibodies		
Oligoclonal bands			

HSV: herpes simplex virus, HHV6: human herpesvirus 6, HHV7: human herpesvirus 7, RSV: respiratory syncytial virus, NMDA: N-methyl-D-aspartate, VGKC: voltage-gated potassium channel complex, SLE: systemic lupus erythematosus, ACE: angiotensin-converting enzyme, MELAS: mitochondrial encephalomyopathy, lactic acidosis, and stroke-like episodes.

• Diagnostic tests guided by history and risk factors for each patient

Neuroimaging

• No consensus on timing of imaging. The American Academy of Neurology Practice Parameter recommends imaging after SE is controlled and the child is stable[7]
• Where the cause of SE is clear, CNS imaging may be obtained at the physician's discretion[8]

INDICATIONS FOR EEG MONITORING

Nonconvulsive seizures occur in up to 30% of critically ill children, require continuous (c) EEG monitoring for detection, and are associated with worse outcomes.[9]

• Among children who present with convulsive SE, one-third have only electrographic seizures[10]
  ○ Consensus criteria for the use of cEEG in children have been established and include[1,11]:
    ▪ Persistent altered mental status following resolution of convulsive SE
    ▪ Acute brain injury including moderate-severe traumatic brain injury, stroke, CNS infection, brain tumors, cardiorespiratory arrest, intracerebral hemorrhage
    ▪ Sepsis with altered mental status
    ▪ During extracorporeal membrane oxygenation[12]
    ▪ Induction of pharmacologic coma for seizure management
• cEEG should be continued for 24 to 48 hours[1,11]

REFERENCES

1. Brophy G, Bell R, Claassen J, et al. Guidelines for the evaluation and management of status epilepticus. *Neurocrit Care*. 2012;17:3-23.
2. Chin R, Neville B, Peckham C, et al. Incidence, cause, and short-term outcome of convulsive status epilepticus in childhood: Prospective population-based study. *Lancet*. 2006;368:222-229.
3. Sanchez Fernandez I, Abend NS, Agadi S, et al. Time from convulsive status epilepticus onset to anticonvulsant administration in children. *Neurology*. 2015;84(23):2304-2311.
4. Chin RF, Neville BG, Peckham C, et al. Treatment of community-onset, childhood convulsive status epilepticus: A prospective, population-based study. *Lancet Neurol*. 2008;7(8):696-703.
5. Abend NS, Bearden D, Helbig I, et al. Status epilepticus and refractory status epilepticus management. *Semin Pediatr Neurol*. 2014;21(4):263-274.
6. Shorvon S, Baulac M, Cross H, et al. The drug treatment of status epilepticus in Europe: Consensus document from a workshop at the first London. *Epilepsia*. 2008;7:1277-1285.
7. Riviello J, Ashwal S, Hirtz D, et al. Practice parameter: Diagnostic assessment of the child with status epilepticus (an evidence-based review). *Neurology*. 2006;67:1542-1550.
8. Smith DM, McGinnis EL, Walleigh DJ, et al. Management of status epilepticus in children. *J Clin Med*. 2016;5(47).
9. Payne E, Zhao X, Frndova H, et al. Seizure burden is independently associated with short term outcome in critically ill children. *Brain*. 2014;137:1429-1438.
10. Sanchez Fernandez I, Abend NS, Arndt DH, et al. Electrographic seizures after convulsive status epilepticus in children and young adults: A retrospective multicenter study. *J Pediatr*. 2014;164(2):339-346.
11. Herman ST, Abend NS, Bleck TP, et al. Consensus statement on continuous EEG in critically ill adults and children, part I: Indications. *J Clin Neurophysiol*. 2015;32(2):87-95.
12. Piantino J, Wainwright M, Grimason M, et al. Nonconvulsive seizures are common in children treated with extracorporeal cardiac life support. *Pediatr Crit Care Med*. 2013;14:601-609.

BACKGROUND AND EPIDEMIOLOGY

DIFFERENCES FROM STROKE IN ADULTS

- Immature neuraxis
  - Causes subtle exam findings, leading to delay in diagnosis
    - Stroke must be considered in any patient with acute neurologic deficit
- Risk factors for stroke are different compared to adults
  - Atherosclerosis is not common cause of stroke in children
  - There are no randomized, controlled therapeutic trials in children
- Type of stroke: Arterial ischemic stroke (AIS), hemorrhagic stroke (HS), cerebral venous sinus thrombosis (CVST)
- Prompt recognition: Allows for optimization of cerebral perfusion and can minimize secondary injury

EPIDEMIOLOGY

- Pediatric stroke (age 30 days–18 years): annual average incidence of 1.6 to 13/100,000[1,2]
- Arterial ischemic stroke (including CVST):
  - 50% to 70% of pediatric strokes
  - Comprises 15% of all ischemic strokes that occur in young adults and adolescents
  - Mortality after AIS ranges from 10% to 15% with 50% of survivors left with a neurologic deficit
  - Risk for recurrence ranges from 1% to 20%[3]
- Hemorrhagic stroke:
  - 41% to 49% of pediatric strokes
  - Two to three times the incidence of adults
  - Median age is 5 to 10 years
  - Males are at slightly higher risk (55% to 60%)
  - Mortality is lower in children than adults. While survival is greater, morbidity among survivors is high

RISK FACTORS (TABLE 43-1)

CONSIDERATIONS

- Many patients have multiple risk factors, whereas 10% to 38% have *no* risk factor identified[2,4]
- Recurrent stroke increased if multiple risk factors identified[5]
- Chromosomal mutations (trisomy 21), genetic syndromes (Sturge Weber), and single-gene disorders (sickle cell) may predispose to stroke

AIS

- Arteriopathies: Identified in 31% to 60% of patients[6]
  - Nontraumatic dissections, vasculitis, moyamoya, postvaricella arteriopathy, primary vascular disorder, sickle cell disease, transient arteriopathies (recent viral infections)
  - *Vasculopathy:* Increases risk of stroke recurrence, especially in the first 6 months after stroke presentation[7]

TABLE 43-1	Risk Factors Identified in Pediatric Stroke
Risk Factor	**% Patients Affected**
Acute Ischemic Stroke	
All arteriopathies	31–60
Moyamoya arteriopathy	4.6–22
Postvaricella arteriopathy	1.5–7
Nontraumatic dissection	1–20
SCD arteriopathy	8–17
CNS lupus arteriopathy	3.1
Nonspecific vasculitides	12
Cardiac etiology	2–27
Infection	2.9–40
Hypercoagulable condition	11.4–25.6
Prothrombotic state	Undefined
Trauma	7.7–12
Malignancy	1–2.3
Mitochondrial	2.9–6.4
No identified risk factor	10–38
Cerebral Venous Sinus Thrombosis	
Nonspecific infection	40
Chronic otitis media and orbital cellulitis	28
Prothrombotic state	14
Hematologic or metabolic disorder not otherwise specified	60
No factor identified	0–57
Hemorrhagic Stroke	
Vascular abnormalities	48–67
Hematologic disorder	10
Bleeding into intracranial tumor	10
Cavernous venous malformation	6.4
Vertebral artery dissection	6.4
No risk factor identified	14–40

Data summarized from references.[2,6,8] SCD: Sickle cell disease, CNS: central nervous system.

- Congenital heart disease[8]
  - ○ Highest stroke risk after cardiac catheterization or surgery
  - ○ Most likely cardioembolic rather than vascular
- Hypercoagulable states
  - ○ Methylene tetrahydrofolate reductase (MTHFR), factor V Leiden, protein C/S deficiency, homocystinuria, malignancy, iron-deficiency anemia, oral contraceptive use, autoimmune disease

- Trauma
  - Arterial dissection: Most commonly involving the internal carotid artery (usually intracranial) or vertebral artery (usually extracranial)[9]
  - Mechanism may seem minor (i.e., wrestling with friends or jumping off a bed)

HS

- Intracranial vascular abnormalities (aneurysms, arterial venous malformations, cavernous malformations), brain tumors, hematologic disorder

CVST

- Systemic or central nervous system (CNS) infection, chronic otitis media and orbital cellulitis, prothrombotic state, hematologic or metabolic disorder
- Dehydration and anemia

PRESENTATION

PHYSICAL EXAM

- AIS: Focal neurologic deficits 60% to 80%[2,4,5]
  - Acute hemiplegia 50% to 70%; cranial nerve palsies, visual and speech impairments in 29% to 47%; seizures in 25% to 33%; altered consciousness in 32% to 52%; headache with posterior circulation strokes or larger lesions
  - Acute systemic conditions associated with more diffuse symptoms, whereas arteriopathies have more focal findings[8]
- HS: Similar presentation to AIS
  - Headache, vomiting, alteration in mentation, and vertigo more common in HS than AIS[5]
  - Focal weakness only in 35% to 38%, compared to 50% to 70% in AIS[5]
- CVST: Stiff neck and loss of consciousness or ataxia most common presenting signs

DELAY IN DIAGNOSIS

- Remains a significant challenge in pediatric stroke[4,5]
- Immature neuraxis: Limited expression of focal neurologic deficits clinically coupled with inability for many patients to report symptoms
- Challenging to examine an uncooperative child
- Stroke mimics: 11% to 21% of suspected strokes are due to other causes[10] (Table 43-2)

TABLE 43-2 Common Stroke Mimics	
Medical Emergencies	**Benign Disorders**
Postictal (Todd's) paralysis	Migraine
Demyelinating disorder (ADEM, MS)	Conversion disorder
PRES	Musculoskeletal disorder
Tumor	
CNS infection	
Drug toxicity	
Metabolic stroke	

PRES: Posterior reversible leukoencephalopathy syndrome; ADEM: acute demyelinating encephalomyelitis: MS, multiple sclerosis.

- ○ Cannot reliably differentiate mimics from stroke on basis of neurologic examination alone
- ○ Focal symptoms: Focal weakness with episode of demyelination, transient paresis following seizure, hemiplegic migraine
- Hospital delay[4]:
  - ○ Median time from presentation to diagnosis is almost 24 hours, with in-hospital delays accounting for largest proportion of time
  - ○ Failure of clinicians to recognize subtle neurologic deficits in children or to consider stroke in the differential diagnosis
  - ○ Nonspecific symptoms like seizures, headache, ataxia
- Education of the general public: Remind that children have strokes too, incorporating into current campaigns ("FASTR – Face drooping-Arm weakness-Speech difficulty-Time to call 911-and 'Remember children have stroke too'")[11]

USE OF NEUROIMAGING

- Imaging required due to frequency of stroke mimics in children
- Study of choice: Magnetic resonance imaging (MRI)
  - ○ Noncontrast computerized tomography (CT) if MRI not immediately available
    - May miss early ischemia or posterior circulation involvement
  - ○ *"Fast"* MRI: Diffusion-weighted imaging (DWI), axial T2 fluid-attenuated inversion recovery (FLAIR), susceptibility-weighted imaging (SWI) or gradient echo (GRE) with time-of-flight (TOF) magnetic resonance angiogram (MRA) of head and neck[11]
    - 20 to 25 minutes to complete in most centers
  - ○ MRA (magnetic resonance angiography): Perform concurrently with MRI, given the increased incidence of underlying arteriopathies
    - Good screening tool, but less sensitive than CT angiography in diagnosis of vertebral or internal carotid artery dissection[12]
    - Conventional cerebral angiography; gold standard for suspected arteriopathies

TREATMENT (FIGURE 43-1)

ACUTE TREATMENT AND SUPPORTIVE CARE

- Goal is to minimize injury and prevent early complications such as extension of penumbra and recurrent stroke
- Neuroprotection: Head flat to optimize cerebral perfusion (unless HS or CVST is of concern); maintain adequate oxygenation, isotonic fluids with dextrose, blood pressure 50% to 95% for height and age with permissive hypertension up to 20% above 95%, nothing by mouth for possible sedation and to avoid choking, avoid electrolyte abnormalities/hypoxemia/hyperthermia/hypo- or hyperglycemia (goal 80–180 mg/dL), as all are deleterious to preischemic brain tissue[7]
- Other considerations: Airway monitoring, as alteration in mentation may require intubation; exchange transfusions for sickle cell patients; anticonvulsant medication for any patients with seizures, as further seizures may compromise the vulnerable ischemic penumbra
- Aspirin: 3 to 5 mg/kg once hemorrhage is ruled out by imaging or history[1]
- Laboratory evaluation (see Table 43-3)
- Neurology consult
- Consider electroencephalogram (EEG) monitoring: Clinical and subclinical seizures common in children with acute neurologic injuries

CONFIRMED STROKE

- Treatment with aspirin (ASA) or anticoagulation (low-molecular-weight heparin or unfractionated heparin) for up to 1 week after ischemic stroke[1]; newer anticoagulants (dabigatran, rivaroxaban, apixaban) not yet studied in pediatric stroke
  - *Cardioembolic source or acute extracranial dissection*: Anticoagulation rather than antiplatelet therapy[1,9]

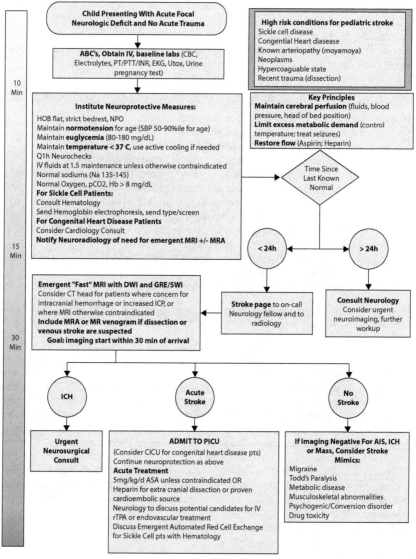

FIGURE 43-1 Recommended diagnostic studies and approach to acute stabilization in a child with suspected stroke. AIS, arterial ischemic stroke; ICH, intracerebral hemorrhage; DWI, diffusion-weighted imaging; GRE, gradient echo; HOB, head of bed.

TABLE 43-3 Laboratory Evaluation in Acute Stroke

Common Tests

Head CT, brain MRI

CTA, MRA, conventional angiogram

Complete blood count with differential

Serum electrolytes, liver and renal function tests

Blood glucose

Erythrocyte sedimentation rate, C-reactive protein

Coagulation profile (PT, APTT, D-dimer, fibrinogen)

Lipid panel, lipoprotein (a) level

Urinalysis

Urine or serum pregnancy test in women of childbearing age

Selected tests

Transthoracic and/or transesophageal echocardiography, ECG – history of congenital heart disease, clinical signs of heart disease

Serum and urine toxicology screen – amphetamine, cocaine, marijuana, opiate abuse

CSF studies: viral including varicella zoster virus testing, fungal, bacterial, parasitic – recent fever, headache, meningeal signs

Rheumatologic tests: antinuclear antibody, antibody to double-stranded DNA, rheumatoid factor, anticardiolipin antibodies, complement levels, neutrophil cytoplasm antibody (cANCA, pANCA), anti-Ro (SSA) and anti-La (SSB) cytoplasmic antibodies, serum angiotensin-converting enzyme – central nervous system vasculitis

Infectious disease tests: varicella-zoster virus, herpes simplex virus, Epstein-Barr virus, HIV, hepatitis B and C viruses, tuberculosis, syphilis, Lyme

Hypercoagulable tests: protein C, protein S, prothrombin gene mutation, 5, 10 Methylene tetra-hydrofolate reductase (MTHFR) mutation, homocysteine, antithrombin III activity, Factor V Leiden mutation

Antiphospholipid antibodies: anticardiolipin antibody IgM, IgG, and IgA; anti-beta-2 glycoprotein-1 IgM, IgG, IgA; lupus anticoagulant – antiphospholipid antibody syndrome

CTA=Computed tomography angiogram, MRA=magnetic resonance angiogram, PT=prothrombin time, APTT=activated Partial thromboplastin time, ECG=echocardiogram,

- ○ *Large territory MCA strokes* (>30%–50% of MCA territory): Anticoagulation contraindicated due to risk for hemorrhagic conversion
  - ▪ Consider ASA for 2 to 3 days followed by anticoagulation if exam not improving
- Aspirin 3 to 5 mg/kg/day: Start if antithrombotic or thrombolytic medication not used and there is no contraindication such as intracranial hemorrhage[1]
  - ○ Decrease dose to 1 to 3 mg/kg/day if excessive bleeding or bruising
  - ○ Treatment duration of 3 to 5 years, may extend indefinitely in high-risk patients
  - ○ For extracranial dissection, mean treatment duration of 12 months
- Intravenous tissue plasminogen (IV tPA)[11]
  - ○ *Mechanism of action*: Facilitates degradation of fibrin in thrombus and can lead to early recanalization of an artery occluded by a thrombus
  - ○ Currently no standards in pediatric stroke
  - ○ May be considered in consulation with a stroke neurologist within 4.5 hours of symptom onset
- Intra-arterial thrombolysis[7]: Case reports in children with middle cerebral artery and basilar artery occlusion, but several potential complications (iatrogenic arterial dissection, intracranial hemorrhage, recurrent stroke distal to site of thrombosis)

- Decompressive hemicraniectomy: May be considered for large MCA territory stroke with declining mental status and cerebral edema
- Neurosurgery consult: If confirmation of hemorrhagic stroke
- Transthoracic echocardiogram (TTE): Indicated in all children with stroke due to congenital and acquired heart disease as a common cause of pediatric stroke

KEY PRINCIPLES FOR MANAGEMENT OF ACUTE STROKE

- High index of suspicion for stroke as etiology of neurologic deficit
- Needs immediate access to MRI for confirmation of ischemia
- Multidisciplinary management between Critical Care, Neurology, and Neurosurgery
- Optimize flow
  - Head of bed (HOB) flat and give fluids (AIS)
  - Reduce intracranial pressure (ICP) (HS)
  - Decompressive hemicraniectomy
- Limit excess metabolic demand (fever, seizures)
- Limit clot formation or restore patency of occluded vessel in AIS
  - Anticoagulation or antiplatelet therapy
  - Use of thrombolysis or thrombectomy on case-by-case basis

REFERENCES

1. Roach ES, Golomb MR, Adams R, et al. Management of stroke in infants and children: A scientific statement from a Special Writing Group of the American Heart Association Stroke Council and the Council on Cardiovascular Disease in the Young. *Stroke*. 2008;39(9):2644-2691.
2. Mallick AA, Ganesan V, Kirkham FJ, et al. Childhood arterial ischaemic stroke incidence, presenting features, and risk factors: A prospective population-based study. *Lancet Neurol*. 2014;13(1):35-43.
3. Mallick AA, Ganesan V, Kirkham FJ, et al. Outcome and recurrence one year after paediatric arterial ischaemic stroke in a population-based cohort. *Ann Neurol*. 2016;79(5):784-793. doi:10.1002/ana.24626.
4. Rafay MF, Pontigon AM, Chiang J, et al. Delay to diagnosis in acute pediatric arterial ischemic stroke. *Stroke*. 2009;40(1):58-64.
5. Yock-Corrales A, Mackay MT, Mosley I, et al. Acute childhood arterial ischemic and hemorrhagic stroke in the emergency department. *Ann Emerg Med*. 2011;58(2):156-163.
6. Elbers J, deVeber G, Pontigon AM, et al. Long-term outcomes of pediatric ischemic stroke in adulthood. *J Child Neurol*. 2013;29(6):782-788.
7. Elbers J, Wainwright MS, Amlie-Lefond C. The pediatric stroke code: Early management of the child with stroke. *J Pediatr*. 2015;167(1):19-24.
8. Mackay MT, Wiznitzer M, Benedict SL, et al. Arterial ischemic stroke risk factors: The International Pediatric Stroke Study. *Ann Neurol*. 2011;69(1):130-140.
9. Stence NV, Fenton LZ, Goldenberg NA, et al. Craniocervical arterial dissection in children: Diagnosis and treatment. *Curr Treatment Options Neurol*. 2011;13(6):636-648.
10. Shellhaas RA, Smith SE, O'Tool E, et al. Mimics of childhood stroke: Characteristics of a prospective cohort. *Pediatrics*. 2006;118(2):704-709.
11. Rivkin MJ, Bernard TJ, Dowling MM, et al. Guidelines for urgent management of stroke in children. *Pediatr Neurol*. 2016;56:8-17.
12. Lall NU, Stence NV, Mirsky DM. Magnetic resonance imaging of pediatric neurologic emergencies. *Topics Mag Res Imaging*. 2015;24(6):291-307.

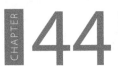

44 Meningitis/Encephalitis

DEFINITIONS

Meningitis: Inflammation of the meninges, the membranes covering the brain and spinal cord

Encephalitis: Inflammation of the brain parenchyma

ETIOLOGY

NEONATES <2 MONTHS

- Bacteria:
  - Group B *Streptococcus* (52%)
  - *Escherichia coli* and other gram-negative bacilli (rods) (27%)
  - *Listeria monocytogenes* (6%)
  - Anaerobes (3%)
  - Other gram-positive organisms (7%): enterococci, *Streptococcus pneumoniae*, staphylococci
  - Other gram-negative organisms (5%): *Haemophilus influenzae, Neisseria meningitides, Pseudomonas*
- Viruses: Herpes simplex virus (HSV), human herpesvirus 6 (HHV-6), enteroviruses, arboviruses, human immunodeficiency virus (HIV), adenovirus, varicella zoster virus (VZV), Epstein-Barr virus (EBV), cytomegalovirus (CMV), measles, mumps, rubella, influenza, parainfluenza, parvovirus B19, rotavirus, others

INFANTS >2 MONTHS AND CHILDREN

- Bacteria:
  - *S. pneumoniae* and *N. meningitidis* (90%–95%)
  - Other organisms: *H. influenzae, Salmonella species, group B Streptococcus, L. monocytogenes,* anaerobes
- Viruses: Enteroviruses, arboviruses, HSV, HHV-6, HIV, adenovirus, VZV, EBV, CMV, measles, mumps, rubella, influenza, parainfluenza, parvovirus B19, rotavirus, zoonotic diseases, arthropod-borne diseases, others

SPECIAL POPULATIONS

- *Mycoplasma tuberculosis*: Consider based on history of exposure
- Fungi: Immunocompromised patients
- Parasites and protozoa: Consider based on history of exposure
- Rabies: Consider based on history of exposure

Enteroviruses account for 85% to 95% of viral meningoencephalitis in which an etiologic agent is identified.

CLINICAL MANIFESTATIONS

NEONATES/INFANTS

- Fever of unknown origin
- Vomiting, poor feeding, failure to thrive (FTT)

- Apnea or respiratory distress
- Altered mental status: irritability or lethargy
- Signs of increased intracranial pressure (ICP): bulging fontanelle
- Focal neurologic deficits
- Seizures
- Petechiae/purpura or rash
- Shock

OLDER CHILDREN

- Fever: almost always present
- Nausea/vomiting
- Headache, photophobia
- Back pain
- Altered mental status
- Focal neurologic deficits
- Seizures
- Signs of increased ICP: papilledema (if present, look for brain abscess, venous sinus thrombosis, and subdural fluid collection/empyema)
- Signs of meningeal irritation: positive Kernig's and Brudinski's signs
- Petechiae/purpura or rash
- Shock

DIAGNOSIS

LABORATORY EVALUATION

- Serum tests: abnormal white blood cell (WBC) count (leukocytosis or leukopenia), prominence of atypical lymphocytes (EBV), viral studies
- Cerebrospinal fluid (CSF) studies: cell count, WBC differential, glucose, protein, Gram stain, culture, viral studies (enterovirus polymerase chain reaction [PCR], HSV PCR, etc.), acid-fast bacillus AFB stain, tuberculosis culture – See Table 44-1

TABLE 44-1	Cerebrospinal Fluid Analysis		
TEST	**BACTERIAL**	**VIRAL**	**FUNGAL/TB**
Opening pressure	Elevated	Usually normal	Normal or elevated
Appearance	Turbid/purulent or bloody	Clear/cloudy	Clear, turbid, or with fibrin cobweb formation
White blood cell count	≥ 1000 per mm^3	<100 per mm^3	Variable
Cell differential	Neutrophils predominate (lymphocytosis present 10% of the time)	Lymphocytes predominate (neutrophils may predominate early in the course)	Lymphocytes predominate
Protein	Markedly elevated	Normal	Elevated
CSF-to-serum glucose ratio	Decreased	Usually normal	Normal to decreased

- Blood culture: positive in 80% to 90% of patients with suspected bacterial meningitis who were not pretreated with antibiotics
- Nasopharyngeal swab: For viral studies

IMAGING

- Head computerized tomography (CT) or magnetic resonance imaging (MRI): may be useful in identifying complications (hemorrhage, mass, cerebral edema, hydrocephalus, abscess, subdural fluid collection/empyema, etc.)
- MR venogram: cerebral sinus venous thrombosis
- HSV: temporal involvement

EEG

- HSV: PLED (periodic lateralized epileptiform discharges) over the temporal region
- Rule out subclinical seizures

TREATMENT

See *Surviving Sepsis Guidelines* to reverse shock.

Additional medical management

- Frequent neurologic checks
- Monitor head circumference daily in neonates/infants
- Aggressively treat seizures and increased ICP
- Avoid overhydration because it may worsen cerebral edema
- Monitor and treat sodium dysregulation and disseminated intravascular coagulopathy (DIC)

ANTIMICROBIAL THERAPY

- Empiric IV antimicrobials:
  - Neonates <1 month: ampicillin + cefotaxime or ampicillin + gentamicin
  - Neonates 1 to 3 months: vancomycin + cefotaxime or ceftriaxone; consider ampicillin for *Listeria* coverage
  - Infants >3 months and children: third-generation cephalosporin + vancomycin
  - Consider acyclovir for anyone in which HSV is suspected
  - Special populations: additional antimicrobial coverage based on etiologic suspicion
- Switch to enteral antimicrobial: afebrile and able to tolerate enteral medications
- Narrow antimicrobial therapy: based on culture results
  - For meningococcus: use penicillin, cefotaxime, or ceftriaxone for a minimum of 7 days
- Pediatric ID consultation is recommended
- Duration: minimum of 10 to 14 days, sometimes up to 21 days
- May need to repeat lumbar puncture to see if CSF is being adequately treated

ANTI-INFLAMMATORY THERAPY

- Dexamethasone: give shortly before or at the time of first IV antibiotic administration
  - Reduces the frequency of hearing loss and neurologic sequelae in patients with *H. influenzae* type B meningitis
  - Reduces overall unfavorable outcomes and mortality in adults with pneumococcal meningitis
  - Benefits not conclusive in pneumococcal or meningococcal meningitis in children
  - No data for use in children <6 weeks old

SURGICAL INTERVENTION

• Drainage of abscess or subdural fluid collection/empyema
• Insertion of external ventricular drain (EVD) for hydrocephalus

OTHER

• Chemoprophylaxis for household and other close contacts of meningococcal disease

COMPLICATIONS

ACUTE

• Brain abscess
• Cerebral sinus venous thrombosis resulting in stroke or ischemia
• Hydrocephalus +/− increased ICP
• Subdural fluid collection/empyema
• Sodium dysregulation (syndrome of inappropriate antidiuretic hormone [SIADH] most common)

LONG-TERM NEUROLOGIC SEQUELAE (UP TO 50% OF PATIENTS)

• Hearing loss
• Seizures
• Motor abnormalities, including paralysis
• Language disorders or delay
• Cognitive impairment
• Cerebral palsy
• <1% relapse rate of infection after antibiotic therapy

OUTCOMES

• Mortality rates for bacterial meningitis is 1% to 5% in all pediatric patients, but is 15% to 20% for neonates.

SUGGESTED READINGS

Fishman RA. *Cerebrospinal Fluid in Diseases of the Nervous System.* 2nd ed. Philadelphia, PA: Saunders; 1992.
Wubbel L, McCracken GH Jr. Management of bacterial meningitis: 1998. *Pediatr Rev.* 1998;19:78-84.
Zunt JR, Marra CM. Cerebrospinal fluid testing for the diagnosis of central nervous system infection. *Neurol Clin.* 1999;17:675-689.

45   Weakness in the ICU

INTRODUCTION

Weakness presenting to the ICU is either due to an acute/acquired cause or is a complication of chronic weakness, such as acute on chronic respiratory failure. This chapter will focus on the physical exam of a patient with new-onset weakness and summarize chronic neuromuscular diseases that could lead to ICU presentation.

LOCALIZATION OF WEAKNESS

Weakness can arise from pathology at any point along the neuroaxis from brain to muscle. It can be a single discrete lesion causing a focal deficit or a generalized process causing more disseminated signs. Physical exam is one of the key tools for localizing the lesion and narrowing the differential diagnosis. Table 45-1 describes the typical exam findings based on a lesion at each level of the neuroaxis and examples of associated disease states. Table 45-2 lists neurologic signs that are characteristic of specific lesions or disease processes.

TABLE 45-1	Physical Exam Findings and Disease Processes Based on Site of Lesion	
	Typical Physical Exam Findings	**Prototypical Diseases**
Spinal cord	Acute: flaccid, hyporeflexic	Transverse myelitis
	Subacute/chronic: spastic, hyperreflexic	Acute flaccid myelitis (AFM)
	Mixed sensory and motor deficits	Infectious myelitis
	Acute neurologic change at discrete spinal level	Cord ischemia
	Bowel and bladder dysfunction	Spinal cord tumor
Anterior horn cell	Flaccid tone	Spinal muscular atrophy (SMA)
	Reflexes decreased or absent	Poliomyelitis
	Sensation intact	
Peripheral nerve	Distal > proximal weakness	Guillain-Barre syndrome (GBS)
	Flaccid tone	
	Reflexes decreased or absent	
	Sensory and motor deficits	
	Fasciculations	
Neuromuscular junction (NMJ)	Cranial nerve dysfunction	Botulism
	Flaccid tone	Myasthenia gravis (MG)
	Reflexes decreased or absent	Organophosphate Intoxication
	Sensation intact	
Muscle	Proximal > distal weakness	Rhabdomyolysis/myositis
	Reflexes normal or decreased	Muscular dystrophy
	Muscle atrophy or tenderness	Congenital myopathy
	Sensation intact	

TABLE 45-2	Physical Exam Findings with the Associated Pathologic Process
Physical Exam Finding	**Lesion/Disease**
Flaccid tone, areflexia	Lower motor neuron lesion
Spastic/increased tone, hyperreflexia	Upper motor neuron lesion
Proximal weakness	Myopathy, neuromuscular junction
Distal weakness	Neuropathy
Cranial neuropathies	MG, GBS (Miller Fisher variant), botulism, tick paralysis
Ascending paralysis, symmetric	GBS, tick paralysis
Descending paralysis, symmetric	Botulism
Asymmetric paralysis	Spinal cord tumor, transverse myelitis, polio-like viruses
Respiratory muscle weakness	Cervical spinal cord injury from any cause, GBS, MG, botulism, polio-like illness, organophosphates, ticks
Fasciculations	Anterior horn cell – SMA
	NMJ stimulation – organophosphate intoxication
Sensation intact	Anterior horn cell, myopathy
Autonomic dysfunction	GBS, botulism, organophosphate intoxication, transverse myelitis

ACUTE WEAKNESS

Acute weakness can be caused by ischemia/hypoperfusion, inflammation, toxin, or metabolic derangements affecting the neuroaxis. The following are summaries of pathologic conditions, starting at the spinal cord and moving distally, that could lead to ICU presentations of acute weakness. Other chapters in this handbook address brain pathology, including stroke.

SPINAL CORD

- Transverse myelitis (TM)[1,2]: TM is classically thought to be an immune-mediated demyelinating disorder of the spinal cord. It can be idiopathic or the initial presentation of an underlying demyelinating disorder such as multiple sclerosis, neuromyelitis optica, or a manifestation of another systemic disease such as systemic lupus erythematosus (SLE).
  - *Clinical features:* TM affects children less frequently than adults in a bimodal distribution (<5 yr and >10 yr). Two-thirds have a history of infection in the previous month. It can present initially with back pain, followed by symmetric or patchy sensory changes such as paresthesias or numbness, flaccid motor deficits, and bowel/bladder dysfunction such as urinary retention requiring catheterization.
  - *Diagnosis: Refer to Table 45-3*
  - *Evaluation:* Magnetic resonance imaging (MRI) with and without contrast of entire spine and brain. Obtain cerebrospinal fluid (CSF) for cell count, protein, glucose, IgG index, oligoclonal bands, bacterial/viral culture, and polymerase chain reaction (PCR).
  - *Treatment:* Corticosteroids 30 mg/kg/day for 3 to 5 days (max 1000 mg/day). Consider plasma exchange for five to seven sessions. Consider IVIg 2 gm/kg divided over 2 to 5 days.
  - *Prognosis:* 50% have full recovery by 2 years, 25% are nonambulatory or require walking aids, 10% to 20% never regain mobility or normal bladder function. High cervical cord lesions and respiratory failure are associated with increased risk for mortality.

TABLE 45-3	Diagnostic Criteria Proposed by the Transverse Myelitis Consortium Working Group[2]
Inclusion Criteria	**Exclusion Criteria**
1. Sensory, motor, and/or autonomic dysfunction attributable to the cord	1. Previous radiation to the spine within the last 10 yr
2. Bilateral signs/symptoms ± symmetric	2. Clear arterial distribution of clinical deficit consistent with anterior spinal artery thrombosis
3. Clearly defined sensory level	
4. Exclusion of extra-axial compressive etiology by MRI or myelography	3. Abnormal flow voids on the surface of the spinal cord consistent with AVM
5. Inflammation within the spinal cord by CSF pleocytosis or elevated IgG index or gadolinium enhancement (if negative, repeat in 2–7 days)	4. Serologic or clinical evidence of connective tissue disease
	5. CNS manifestations of syphilis, Lyme disease, HIV, HTLV-1, *Mycoplasma*, other viral infection (e.g., HSV, VZV, EBV, CMV, HHV-6, enteroviruses)
6. Progression to nadir between 4 hr and 21 days from symptom onset	6. Brain MRI abnormalities suggestive of MS
	7. History of clinically apparent optic neuritis

- Anterior spinal artery infarction[3,4]: The anterior spinal artery supplies the anterior two-thirds of the spinal cord, which contains the corticospinal (motor) and spinothalamic (pain and temperature sense) tracts. The dorsal columns (proprioception and vibration) are supplied by the posterior spinal arteries. Anterior spinal artery infarction is a rare neurologic emergency in children and can be difficult to differentiate from transverse myelitis. Risk factors/causes include aortic surgery, trauma, umbilical artery catheter, thrombophilia, fibrocartilaginous embolism, cerebellar herniation, CNS vasculitis secondary to infection, lupus, arteriovenous malformation (AVM), and hypotension/cardiac arrest.
  - *Clinical Features:* Patients may have preceding back pain at the site of infarction followed by an abrupt onset of bilateral weakness. Classically there is also a loss of pain and temperature sensation while maintaining vibratory and proprioception sensation; however, case series have shown varying degrees of sensory dysfunction, including complete sensory loss. Bowel and bladder function is often affected. Cord infarction due to fibrocartilaginous embolism may differ in time course, causing a more slowly progressive neurologic deterioration over hours to 1 to 2 days.
  - *Diagnosis:* MRI of the spinal cord with diffusion-weighted and T2-weighted imaging in axial and sagittal planes.
  - *Treatment:* Treat the underlying mechanism for injury. Optimize oxygen and blood supply to the cord with supportive care. Consider anticoagulation and/or aspirin.
  - *Prognosis:* The majority of patients will have some degree of motor and bowel/bladder recovery, including a minority with complete recovery.

ANTERIOR HORN CELL

- Acute flaccid paralysis[5-7]: Enteroviruses, of which poliomyelitis is the most notorious, can infect the anterior horn motor neurons leading to cell death and subsequent weakness. In some patients, infection is not restricted to the anterior horn and can involve the brainstem causing cranial neuropathies and bulbar weakness. Nonpolio enteroviruses generally have a milder clinical course; however, an entity called acute flaccid myelitis (AFM), first described in 2012-2014, is a syndrome of acute flaccid paralysis with anterior myelitis, which can cause a prolonged polio-like weakness, and was associated with an outbreak of enterovirus D68 infections, although the etiology is still unclear. Arboviruses such as West Nile virus can also cause an asymmetric flaccid paralysis.

- ○ *Clinical Features*: Patients may have a few days of prodromal symptoms such as fever, sore throat, headache, nausea, constipation, and malaise. After resolution of these symptoms, patients can develop a rapidly progressive, flaccid, asymmetric weakness involving the limbs. It is classically proximal, with the legs usually involved in polio and arms with AFM. Cranial nerves and muscles of respiration can also be involved, leading to respiratory failure. Sensation is usually preserved, and patients may experience myalgias and/or arthralgias. Autonomic dysfunction, especially bowel and bladder dysfunction, may be present.
- ○ *Diagnosis:* CSF may show pleocytosis with lymphocytic predominance (PMNs may predominate early on), normal to slightly elevated protein, and normal glucose. Polio can be confirmed by stool or throat culture. Suspected cases of polio should be reported to the state health department. For AFM, MRI of brain and spinal cord shows T2, non-enhancing, confluent, and longitudinally involved lesions of the gray matter of the cord +/− brainstem.
- ○ *Treatment:* Provide supportive care. For AFM, IVIg, plasmapheresis, and corticosteroids have been used. There are no current guidelines for immunomodulatory therapies.
- ○ *Prognosis*: For polio, 50% of patients with paralysis will have some residual deficits. For AFM, most patients will show improvement in strength; but only a minority will have full recovery. Some have ventilator dependence at time of hospital discharge.

PERIPHERAL NERVE

- Guillain-Barre syndrome (GBS)[8,9]: GBS is an acute inflammatory demyelinating polyneuropathy or an acute axonal motor (+/− sensory) neuropathy. Preceding infection, classically *Campylobacter jejuni*, or immune stimulation, such as vaccines, leads to an autoimmune response by molecular mimicry in a susceptible host.
  - ○ *Clinical Features:* Patients may have a respiratory or gastrointestinal illness in the month prior to symptom onset. Ascending, progressive, and generally symmetric flaccid weakness with areflexia then follows. Mild sensory symptoms and pain may be present. Autonomic dysfunction such as cardiac arrhythmias, blood pressure lability, ileus, and urinary retention should be monitored. Weakness can progress to respiratory failure. The Miller-Fisher variant has the triad of ophthalmoplegia, ataxia, and areflexia.
  - ○ *Diagnosis:* GBS is a clinical diagnosis. Physical exam should show a progressive, relatively symmetric weakness in upper and lower extremities with areflexia. Nerve conduction studies can be helpful in supporting the diagnosis early in the course as evidenced by prolongation or loss of F-wave responses. It can also help in differentiating between demyelinating and axonal subtypes. MRI of spine may show enhancement of nerve roots. CSF analysis often reveals an albuminocytologic dissociation.
  - ○ *Treatment:* IVIg 2 g/kg over 2 to 5 days or plasmapheresis for five cycles over 2 weeks. Provide supportive care, with close monitoring of respiratory function, including negative inspiratory force (NIF) and vital capacity (VC). Consider intubation if NIF > −30 or VC <20 cc/kg. Should also monitor for autonomic dysfunction leading to cardiac rhythm disturbances.
  - ○ *Prognosis:* Recovery can take months to years.

NEUROMUSCULAR JUNCTION (NMJ)

- Myasthenia gravis (MG)[10–12]: MG is an autoantibody-mediated disorder against acetylcholine receptor (AChR-Ab) and/or muscle-specific tyrosine kinase (anti-MuSK Ab) in most patients. These antibodies lead to direct blocking of acetylcholine at the receptor, receptor degradation, and NMJ membrane damage.

- ○ *Clinical Features*: The characteristic findings are fatigability, ptosis, ophthalmoplegia, and bulbar dysfunction. Weakness of the limbs is proximal and usually does not occur without ocular findings. Some patients may have isolated ocular findings. Myasthenic crisis is a rapid and life-threatening worsening of MG leading to airway compromise from ventilatory or bulbar dysfunction. Exacerbations can be triggered by heat, illness, stress, or medications (e.g. aminoglycosides, fluoroquinolones, neuromuscular blockade, magnesium sulfate, etc.)
- ○ *Diagnosis*: Diagnosis is made by a combination of history, physical exam, decrement on repetitive nerve stimulation, abnormal jitter on single-fiber electromyography, and positive AChR-Ab or anti-MuSK Ab. Absence of autoantibodies does not exclude the diagnosis.
- ○ *Treatment for myasthenic crisis*: Provide respiratory support if needed: noninvasive positive pressure ventilation (NIPPV) vs. endotracheal intubation. Administer IVIg 1 g/kg/day × 2 days OR plasma exchange × five cycles. Consider prednisone/methylprednisolone (1 mg/kg/day, max 100 mg/day), although its use can cause a transient exacerbation of weakness.
- ○ *Chronic treatment*: Titrate pyridostigmine (mestinon) to effect while monitoring for cholinergic side effects. Chronic immunomodulation should be managed by an expert (corticosteroids, azathioprine, cyclosporine, mycophenolate, tacrolimus, rituximab, chronic IVIg, or PLEX)
- ○ *Prognosis*: Variable.
- Botulism[13]: Botulism is caused by a neurotoxin released by *Clostridium botulinum* that disrupts presynaptic acetylcholine release. In infants, ingested spores from raw honey or environmental dust/soil develop into toxin-secreting bacteria, which leads to disease. Adults require ingestion of preformed toxin from improperly canned foods to cause disease.
- ○ *Clinical Features:* In infants, constipation is followed by symmetric descending weakness with cranial neuropathies such as dilated unreactive pupils and facial weakness. About half will require respiratory support during hospitalization. Adults present similarly with cranial neuropathies and descending symmetric weakness. Either age group may have bradycardia.
- ○ *Diagnosis:* Positive stool botulinum toxin. Repetitive nerve conduction studies can be helpful while waiting for stool studies to result.
- ○ *Treatment:* For infant botulism: BabyBIG (intravenous botulism immunoglobulin). For botulism in patients >1yo: equine serum botulism antitoxin. Provide supportive care, including possible need for mechanical ventilation.
- ○ *Prognosis:* Excellent prognosis for full recovery although it may take weeks to months. The mortality rate for infant botulism is <1% in the United States.
- Organophosphate and carbamate intoxication[14]: Organophosphates and carbamates are acetylcholinesterase inhibitors and are generally used as pesticides. Exposure to these compounds leads to excessive cholinergic stimulation at muscarinic and nicotinic receptors.
- ○ *Clinical Features:* Muscarinic stimulation leads to diarrhea, urination, miosis, bronchorrhea/bronchospasm/bradycardia, emesis, lacrimation, salivation ("DUMBELS"). Nicotinic stimulation leads to fasciculations, muscle weakness, and paralysis, which can cause respiratory arrest. Nicotinic stimulation of sympathetic ganglia can lead to tachycardia and hypertension, making the diagnosis of cholinergic poisoning challenging. CNS effects can lead to anxiety, ataxia, seizures, and coma.
- ○ *Diagnosis:* Diagnosis is made by clinical signs and symptoms.
- ○ *Treatment:* Decontaminate the patient by removing clothing and washing with soap and water. For muscarinic toxicity, atropine 2 to 5 mg IV for adults, 0.05 mg/kg IV

for children. The dose should be doubled every 5 minutes until respiratory secretions and bronchoconstriction are alleviated and hemodynamics are acceptable. An atropine continuous infusion then should be initiated at 10% to 20% of the total given dose. For nicotinic toxicity, pralidoxime 1 to 2 G IV for adults, 20 to 50 mg/kg IV for children (max 2 G). Repeat dose at 1 hour, then every 10 to 12 hours until weakness resolves. For seizures, use benzodiazepines.

○ *Prognosis:* Variable depending on severity of poisoning.

• Tick paralysis[15]: Female gravid ticks secrete a salivary neurotoxin that can induce paralysis of the host during blood feeding. In North America, *Dermacentor andersoni* (most common), *Dermacentor variabilis, Amblyomma americanum, Amblyomma maculatum,* and *Ixodes scapularis* are the causal ticks.

○ *Clinical Features:* After the initial tick bite, which may go unnoticed by the patient, the patient can develop ataxia followed by rapid ascending symmetric weakness with areflexia, progressing to cranial nerve involvement and ultimately respiratory muscle failure.

○ *Diagnosis:* Careful inspection to locate the tick on the patient.

○ *Treatment:* Remove tick. Provide supportive care.

○ *Prognosis:* Improvement in weakness can be observed within hours and full recovery within 1 to 2 days.

MUSCLE

• Rhabdomyolysis/myositis[16]: Muscle injury, ischemia, and/or inflammation leads to necrosis, which results in release of intracellular contents of myocytes into the systemic circulation. It can be triggered by a preceding viral infection, trauma, strenuous exercise, heat stroke, metabolic myopathy, and medications such as statins.

○ *Clinical Features:* Myalgias, weakness, and dark urine are classic findings. Complications of rhabdomyolysis are acute kidney injury, electrolyte disturbances, and rarely compartment syndrome.

○ *Diagnosis:* Elevated creatine kinase, typically at least five times the upper limit of normal. Urinalysis with positive blood and absence of red blood cells (RBCs), consistent with myoglobinuria.

○ *Treatment:* Treat the underlying cause of muscle injury. Supportive care with aggressive intravenous hydration and close monitoring of electrolytes and kidney function. Consider urine alkalinization with a goal urine pH >6.5 for the theoretical benefit of preventing acute kidney injury (AKI) from myoglobin toxicity. Renal replacement therapy may be necessary to treat hyperkalemia, acidosis, fluid overload, and anuria.

METABOLIC

• Electrolyte derangements such as hypokalemia/hyperkalemia, hypercalcemia, hypoglycemia, hypermagnesemia, and hypophosphatemia can precipitate weakness. Generally, correction of the derangement will lead to a rapid resolution of weakness.

CHRONIC WEAKNESS

Chronic weakness in pediatrics can be caused by congenital/genetic changes leading to disruption of neuromuscular function. Presentation to the ICU is generally a consequence of acute or chronic respiratory failure, cardiomyopathy, or postsurgical management.

ANTERIOR HORN CELL DISORDER

• Spinal muscular atrophy (SMA)[17]: SMA is caused by a mutation/deletion of the SMN1 gene (survival motor neuron) and is traditionally inherited in an autosomal-recessive pattern.

Loss of SMN1 gene function results in degeneration of alpha motor neurons in the spinal cord and motor nuclei in the brainstem causing a lower motor neuron pattern of weakness. SMA, in order of decreasing weakness/morbidity, is most commonly categorized into type 1 (cannot sit), 2 (sit but cannot walk), and 3 (walk but is weak). SMA0 kids are weak at birth and do not survive into infancy. Pulmonary complications cause significant morbidity and mortality for these patients.

○ *Clinical Features:* SMA is characterized by a progressive, symmetric flaccid weakness that is proximal > distal and involves the lower extremities > upper extremities, paradoxical breathing due to weak intercostal muscles with initially preserved diaphragmatic strength, and absence of deep tendon reflexes. Bulbar dysfunction increases the risk for aspiration. Respiratory insufficiency is most pronounced for type 0 to 2 SMA and causes impaired cough and secretion clearance, nocturnal hypoventilation that progresses to continuous hypoventilation, chest wall and lung underdevelopment, and recurrent infections that exacerbate muscle weakness.

○ *Treatment:* For respiratory insufficiency: cough assistance, chronic noninvasive positive pressure ventilation, and consideration for tracheostomy, depending on family's goals for care. Involving primary care and palliative care teams early on in the process of respiratory failure helps support the family. For malnutrition/aspiration, consider early gastrostomy placement (no consensus guideline). When placing a G-tube, Nissen fundoplication should be strongly considered. Orthopedic care includes management of scoliosis, hip subluxation, and joint contractures. Nusinersen, an antisense oligonucleotide delivered by intrathecal injection that increases production of full-length SMN protein by the SMN2 gene, was approved by the Food and Drug Administration (FDA) in December 2016 and is available at some institutions.

○ *ICU Considerations:* For acute-on-chronic respiratory failure, management should include cough assistance and airway clearance therapies, escalation of NIPPV, and possible intubation, if family goals for care align. Factors to consider for extubation readiness include low secretion burden, lack of atelectasis on chest x-ray, minimal ventilator support, and ability to extubate to NIPPV.

MUSCULAR DYSTROPHY

• Duchenne muscular dystrophy (DMD)[18,19]: DMD is the most common and most severe muscular dystrophy. It is caused by an X-linked recessive mutation in the dystrophin gene. The resultant lack of functional dystrophin protein causes degeneration of striated muscle, elevated creatine kinase levels, progressive weakness, and cardiomyopathy. It overwhelmingly affects males; however, female carriers may also develop weakness and cardiomyopathy.

○ *Clinical Features:* Weakness onset is in early childhood with eventual progression to being nonambulatory. It initially involves proximal > distal and lower extremities > upper extremities. Neuromuscular scoliosis often results. Other classic findings are Gower's sign and calf pseudohypertrophy. Respiratory insufficiency is progressive and may begin with sleep-disordered breathing. Symptoms of dilated cardiomyopathy and cardiac conduction defects usually begin in early adolescence. Varying degrees of intellectual disability are present.

○ *Treatment:* Chronic corticosteroids have been shown to improve strength and pulmonary function and delay cardiomyopathy.[20] Chronic NIPPV can ameliorate sleep-disordered breathing and hypoventilation. Heart failure can be managed with angiotensin-converting enzyme (ACE) medications and/or beta blockers. Arrhythmia management may require antiarrhythmics and possible implantable cardioverter defibrillator (ICD) placement.[21] Orthopedics can address scoliosis, contractures, and fractures.

○ *ICU Considerations:* Heart failure and respiratory failure are the leading causes of death. DMD-associated dilated cardiomyopathy is a cardiomyopathy out of proportion to weakness and respiratory dysfunction. It increases the risk for ventricular arrhythmias causing sudden death. For treatment of acute on chronic respiratory failure, consider escalation of airway clearance therapies, NIPPV, and possible endotracheal intubation if in line with the patient's goals of care. The following precautions should be observed with anesthesia[22]: depolarizing muscle relaxants are contraindicated due to risk for rhabdomyolysis, hyperkalemia, and cardiac arrest; and inhalational anesthetics are associated with a risk for malignant hyperthermia.

CONGENITAL MYOPATHIES

Congenital myopathies are a clinically heterogeneous group of disorders that cause generalized weakness that result from mutations in multiple genes that code for and support the contractile apparatus of the muscle. These can include actin, tropomyosin, and ryanodine receptors, to name a few. A characteristic phenotype can help with focused genetic testing, or sometimes a muscle biopsy may be done prior to genetic testing to help narrow the differential. Genetic testing can elucidate the specific gene mutation; however, mutations in the same gene can lead to different types of congenital myopathies, and different myopathies can be caused by mutations in overlapping genes. Weakness generally does not progress after the neonatal/infantile period, and some patients may even gain strength and mobility. Patients with severe respiratory failure in the neonatal/infantile period are also at the highest risk for mortality. Multidisciplinary subspecialty care is recommended to manage the pulmonary, nutritional, orthopedic, and neurologic complications of these diseases. Following is a summary of clinical complications of interest to an intensivist that may arise in congenital myopathies.[23]

- Respiratory failure: All patients with congenital myopathy are at risk for respiratory insufficiency. Respiratory failure presenting in the neonatal period is common in X-linked tubular myopathy and severe cases of nemaline myopathy with ACTA1 mutations. Respiratory weakness out of proportion to overall muscle weakness can be seen in multiminicore disease with SEPN1 mutations, nemaline myopathy with NEB or ACTA1 mutations, and selected patients with TPM3 mutation. Patients who did not have respiratory failure during infancy who then develop progressive respiratory failure during adolescence and adulthood generally carry the following mutations: SEPN1, TPM3, ACTA1, NEB, DNM2, MTM1.
- The most common phenotype of respiratory insufficiency is sleep disordered breathing. Respiratory failure can also develop from progressive hypoventilation and progressive atelectasis that is not initially clinically apparent, or restrictive lung disease from scoliosis. Decompensations during intercurrent illness may require escalation of cough assistance, airway clearance, and noninvasive positive pressure ventilation, and if unsuccessful, endotracheal intubation if within the patient's goals of care.
- Cardiomyopathy: Primary cardiomyopathies are unusual in congenital myopathies. There have been observed cases with actin α1 (ACTA1), dynamin 2 (DNM2), and tropomyosin 2 (TPM2) mutations. Secondary right ventricular dysfunction may be present in patients with significant pulmonary disease.
- Orthopedic: Scoliosis can develop in all congenital myopathies, especially when axial weakness is a prominent feature. Scoliosis correction with risk for postoperative respiratory failure may necessitate ICU admission and monitoring.
- Anesthesia Risk: As a general rule, inhalational anesthetics and depolarizing muscle relaxants should be avoided in patients with congenital myopathies and are contradindicated in patients with RYR1 mutation due to the risk for malignant hyperthermia.

- Bulbar Dysfunction: Bulbar dysfunction is commonly present in nemaline myopathy and can also be seen with recessive mutations in RYR1 causing multiminicore disease and subgroups of centronuclear myopathy. Gastric or jejunal feeding may be required due to poor handling of oral contents and the risk for aspiration. Anticholinergic agents may be trialed to treat sialorrhea while monitoring for the side effects of constipation and creation of thick tenacious secretions.
- Cognitive Impairment: Cognitive impairment is unusual in congenital myopathies, unless respiratory failure led to hypoxic-ischemic brain injury. Alternative or additional diagnoses should be explored if this is a prominent feature.

CONCLUSION

Weakness is a relatively common clinical entity requiring admission to the intensive care unit. Acute weakness should start with localization of the lesion in order to focus the differential diagnosis and diagnostic evaluation. Patients with chronic weakness are often cared for by intensivists in the setting of respiratory complications of their disease, but may have multiorgan involvement, including cardiac, gastrointestinal, and orthopedic.

REFERENCES

1. Absoud MA, Greenberg BM, Lim M, et al. Pediatric transverse myelitis. *Neurology.* 2016;87(9):S46-S52.
2. Transverse Myelitis Consortium Working Group. Proposed diagnostic criteria and nosology of acute transverse myelitis. *Neurology.* 2002;59:499-505.
3. Nance JR, Golomb MR. Ischemic spinal cord infarction in children without vertebral fracture. *Pediatr Neurol.* 2007;36(4):209-216.
4. Stettler S, El-Koussy M, Ritter B, et al. Non-traumatic spinal cord ischaemia in childhood – clinical manifestation, neuroimaging and outcome. *Eur J Paediatr Neurol.* 2013;17(2):176-184.
5. Weimer MB, Reese JJ Jr, Tilton AH. Acute neuromuscular disease and disorders. In: Fuhrman BP, Zimmerman JJ, Carcillo JA, et al., eds. *Pediatric Critical Care.* 4th ed. Philadelphia, PA: Mosby; 2011:907-917.
6. American Academy of Pediatrics. Poliovirus infections. In: Kimberlin DW, Brady MT, Jackson MA, et al., eds. *Red Book: 2015 Report of the Committee on Infectious Diseases.* 30th ed. American Academy of Pediatrics; 2015:644-650.
7. Messacar K, Schreiner TL, Van Haren K, et al. Acute flaccid myelitis: A clinical review of US cases 2012-2015. *Ann Neurol.* 2016;80(3):326.
8. Willison HJ, Jacobs BC, van Doorn PA. Guillain-Barre syndrome. *Lancet.* 2016;388:717-727.
9. Lawn ND, Fletcher DD, Henderson RD, et al. Anticipating mechanical ventilation in Guillain-Barre syndrome. *Arch Neurol.* 2001;58(6):893-898.
10. Barth D, Nabavi Nouri M, Ng E, et al. Comparison of IVIg and PLEX in patients with myasthenia gravis. *Neurology.* 2011;76(23):2017-2023.
11. Trouth AJ, Dabi A, Solieman N, et al. Myasthenia gravis: A review. *Autoimmune Dis.* 2012;2012:874680.
12. Sanders DB, Wolfe GI, Benatar M, et al. International consensus guidance for management of myasthenia gravis: Executive summary. *Neurology.* 2016;87(4):419-425.
13. Rosow LK, Strober JB. Infant botulism: Review and clinical update. *Pediatr Neurol.* 2015;52(5):487-492.
14. King AM, Aaron CK. Organophosphate and carbamate poisoning. *Emerg Med Clin North Am.* 2015;33(1):133-151.

15. Pecina CA. Tick paralysis. *Semin Neurol*. 2012;32(5):531-532.

16. Chavez LO, Leon M, Einav S, et al. Beyond muscle destruction: A systematic review of rhabdomyolysis for clinical practice. *Crit Care*. 2016;20(1):135.

17. Farrar MA, Park SB, Vucic S, et al. Emerging therapies and challenges in spinal muscular atrophy. *Ann Neurol*. 2017;81(3):355-368.

18. Yiu EM, Kornberg AJ. Duchenne muscular dystrophy. *J Paediatr Child Health*. 2015;51(8):759-764.

19. Emery AEH. The muscular dystrophies. *Lancet*. 2002;369(9307):687-695.

20. Gloss D, Moxley RT 3rd, Ashwal S, et al. Practice guideline update summary: Corticosteroid treatment of Duchenne muscular dystrophy. *Neurology*. 2016;86(5):465-472.

21. Punnoose AR, Kaltman JR, Pastor W, et al. Cardiac disease burden and risk of mortality in hospitalized muscular dystrophy patients. *Pediatr Cardiol*. 2016;37(7):1290-1296.

22. Birnkrant DJ. The American College of Chest Physicians consensus statement on the respiratory and related management of patients with Duchenne muscular dystrophy undergoing anesthesia or sedation. *Pediatrics*. 2009;123(Supp 4):S242-S244.

23. Wang CH, Dowling JJ, North K, et al. Consensus statement on standard of care for congenital myopathies. *J Child Neurol*. 2012;27(3):363-382.

DEFINITION AND SUBTYPES

- Delirium: A form of acute and fluctuating global cerebral dysfunction caused by the direct physiologic consequences of a general medication condition and characterized by disturbances in attentiveness and awareness and cognitive impairment affecting memory, cerebral orientation, language, perception, and/or visual or auditory hallucinations. Four current subtypes exist:
  - Hyperactive: The "classic" form of delirium and intensive care unit psychosis featuring episodic or progressive agitation, restlessness, hallucinations, delusions, and/or emotional lability. Most easily recognized subtype by providers and family members.
  - Hypoactive: Can also be referred to as "encephalopathy of critical illness" with decreased responsiveness, blunted levels of consciousness, quiet confusion, and apathy. Oftentimes can be confused with depressive symptoms or acute stress disorders.
  - Mixed: Waxing and waning occurrences of both hyperactive and hypoactive delirium throughout its fluctuating course.
  - Subacute: Usually related to an indolent, progressive medical condition over time with occasional occurrences of either hyperactive delirium or hypoactive delirium or both that is not defined by an additional psychiatric diagnosis.

ETIOLOGY

- Often is multifactorial. Care should be made to evaluate for all of the following etiologies as a possible cause:
  - Underlying disease processes – most often associated with compensated or uncompensated shock; systemic or localized infection; acute or chronic hypoxia/hypoxemia; neoplasms; seizures; and/or electrolyte, renal, or endocrine derangements
  - Environmental exposures – prolonged states of immobilization or paralysis, day and night lighting disturbances, and sleep deprivation
  - Iatrogenic – suspected to be related to certain acute or prolonged drug exposures (i.e., sedative medicines like benzodiazepines, barbiturates, or opioids or anticholinergic medications) or withdrawal from previously utilized medications

IMPACT AND RECOGNITION

- Delirium is widely accepted as a negative predictor for clinical outcomes in adult patients, particularly those on mechanical ventilation and prolonged sedative infusions.
- Although pediatric data remains limited, emerging literature suggests similar risk factors for developing delirium and an impact on short- and long-term outcomes for children.
- Diagnosing and recognizing delirium in pediatric patients is difficult and is complicated by variations in pediatric development and age.
- Once diagnosed, delirium has been shown to predispose adult patients to:
  - Increased in-hospital mortality
  - Longer lengths of stay, both in the ICU and general hospital
  - Higher medical costs
  - Long-term cognitive impairments
  - Developing post-intensive care syndrome (PICS)

SCREENING TOOLS

- Utilization of quick, reliable, feasible, and observational screening tools for pediatric patients aids physicians in diagnosing all four delirium subtypes.
- Three tools are currently in use:
  - Preschool Confusion Assessment Method for the ICU (psCAM-ICU)
  - Pediatric Confusion Assessment Method for the ICU (pCAM-ICU)
  - Cornell Assessment of Pediatric Delirium (CAPD) - See Figure 46-1
- The psCAM-ICU and pCAM-ICU cannot be fully utilized on developmentally delayed children, which is a recognized limitation of these tools. The CAPD scale can be applied to all children regardless of delay.

PROCEDURAL APPROACH TO DIAGNOSIS

- When referencing one of these screening tools, physicians and nurses should apply the CAPD questionnaire at the end of each shift to every ICU patient who exhibits a Richmond Agitation-Sedation Scale (RASS) of ≥ -3 (or for simplification purposes has spontaneous eye opening) See Figure 46-2.
- Each question is scored according to physician and/or nursing observation over the course of the shift.

RASS Score _____ (if -4 or -5 do not proceed)						
Please answer the following questions based on your interactions with the patient over the course of your shift:						
	Never	Rarely	Sometimes	Often	Always	Score
	4	3	2	1	0	
1. Does the child make eye contact with the caregiver?						
2. Are the child's actions purposeful?						
3. Is the child aware of his/her surroundings?						
4. Does the child communicate needs and wants?						
	Never	Rarely	Sometimes	Often	Always	
	0	1	2	3	4	
5. Is the child restless?						
6. Is the child inconsolable?						
7. Is the child underactive—very little movement while awake?						
8. Does it take the child a long time to respond to interactions?						
					TOTAL	

FIGURE 46-1 **Cornell Assessment of Pediatric Delirium (CAPD) revised.**

Richmond Agitation and Sedation Scale (RASS)		
+4	Combative	Violent, immediate danger to staff
+3	Very Agitated	Pulls or removes tube(s) or catheter(s): aggressive
+2	Agitated	Frequent non-purposeful movement, fights ventilator
+1	Restless	Anxious, apprehensive but movements not aggressive or vigorous
0	Alert & calm	
−1	Drowsy	Not fully alert, but has sustained awakening to *voice* (eye opening & contact ≥ 10 sec)
−2	Light sedation	Briefly awakens to *voice* (eye opening & contact < 10 sec)
−3	Moderate sedation	Movement or eye-opening to *voice* (but no eye contact)
−4	Deep sedation	No response to voice, but movement or eye opening to *physical* stimulation
−5	Unarousable	No response to *voice or physical* stimulation

FIGURE 46-2 **Richmond Agitation and Sedation Scale (RASS).**

- A score ≥9 is usually diagnostic of delirium in developmentally appropriate children.
- Children with developmental delay must be viewed on a spectrum to establish a change from their baseline, making diagnosis possible in these children but more difficult.

TREATMENT

- A three-tiered approach to the treatment of delirium should be applied for every patient:
  - Address the underlying disease process
    - Assess for infection, hypoxemia, and medication withdrawal
    - Achieve adequate pain control
  - Optimize the clinical environment
    - Clear and direct communication with the patient
    - Creation of a quiet, well-lit, controlled space
    - Frequent reorientation of the patient to their surroundings
  - Minimize iatrogenia
    - Reduce sedative exposure when possible
    - Avoid anticholinergics
    - Avoid physical restraints
    - Facilitate sleep through bundled nursing care and assessments
- Pharmacologic agents:
  - There currently are no studies on pharmacologic prevention of delirium in pediatrics, and treatment response is, at best, anecdotal.
  - Treatment for hyperactive delirium may include the use of typical (e.g., haloperidol) or atypical antipsychotics (risperidone, olanzapine) but should only be utilized in consultation alongside a clinical pharmacist and after discussion of the risks and benefits of these medications.

○ There are no current pharmacologic recommendations for the treatment of hypoactive delirium.

SUGGESTED READINGS

Silver G, Traube C, Kearney J, et al. Detecting pediatric delirium: Development of a rapid observational assessment tool. 2012. http://www.icudelirium.org/pediatric.html.Access date: April 2017.

Traube C, Silver G, Kearney J, et al. Cornell assessment of pediatric delirium: A valid, rapid, observational tool for screening delirium in the PICU. *Crit Care Med.* 2013;42:656-663.

47 Brain Death Evaluation

BRAIN DEATH DETERMINATION AND GUIDELINES

Brain death in infants and children according to current guidelines[1]:

- Brain death guidelines: Defining brain death originates from the President's Commission of the Study of Ethical Problems in Medicine and Biomedical and Behavioral Research. For pediatric patients, the most recent brain death guidelines were published in 2011 by a multidisciplinary taskforce and are endorsed by the Society of Critical Care Medicine, the American Academy of Pediatrics, American Association of Critical Care Nurses, Child Neurology Society, and Society of Pediatric Neuroradiology. This definition of death is affirmed by the American Bar Association. Despite wide acceptance, no federal brain death law exists, so providers must review their state and institutional statutes and policies that may restrict this definition.
- Brain death: **Cessation of all neurologic functions of the brain due to a known, irreversible cause.**
  - *Clinical Diagnosis:* This is a clinical diagnosis and must be made by a physician who has taken the history and completed the exam. Coma and apnea must coexist.
  - *Clinical examination*: Includes evaluation of coma, loss of brainstem functioning, and apnea.
- Prerequisites for initiating brain death evaluation:
  - *Irreversible coma with known cause:* Although not considered ancillary studies, magnetic resonance imaging (MRI) or computerized tomography (CT) findings should show evidence of acute injury consistent with significant neurologic damage.
  - *Hemodynamic and metabolic stability:* Shock, hypotension, hypothermia, and severe metabolic disturbances that could affect neurologic function (i.e., glucose and electrolytes) must be corrected before initiating the exam.
  - *Pharmacologic agents:* Neuromuscular blockades, sedatives, barbiturates, opioids, and antiepileptics must be discontinued prior to the examination. For recently administered medications, adequate clearance should be allowed (based on half-life, organ dysfunction, and patient age).
  - *Cardiopulmonary resuscitation:* It may be necessary to wait 24 to 48 hours after cardiopulmonary arrest or severe acute brain injury due to patient instability or inconsistencies in neurologic examinations, as assessed by clinical judgment.
- Number of examinations: Two examinations should be performed, separated by an observation period.
  - *Neonates:* For patients 37 weeks up to 30 days of age, the observation period between two exams should be 24 hours. Due to open sutures and fontanelles, neonates are less likely to have as significant intracranial hypertension, leading to cerebral ischemia and herniation, as older children.
    - Current guidelines do not include information for preterm infants.
  - *Infants and children:* For infants older than 30 days of age and children up to 18 years of age, the observation period between two exams should be 12 hours.
  - *Special considerations:* Should there be a desire to decrease the period of observation, an ancillary test may be considered.

- Examiners: The clinical examinations should be performed by two different attending physicians, each with expertise in neurocritical care. Because the apnea exam is an objective exam, it may be performed by the same attending physician.
- Neurologic examination: To assess loss of all brainstem reflexes. The following are consistent with cessation of brainstem function:
  ○ *Absence of pupillary response:* Midposition or fully dilated pupils that are nonreactive to bright light.
  ○ *Absence of bulbar musculature:* Deep pressure on the condyles at the level of the temporomandibular joints and at the supraorbital ridge produce no movement of the facial and oropharyngeal muscles.
  ○ *Absence of gag, cough, sucking, and rooting reflexes:* Using a tongue blade or suction device for posterior pharynx and endotracheal suctioning at the level of the carina does not illicit a cough.
  ○ *Absence of corneal reflexes:* A soft tissue, cotton, or water to the cornea does not illicit eyelid movement.
  ○ *Absence of oculovestibular reflexes:* Cold caloric testing (irrigating each ear with 10–50 mL of ice water) into patent auditory canals does not produce movement of the eyes within 1 minute.
- Apnea test: The patient must have absence of respiratory effort coinciding with $PaCO_2 \geq 60$ mmHg and ≥ 20 mmHg above baseline.
  ○ *Prerequisites for testing:* Normalized pH, $PaCO_2$, blood pressure, and temperature; preoxygenation with FiO_2 of 1.0 for 5 to 10 minutes prior to beginning the exam.
  ○ *Apnea test:* Patient should be removed from mechanical ventilation to T-piece or self-inflating bag with oxygen. Closely monitor for spontaneous respiratory effort and hemodynamic instability. If SpO_2 falls below 85% or patient has hemodynamic instability, the test should be stopped and patient should be placed back on mechanical ventilation.
  ○ *Special consideration:* If a patient has chronic lung disease and may only respond to supranormal $PaCO_2$, may start at baseline $PaCO_2$ and observe for rise ≥ 20 mmHg above baseline.
- Challenges to diagnosis of brain death
  ○ *Spontaneous and reflex movements:* May be noted in patients meeting criteria for brain death. These can either be spontaneous or triggered by a stimulus. These movements are known as spinal reflexes.[2] See Table 47-1.

TABLE 47-1 Reflexes in Brain Death[1,2]	
- Occur in response to a trigger and are often reproducible	Examples include:
- Nonpurposeful	▪ Small finger movements
- Often seen within the first 24 hours, but can be present longer	▪ Deep tendon reflexes
- May mimic clinical patterns not consistent with brain death	▪ Triple flexion
	▪ Respiration-like movements
	▪ Superficial abdominal reflexes
	▪ Babinski's sign
	▪ Head turning
	▪ Lazarus' sign
	▪ Facial myokymia

- Ancillary studies: Used when components of the neurologic examination or apnea test are unable to be performed, results are not definitive, medications are present, or to reduce observation period. Otherwise, not required for a patient to meet brain death criteria. In pediatrics should be performed and interpreted by trained and qualified individuals.
  - *Four-vessel cerebral angiography*: Demonstrates absence of cerebral blood flow; gold standard but may be difficult to perform in a child due to need for transport, thereby affecting hemodynamic stability.

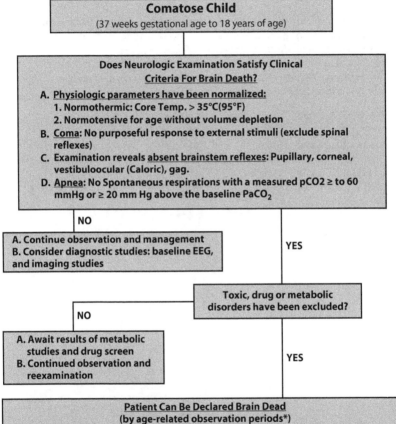

FIGURE 47-1 **Algorithm to Diagnose Brain Death in Infants and Children**[1]

- ○ *Radionuclide cerebral blood flow:* Demonstrates absence of cerebral blood flow.
- ○ *Electroencephalography (EEG):* Documents electrocerebral silence (ECS).
- ○ If cerebral blood flow is present or EEG shows electrical activity, the patient cannot be pronounced brain dead and should be observed before clinical examination can confirm cessation of neurologic function. Waiting period of 24 hours is recommended prior to repeat testing.
- • Declaration of brain death: Occurs after the second neurologic exam and apnea test are consistent with cessation of neurologic function. See Figure 47-1.
- • Supporting the family: Communication with families must be supportive, clear, and concise.
  - ○ Parental presence during testing may be helpful in understanding that the child has died.
  - ○ Families must understand that once a child meets criteria for brain death, the patient meets legal criteria for death.
  - ○ Clinicians should avoid discussions of "withdrawal of support" after declaration of brain death, as this is confusing to families. Rather, discontinuation of medical equipment must occur unless there is a consideration of organ donation.

REFERENCES

1. Nakagawa TA, Ashwal S, Mathur M, et al. Guidelines for the determination of brain death in infants and children: An update of the 1987 task force recommendations. *Pediatrics.* 2011;128(3):e720-e740.
2. Busl KM, Greer DM. Pitfalls in the diagnosis of brain death. *Neurocrit Care.* 2009;11(2):276-287.

4

Renal/Fluids and Electrolytes

48 Maintenance Fluids

PURPOSE OF INTRAVENOUS (IV) FLUID THERAPY: WHY "MAINTENANCE"?

Parenteral fluids are typically administered to patients whose spontaneous and/or enteral intake is insufficient to meet physiologic needs. Delivering a particular quantity of water, dextrose, and electrolytes every hour at a weight-based "maintenance rate" is intended to meet the cellular requirements for basic functionality. The widely used formula for calculating this rate (the "4-2-1 rule") was developed in 1957 and was popularized as much for simplicity as for accuracy. Its original proponents utilized a rough estimate of patient energy requirements to extrapolate fluid needs, escalating stepwise with increases in weight, to arrive at the "4-2-1" progression. This approximation results in a "maintenance" hourly value providing the necessary intake to meet a minimum of one's basal metabolic needs, but likely not those accompanying routine physical activities. It is worth noting that this formula was developed based on data from hospitalized, bedridden patients.[1]

CALCULATION OF THE MAINTENANCE FLUID RATE

Based on the estimations of the rising energy requirement with each kilogram of body weight, a patient's maintenance IV rate is calculated as shown in Table 48-1.

As stated earlier, calculations are done according to the "4-2-1" rule. This rate can be used solely for parental fluid administration or as a goal for the *total* hourly fluid intake (also taking into account continuous infusions and/or high-volume medications). Patients with normal end-organ function (e.g., those children simply *nil per os* [NPO] prior to surgery) may tolerate delivery of a full "maintenance" IV fluid volume in addition to other medications, infusions, and flushes without complication. Contrast this with a fluid-overloaded child with multiorgan dysfunction, who may not tolerate much "surplus" IV volume without cardiopulmonary consequences. In this instance, it may be beneficial to limit *total* hourly intake to the calculated maintenance rate, delivering only a portion of the total via continuous IV fluids. Fluid restriction, even to intake rates below maintenance, can be appropriate in patients with impaired renal function, pulmonary pathology, or fluid overload.

CHOOSING IV FLUID COMPOSITION

Choice of intravenous fluids should be made with an understanding of both the clinical situation and the respective risk–benefit profile.

The three major components of IV fluids are as follows:

- Base sodium content: One of the primary determinants of serum osmolality. All intravenous fluids use sodium and chloride as the primary contributors to solution tonicity in order to allow for safe intravenous administration. IV fluids can be isotonic (similar

TABLE 48-1	Weight-Based Estimation of Pediatric Maintenance Fluid Requirements[1]
Weight (kg)	**Maintenance Rate**
0–10	4 mL/kg/hr
11–20	40 mL/hr + 2 mL/kg/hr
>20	60 mL/hr + 1 mL/kg/hr

tonicity to plasma), hypotonic, or hypertonic, depending primarily on their respective sodium and dextrose content.

$$\text{Serum osmolality} = (2 \times \text{serum sodium}) + (\text{blood urea nitrogen} \div 2.8)$$
$$+ (\text{serum glucose} \div 18)$$

Hypotonic fluid administration, using relatively low sodium concentrations, has been implicated in the development of iatrogenic hyponatremia and a similarly hypotonic serum.[2]

- Dextrose: Provides some nutritional value, typically expressed as a percentage (% = grams of solute /100 mL of fluid volume)
  - **Glucose Infusion Rate (GIR):** Key to avoiding a catabolic state and maintaining euglycemia when IV fluids are the only source of calories. GIR calculation requires the following formula:

$$\text{Glucose infusion rate} = \frac{\left[\% \, \text{dextrose} \times \text{intravenous fluid rate} \left(\dfrac{mL}{hr} \right) \right]}{[6 \times \text{Wt(kg)}]}$$

  - Recommendations for a minimum GIR are based on age:
    5 mg/kg/min for <6 years of age; 2.5 mg/kg/min for ≥6 years old
  - "D5" (5 g/100mL volume) given at maintenance rate does not deliver an adequate GIR in children under 6 years of age
- Additives: Provide essential electrolytes for cellular function and compensate for ongoing losses

  - *Potassium*: Most effectively delivered as potassium chloride. Daily potassium requirement related to 24-hour fluid needs; amounts to approximately 1 to 2 mEq/100 mL water. This is typically provided using IV fluids with a potassium concentration of 20 to 40 mEq/L. Potassium acetate and potassium phosphate are also used, most often in diabetic ketoacidosis.
  - *Sodium bicarbonate*: Indicated in normal anion gap metabolic acidosis caused by renal or gastrointestinal losses of bicarbonate and in certain drug exposures or toxidromes.
  The content of the most commonly used IV fluid preparations is illustrated in Table 48-2.

TABLE 48-2	Electrolyte Composition and Osmolality of Commonly Used IV Fluids			
Fluid	% Sodium Chloride, Dextrose*	Sodium (mEq/L)	Chloride (mEq/L)	Osmolality (mOsm/L)
Normal saline	0.9% NaCl	154	154	308
D5 normal saline	D 5%, 0.9% NaCl	154	154	560
Hypertonic saline	3% NaCl	513	513	1026
D5 half-normal saline	D 5%, 0.45% NaCl	77	77	406
D5 quarter-normal saline	D 5%, 0.225% NaCl	34	34	321
D5W	D5%, 0% NaCl	–	–	272
Lactated Ringer's	0.6% NaCl†	130	109	273
Plasma	**–**	**135–145**	**95–105**	**285–295**

NS = normal saline, D = dextrose, W = water
*% = grams of solute /100 mL of fluid volume
†Also contains 0.31% sodium lactate, 0.03% potassium chloride, and 0.02% calcium chloride for total of 4 mEq potassium, 3 mEq calcium, and 2 8mEq lactate per liter of lactated Ringer's

Note the osmolality of 0.9% (normal) saline and lactated Ringer's (LR), two formulations considered isotonic to serum despite having higher and lower osmolality than blood. In general, isotonic crystalloids (without dextrose) are appropriate for rapid administration to provide urgent intravascular volume expansion during states of hypovolemia and/or shock. Bolus infusion of fluids containing dextrose is avoided as it may cause a transient hyperglycemia, encouraging an osmotic diuresis and contributing to further volume depletion.

Examples of clinical scenarios with specific fluid recommendations:

- Metabolic acidosis: 0.9% normal saline will provide an excess chloride load while running at a maintenance rate, potentially resulting in hyperchloremia and a worsening non-anion gap acidosis
- Renal insufficiency, oliguria: Avoid potassium additives
- Traumatic brain injury, central nervous system (CNS) pathology: Avoid sodium chloride concentrations less than 0.9%, hypotonic fluids and hyponatremia; avoid 5% albumin

ROUTE OF DELIVERY: IS A PERIPHERAL IV SUFFICIENT?

Most preparations are safe to administer through peripheral access, especially at rates approximating maintenance. However, special consideration should be paid to hypertonic formulations, such as 3% saline, which may not be safe to deliver through a peripheral vein. Smaller-diameter vessels can be the setting for local hemolytic reactions when the hypertonic solution contacts the epithelium. Central venous access allows for access of larger-bore vasculature, containing relatively more blood around the entry site of the catheter and its solution. This "excess" local blood serves to "dilute" the infusing fluid before it can contact the vessel wall and promote a reaction. As such, central venous access should be obtained when anticipating a prolonged infusion of hypertonic fluid. A similar access plan is prudent when giving fluids that are significantly hypotonic, such as "half-" or "quarter-normal" saline without dextrose.

An understanding of tonicity again becomes important with higher dextrose concentrations. Preparations containing more than 12.5% dextrose are usually not safe or appropriate to deliver via peripheral access, and a central venous catheter may be required to meet nutritional goals via the parenteral route if higher calories are desired.

- **Central venous access:** All fluids are safe, including hypotonic or hypertonic fluids, dextrose content >12.5%
- **Peripheral access only:** Isotonic fluids (0.9% NaCl or LR without dextrose or dextrose with ½ normal saline [NS] or dextrose with ¼ NS) or any fluid with less than 12.5% dextrose is safe

THE ADVERSE EFFECTS OF INTRAVENOUS FLUIDS

Intravenous fluids are a therapy with an appropriate dose and duration like any other drug. Some side effects of maintenance IV fluids can carry significant morbidity and even mortality.

Side effects of intravenous fluids include:

- Metabolic acidosis
- Tissue edema
- Organ damage to the brain, kidney, and lungs
- Sodium derangements
- Coagulation abnormalities
- Dilutional anemia leading to unnecessary blood transfusions

- Fluid overload: Increasing evidence has shown that excessive fluid administration and subsequent overload can have detrimental effects on the outcomes of all manner of pediatric patients, such as those with septic shock, acute kidney injury, and acute respiratory distress syndrome (ARDS). In such patients, as alluded to earlier, sometimes a set goal of "maintenance fluid delivery" must be adjusted to incorporate all sources of intravenous intake. Additionally, patient fluid status is best viewed as another "vital sign," with cumulative balance reported alongside heart rate and blood pressure. When appropriate, it may be useful to calculate the percentage of overload in a given patient, using the following formula:

$$\text{Fluid overload} = [[\text{Intake(mL)} - \text{Output(mL)}] \div \text{Wt (kg)}] \times 100\%$$

Percentage of fluid overload can be useful to determine management strategy, such as initiation of diuresis or renal replacement therapy for fluid removal.

FOUR PHASES OF INTRAVENOUS FLUID THERAPY

During critical illness, dynamic physiologic changes make fluid needs time-dependent as well. Data suggest up to 20% of critically ill patients receive "inappropriate" intravenous fluids. A recent framework describes the changing role of IV fluids during the course of critical illness by stratifying fluid needs by stage: rescue, optimization, stabilization and de-escalation.

- Rescue: Active (decompensated) shock state, requires rapid isotonic fluid boluses for volume expansion and resuscitation.
- Optimization: Compensated shock states, arrest less likely; fluid given more judiciously, continue to optimize cardiac function, improve perfusion, and avoid (further) organ dysfunction.
  ○ Use gradual fluid challenges instead of rapid boluses.
- Stabilization: Steady state, absence of shock; fluid to replace ongoing losses, support basic metabolism.
- De-escalation: Early recovery, consider cessation of extraneous fluids, work toward fluid removal and a negative fluid balance.

Stabilization and de-escalation seek to avoid the known adverse effects of aggressive fluid management, accumulation, and overload. Not all patients will enter critical illness in the rescue phase, and those without signs of shock may not require any rapid fluid administration at all. Of course, patients may regress at any point, which should prompt a reassessment of fluid needs.[3]

REFERENCES

1. Holliday MA, Segar WE. The maintenance need for water in parenteral fluid therapy. *Pediatrics*. 1957;19(5):823-832.
2. Moritz ML, Ayus JC. Intravenous fluid management for the acutely ill child. *Curr Opin Pediatr*. 2011;23:186-193.
3. Hoste EA, Maitland K, Budney CS, et al. Four phases of intravenous fluid therapy: A conceptual model. *BJA*. 2014;113(5):740-747.

SODIUM ABNOMALITIES

HYPONATREMIA

- Serum sodium (S_{Na}) < 135 mEq/L (mmol/L)
- Prevalence: Up to 40% of pediatric inpatients, often iatrogenic from hypotonic IV fluid
  - Severe symptoms, morbidity, mortality with rapid S_{Na} decline (>1 mEq/hr)
- Pathophysiology: Osmolality of serum largely dependent on sodium, regulated by antidiuretic hormone (ADH), thirst mechanisms
  - In hyponatremia, normal regulatory mechanisms fail to maintain homeostasis
    - Resultant water/sodium imbalance results in hypotonic serum, regardless of total body water, sodium content
- Etiology: Causes of abnormal sodium levels can be differentiated by the total body sodium level (high or low), the response of ADH, and the volume status of the patient (see Table 49-1)
  - *Factitious, pseudohyponatremia*
    - Hyperglycemia creates an osmotic gradient in plasma favoring extracellular water shift out of the cells
    - S_{Na} "diluted" by ≈2 mEq/L for each 100 mg/dL rise in glucose
  - *Normal body sodium*
    - Syndrome of inappropriate antidiuretic hormone (SIADH): ADH *inappropriately high*, patient is typically euvolemic
      - ✓ Caused by many medications, pulmonary infections, increased intrathoracic pressure from mechanical ventilation, oncologic processes
    - Water intoxication (psychogenic polydipsia): ADH *appropriately low*, patient is typically euvolemic
  - *Decreased body sodium*
    - ADH *appropriately elevated* as the patient is hypovolemic from:
      - ✓ Gastrointestinal (GI) tract losses (vomiting, diarrhea)
      - ✓ Sepsis
      - ✓ Diuretics
      - ✓ Salt wasting: Kidney (renal tubule, concentrating defects), central nervous system (injury may alter sympathetic input to kidney), adrenal insufficiency (e.g., 21-hydroxylase deficiency)
      - ✓ Drain output (e.g., external ventricular drain [EVD])
  - *Increased body sodium*
    - ADH *appropriately decreased* as the patient is hypervolemic
      - ✓ Congestive heart failure, renal failure
      - ✓ Nephrotic syndrome
- Clinical signs and symptoms:
  - *Acute hyponatremia*
    - *Rate of decline* dictates symptoms more than specific S_{Na}
      - ✓ No time for compensation mechanisms to deploy
      - ✓ Cannot offset intracellular water shifts
    - Seizures, lethargy, headache, cerebral edema
  - *Chronic hyponatremia*
    - Hyponatremia for >24 hours and/or developing over days

TABLE 49-1	Etiologies of Hyponatremia with Aspects of Diagnosis and Treatment				
Etiology	Total Body Sodium	ADH	Volume Status	Causes	Treatment
Factitious	Normal	Normal	Varies	Hyperglycemia	Treat underlying condition
SIADH	Normal	Elevated (inappropriate)	Normal	Medications, respiratory infections	Restrict fluid, reverse the cause
Water Intoxication	Normal	Low (appropriate)	Normal to hypervolemic	Psychogenic	Restrict water
Renal, GI losses	Low	Elevated (appropriate)	Hypovolemic	Diarrhea, diuretics, CAH	Replace losses
Heart Failure	High	Low (appropriate)	Hypervolemic	Cardiomyopathy	Restrict fluid, ANP analogs
Renal insufficiency				Nephrotic syndrome	

- Compensatory mechanisms change intracellular osmolality, can mitigate risk of cerebral edema
- Vague neurological, GI symptoms (irritability, fatigue, vomiting)
- Treatment:
  - *Key elements:* Tailor therapy to severity of symptoms, underlying cause(s)
  - *Severe central nervous system (CNS) symptoms (seizures)*
    - 3% NaCl to quickly raise S_{Na} to ≈ 125 mEq/L (or lower if symptoms abate)
    - Rapid creation of osmolar gradient favors extracellular water reducing intracellular edema
  - *Shock/hemodynamic instability*
    - 0.9% NaCl to quickly expand intravascular volume, re-establish blood and oxygen delivery to vital organs
  - *Factitious hyponatremia*
    - Treat primary disease process (e.g. insulin infusion for diabetic ketoacidosis [DKA])
  - *Normal total body sodium, euvolemia (SIADH)*
    - Fluid restriction to ≈1/3 to 2/3 of hourly maintenance rate
    - Avoid hypotonic fluids
  - *Decreased total body sodium, hypovolemia*
    - Calculate sodium deficit

$$(\text{Desired serum Na} - \text{Actual serum Na}) \times 0.6 \times \text{Weight(kg)}$$

  - Must consider maintenance needs and any ongoing losses in calculations
    - ✓ Maintenance sodium needs ≈ 2 to 3 mEq/100 mL fluid
  - Replace with 0.9 normal saline (NS) (154 mEq/L) or 3% saline (513 mEq/L) depending on venous access and symptoms
  - Raise S_{Na} by **NO MORE THAN** 0.5 to 1 mEq/hr
    - ✓ Correcting too rapidly can cause central pontine myelinolysis

HYPERNATREMIA

- Serum sodium (S_{Na}) > 145 mEq/L
- Prevalence: Less common than hyponatremia, can cause irreversible pathology
- Pathophysiology: Most often from excessive free water losses, usually via GI tract
  - GI fluids are "hyponatremic" compared to blood
    - Relatively more water (vs. sodium) is lost per unit volume of GI fluid
  - Leads to CNS symptoms as the developing osmolar gradient favors extracellular water movement, "drying out" cerebral tissue (cells shrink, tear the surrounding/bridging vasculature)
- Etiology:
  - *Increased body sodium*
    - Salt intoxication, poisoning
      - ✓ Infant formula improperly prepared, intentional sodium "overdose"
      - ✓ Hyperosmolarity prompts thirst and ADH release, leading to free water intake/ retention will prompt water intake leading to retention and weight gain (opposite of hypernatremic dehydration)
    - Salt water drowning
  - *Normal body sodium*
    - Increased insensible fluid losses with free water losses exceeding sodium losses
      - ✓ Especially smaller children, infants (more surface area per body volume)
    - Diabetes insipidus
      - ✓ Excessive free water lost in dilute, poorly concentrated urine
      - ✓ Central (CNS dysfunction, ADH deficient) vs. nephrogenic (ADH resistant)
  - *Decreased body sodium*
    - GI losses (vomiting, diarrhea)

- Poor intake
  - ✓ Limited access to drinking water
  - ✓ Cannot effectively communicate thirst (infants)
- Osmotic diuresis
  - ✓ Renal excretion of nonelectrolyte solutes, increasing urine osmolality
  - ✓ Free water "trapped" in urine, more water than sodium excreted
- Clinical signs and symptoms:
  - ○ Vomiting, lethargy, irritability, muscle weakness
  - ○ Seizures, coma, intracranial hemorrhage
- Treatment:
  - ○ *Shock/hemodynamic instability*
    - 0.9% NaCl to quickly expand intravascular volume, re-establish renal blood flow
  - ○ *Calculate free water deficit*

$$\text{Free water deficit (mL)} = (\text{Measured SNa} - \text{Desired SNa}) \times \frac{4\,\text{mL}}{\text{kg}} \times \text{Weight (kg)}$$

- - Replace over ≈ 48 hours along with maintenance needs, ongoing losses
    - ✓ Can replace with enteral water or hypotonic fluids
    - ✓ For $S_{Na} > 170$ mEq/L, use "3 mL/kg" in calculations
    - ✓ Avoid correcting by >10 to 15 mEq/L in 24 hours

POTASSIUM ABNORMALITIES

HYPOKALEMIA

- Serum potassium (S_K) less < 3.5 mEq/L
- Overview:
  - ○ Common in hospitalized children, especially ICUs
  - ○ Nearly all (98%) potassium contained inside cells
    - Mediated by Na-K ATPase on cell membrane, pulling in K^+ against its gradient
    - Essential for muscle contraction, nerve conduction, cellular metabolism
    - Excesses excreted in urine, augmented by aldosterone
- Etiology:
  - ○ *Normal body potassium*
    - Alkalosis
      - ✓ K^+/H^+ pump on cell membranes moves H^+ into serum to offset alkalosis, K^+ moves into cells (keeps transition electrically neutral)
    - Medications/hormones (β-agonists, insulin)
      - ✓ Stimulate Na-K ATPase
  - ○ ***Decreased*** *body potassium*
    - Poor intake
    - Renal, GI losses
      - ✓ Emesis: Upper GI fluids have a low K^+ content, but Cl^- loss/metabolic alkalosis enhances renal K^+ excretion
      - ✓ Diarrhea: Lower GI fluids have a high K^+ content (up to 50 mEq/L)
      - ✓ Renal losses enhanced with diuretics, tubular disorders/injury, renal tubular acidosis (RTA)
- Clinical signs and symptoms:
  - ○ Neurologic
    - Weakness, paralysis, ileus, dysrhythmias

- ○ Cardiac (electrocardiogram [ECG] changes)
  - ▪ T waves flat or absent, conduction delays, U waves develop
- Treatment:
  - ○ *Symptomatic*
    - ▪ Intravenous KCl, especially if enteral route is not feasible
      - ✓ 0.5 to 1 mEq/kg, maximum dose 40 mEq, given slowly (<1 mEq/kg/hour)
  - ○ *Asymptomatic, S_K <3 mEq/L*
    - ▪ Enteral route encouraged, lower risk of transient hyperkalemia/dysrhythmia
      - ✓ 1 mEq/kg, can be given every 6 hours
      - ✓ Monitor for nausea and emesis
  - ○ *Asymptomatic, S_K > 3 mEq/L*
    - ▪ Increase dietary/IV fluid content of potassium
  - ○ *Other considerations*
    - ▪ Correct concurrent hypomagnesemia (enhances renal K^+ losses)
    - ▪ Add potassium-sparing diuretic (e.g., spironolactone) to offset aldosterone

HYPERKALEMIA

- S_K > 5.5 mEq/L, severe with S_K > 7 mEq/L
- Etiology:
  - ○ *Factitious*
    - ▪ Hemolysis of red blood cells sample due to delay in testing/difficulty obtaining sample
    - ▪ Leukocytosis or thrombocytosis
      - ✓ K^+ released from the excess cells during sample collection
  - ○ *Increased potassium load*
    - ▪ Iatrogenic
      - ✓ Large-volume red cell transfusion, total parenteral nutrition
  - ○ *Shift/release from intracellular stores*
    - ▪ Acidosis
      - ✓ K^+/H^+ pump moves H^+ into cells to offset acidosis, K^+ out to maintain neutrality
    - ▪ Hemolysis
    - ▪ Crush injury, rhabdomyolysis, burns
    - ▪ Tumor lysis syndrome
  - ○ *Diminished excretion*
    - ▪ Renal failure
    - ▪ Acute kidney injury, renal dysfunction, or chronic kidney disease
      - ✓ Drop in glomerular filtration rate (GFR) brings less Na^+ to collecting ducts for exchange with K^+, less potassium excreted
      - ✓ Tubular dysfunction, pyelonephritis, sickle cell disease
      - ✓ Type 4 RTA, congenital adrenal hyperplasia (hypoaldosteronism)
    - ▪ Medications
      - ✓ ACE inhibitors, spironolactone
- Clinical signs and symptoms:
  - ○ *Generally absent, mild until S_K >7 mEq/L*
  - ○ *Cardiac conduction changes, dysrhythmias*
    - ▪ S_K 6 to 7 mEq/L: Peaked T waves, shortened QT interval
    - ▪ S_K 7 to 8 mEq/L: Prolonged PR interval, widening of QRS complex
    - ▪ S_K >8 mEq/L: P waves disappear, QRS complex merges with T wave to yield "sine wave," ventricular fibrillation, asystole
  - ○ *Neurologic*: Ascending weakness or paralysis (Guillain-Barré–like syndrome), disorientation, paresthesia

- Treatment depends on level and symptoms:
  - $S_K < 6.5 \ mEq/L, \ no \ ECG \ changes:$
    - Discontinue exogenous potassium and any medications decreasing excretion
    - Sodium polystyrene sulfonate (aka Kayexalate) 1 to 2 g/kg/dose PO/PR
  - $S_K > 6.5 \ mEq/L \ and/or \ ECG \ changes:$
    - Stabilize cardiac membranes
      - ✓ IV calcium chloride (10–25 mg/kg) or calcium gluconate (50–100 mg/kg)
    - Shift serum potassium out of bloodstream, into cells
      - ✓ Inhaled beta-agonist (albuterol)
      - ✓ IV insulin (0.2 U/g of glucose) and glucose (1 gm/kg)
      - ✓ IV sodium bicarbonate (1–2 mEq/kg)
    - Decrease total body potassium
      - ✓ Loop diuretics
      - ✓ Sodium polystyrene sulfonate
      - ✓ Dialysis (hemodialysis preferred)

CALCIUM ABNORMALITIES

HYPOCALCEMIA

- Serum ionized calcium (S_{ica}) $\leq$ 4.5 mg/dL (1.3 mmol/L), total calcium < 8.8 mg/dL (2.2 mmol/L)
- Overview:
  - Calcium, phosphate balance maintained by interplay of parathyroid hormone (PTH), vitamin D, and calcitriol on the GI tract, bone, and kidneys
    - PTH prompts kidneys to reabsorb calcium, bones to release calcium, and convert calcidiol to calcitriol
    - Calcitriol and vitamin D enhance calcium absorption in GI tract
  - Ionized calcium is active form, usually correlates well with total calcium
    - Correlation altered by plasma albumin
      - ✓ Roughly half of total body calcium as S_{ica}, remainder binds albumin or plasma anions
      - ✓ Albumin decrease of 1 g/dL will drop total by 0.8 mg/dL, may not affect S_{ica}
      - ✓ No change in S_{ica} = no symptoms
    - Correlation altered by plasma pH
      - ✓ Decreases in pH (acidosis) displaces calcium from albumin leading to more circulating active calcium = S_{ica} increases
- Etiology:
  - *Hypoparathyroidism*
    - Compromised PTH production or release
    - DiGeorge syndrome
    - Mitochondrial disorders
    - Autoimmune polyglandular syndromes
    - Post-thyroid surgery
    - Heavy metal deposits in parathyroid glands (Wilson's disease)
  - *Pseudohypoparathyroidism*
    - Organs show resistance to PTH effects
    - Multiple genetic mutations yield phenotypes/subtypes
    - Elevated serum PTH, hyperphosphatemia
  - *Inappropriate intake, absorption, metabolism of calcium (or vitamin D)*

- Malnutrition
- GI disease, fat malabsorption
- Limited exposure to sunlight
- Liver, kidney dysfunction
- Prolonged antibiotics, which impair calcium absorption
- Hypovitaminosis D
  - *Ongoing electrolyte disturbances*
    - Hyperphosphatemia: suppresses PTH
    - Hypomagnesemia
  - *Drug or therapy side effects*
    - Citrate-containing blood products or continuous renal replacement therapy (CRRT)
    - Bisphosphonates
    - Loop diuretics
- Clinical signs and symptoms:
  - Generally when S_{ica} <4.3 mg/dL (<1.1 mmol/L), total <7 mg/dL (<1.75 mmol/L)
  - *Neuromuscular*
    - Cramping, paresthesia, spasms (carpopedal, laryngeal, bronchial)
    - Effects augmented by alkalosis
  - *Central nervous system*
    - Seizures, altered mental status, psychiatric symptoms (depression, anxiety)
  - *Cardiovascular*
    - Prolongation of QT interval, myocardial dysfunction, hypotension, dysrhythmias
- Treatment:
  - *IV replacement:*
    - For severe hypocalcemia, ECG changes, overt symptoms (tetany, hypotension)
    - Calcium chloride (10–20 mg/kg), requires central venous access
    - Calcium gluconate (50–200 mg/kg), caution with hepatic dysfunction
  - *Correct simultaneous hypomagnesemia* (impedes PTH secretion, fosters resistance)

HYPERCALCEMIA

- Total calcium > 10.5 mg/dL (2.6 mmol/L), ionized calcium > 5.5 mg/dL (1.4 mmol/L)
- Etiology:
  - *Hyperparathyroidism*
    - Parathyroid adenomas, renal disease
  - *Malignancy*
    - Solid tumor, leukemia, bone metastases
    - Relatively uncommon in children (compared to adults)
  - *Increased calcium intake*
  - *Hypervitaminosis A, D*
  - *Immobilization*
  - *Medications*
    - Thiazide diuretics, lithium, theophylline
- Clinical signs and symptoms:
  - *Mild* (<12 mg/dL, 3 mmol/L)
    - Fatigue, constipation, psychiatric disturbances
  - *Moderate* (12–14 mg/dL, 3–3.5 mmol/L)
    - Polyuria, polydipsia, nausea, weakness, kidney injury
  - *Severe* (>14 mg/dL, >3.5 mmol/L)
    - Lethargy, coma, bradycardia, arrhythmias

- Treatment:
  - *Avoid excess intake, adjust/discontinue medications raising serum calcium*
  - *IV hydration, loop diuretics*
  - *Bisphosphonates, calcitonin for severe hypercalcemia*
  - *Many need emergency renal replacement therapy*

PHOSPHATE ABNORMALITIES

HYPOPHOSPHATEMIA

- Normal ranges vary with age, likely due to changes in bone growth. Lower limit of normal approximately 5 mg/dL for neonates, 4 mg/dL for toddlers, 3 mg/dL for older children
- Overview:
  - Serum level determined by the balance between dietary intake, absorption, and excretion by the kidney
  - Renal excretion is normally efficient as very elevated phosphate intake may not alter serum content
  - Most filtered phosphate is reabsorbed in proximal tubules
    - *PTH augments phosphate excretion by inhibiting tubular reabsorption*
    - *Vitamin D increases phosphate (and calcium) absorption*
- Etiology:
  - *Poor/inadequate intake*
- Parenteral nutrition with absent/inadequate supplementation
- Phosphate binders
- GI tract losses
  - *Cellular shifts*
- Correction of metabolic acidosis
- Diabetic ketoacidosis, with correction
- Hyperventilation
- Refeeding syndrome
  - *Increased losses*
- Renal wasting (Fanconi's syndrome)
- Clinical signs and symptoms: Many are manifestations of ATP depletion
  - *Neurologic*
- Encephalopathy, seizures, coma
- Muscle atrophy and weakness
  - *Cardiovascular*
- Myocardial dysfunction, arrhythmias (ventricular)
  - *Respiratory*
- Decreased contractility of diaphragm, dependence on mechanical ventilation
- Cellular hypoxia as red cell 2,3-DPG levels fall = increased affinity of hemoglobin for oxygen, less released to the tissues
  - *Musculoskeletal*
- Proximal myopathy, rhabdomyolysis
- Increased bone resorption
  - *Gastrointestinal*
- Dysphagia, ileus
  - *Renal*: Acute kidney injury (AKI)
  - *Hematologic*
- Rigidity of red blood cells, hemolysis

- Impaired white blood cell phagocytosis, chemotaxis
- Thrombocytopenia, platelet dysfunction
- Treatment:
  - *Serum level >1 mg/dL*
- Enteral route preferred, KPhos or NaPhos 1 mmol/kg divided q6 to q8h
  - *Serum level < 1 mg/dL*
- IV route preferred, 0.1 to 0.5 mmol/kg given over ≈ 6 hours
  - *With resolving metabolic acidosis*
- Treat underlying cause, hypophosphatemia typically resolves
  - *Dipyridamole:* To increase absorption of phosphate by the kidneys

HYPERPHOSPHATEMIA

- Normal ranges vary with age, likely due to changes in bone growth. Upper limit of normal approximately 8 mg/dL for neonates, 6.5 mg/dL for toddlers, 5.5 mg/dL for older children
- Etiology:
  - *Cell/tissue breakdown*
    - Tumor lysis
    - Muscle injury, necrosis, rhabdomyolysis
    - Hemolysis (rarely)
  - *Extracellular shift*
    - Metabolic acidosis
      - ✓ Lactic acidosis, diabetic ketoacidosis (DKA)
      - ✓ Aerobic metabolism/glycolysis compromised, yields intracellular surplus or unused phosphate which is excreted into the serum
  - *Renal insufficiency, failure*
  - *Hypoparathyroidism*
  - *Vitamin D toxicity*
  - *Medications*
    - Bisphosphonates
    - Amphotericin B (liposomal)
- Clinical signs and symptoms: Many due to concurrent refractory hypocalcemia
  - *Cardiovascular*
    - Prolongation of QT interval, hypotension, myocardial dysfunction and failure
  - *Neurological*
    - Altered mental status, seizures, coma
  - *Neuromuscular*
    - Tetany, paresthesias
- Treatment:
  - *Limit exogenous intake*
  - *Phosphate binders*
  - *IV hydration, loop diuretics*
  - *Acetazolamide to augment renal excretion*

MAGNESIUM ABNORMALITIES

HYPOMAGNESEMIA

- Serum magnesium S_{Mg} < 1.5 mg/dL
- Overview:
  - *Homeostasis:* Not hormonally driven, relies on passive reabsorption in loop of Henle
    - Little redistribution between tissue stores and serum

- Symptoms with small deficits, as extracellular magnesium lost
  - ○ Monitor for concurrent hypokalemia, hypocalcemia
- Etiology:
  - ○ *GI tract losses*
    - Diarrhea, vomiting, malabsorption
  - ○ *Renal losses*
    - Augmented by diuretics (loop, thiazide), antibiotics (aminoglycosides)
  - ○ *Pancreatitis*
  - ○ *Chronic use of proton pump inhibitors*
  - ○ *Hypercalcemia*
- *Uncontrolled diabetes mellitus*
- *Post-transplant patients on calcineurin inhibitors*
- *"Hungry bone syndrome" after thyroidectomy, parathyroidectomy, or correction of metabolic acidosis*
- Clinical signs and symptoms:
  - ○ *Neuromuscular*
    - Muscle tremors, tetany, seizures, involuntary (choreoform) movements, nystagmus
    - Apathy, delirium, coma
  - ○ *Cardiovascular*
    - Widening of QRS complex, peaking of T waves, widening of PR interval, dysrhythmias
  - ○ *Electrolyte disturbances*
    - Hypocalcemia, hypokalemia
- Treatment:
  - ○ Magnesium sulfate 25 to 50 mg/kg IV (maximum of 2 g/dose)

HYPERMAGNESEMIA

- $S_{Mg} > 2.3$ mg/dL
- Etiology:
  - ○ *Renal dysfunction*
  - ○ *Significant magnesium load*
  - ○ *Tumor lysis syndrome*
  - ○ *Primary hyperparathyroidism*
  - ○ *Lithium toxicity*
- Clinical signs and symptoms:
  - ○ *Neurologic*
- Nausea, headache, lethargy, flushing
- Abnormal/absent deep tendon reflexes
  - ○ *Cardiac*
- Hypotension, bradycardia, heart block, cardiac arrest
  - ○ *Respiratory*
- Apnea, respiratory failure
- Treatment:
  - ○ *Discontinue exogenous magnesium*
  - ○ *IV hydration, loop diuretics*
  - ○ *Urgent/emergent dialysis for severe neurologic, cardiac abnormalities*
  - ○ *IV calcium for magnesium antagonism*

COMMON ELECTROLYTE DEFICITS, CLINICAL SYMPTOMS, AND DOSING OF IV THERAPIES - SEE TABLE 49-2

TABLE 49-2	Common Electrolyte Deficits, Clinical Symptoms, and Dosing of IV Therapies	
Abnormality	**Symptoms**	**Therapy**
Hyponatremia	Seizures, lethargy, vomiting	3% NaCl: 5 mL/kg for cerebral edema, increased ICP
		0.9% or 3%NaCl for correction of calculated deficit
Hypokalemia	Weakness, ileus, flat T waves	Potassium chloride: 0.5–1 mEq/kg, max 40 mEq
Hypocalcemia	Tetany, numbness, seizures, hypotension	Calcium chloride: 10–20 mg/kg (CVL)
		Calcium gluconate: 50–100 mg/kg
Hypophosphatemia	Respiratory distress, heart failure, encephalopathy	Sodium, potassium phosphate: 0.1–0.5 mmol/kg
Hypomagnesemia	Tremors, seizures, wide QRS	Magnesium sulfate: 25–50 mg/kg, max 2 g

SUGGESTED READINGS

al-Ghamdi SM, Cameron EC, Sutton RA. Magnesium deficiency: Pathophysiologic and clinical overview. *Am J Kidney Dis*. 1994;24:737.

Alsumrain MH, Jawad SA, Imran NB, et al. Association of hypophosphatemia with failure-to-wean from mechanical ventilation. *Ann Clin Lab Sci*. 2010;40:144.

Aubier M, Murciano D, Lecocguic Y, et al. Effect of hypophosphatemia on diaphragmatic contractility in patients with acute respiratory failure. *N Engl J Med*. 1985;313:420.

Cummings BM, Macklin EA, Yager PH, et al. Potassium abnormalities in a pediatric intensive care unit: Frequency and severity. *J Intensive Care Med*. 2014;29:269.

Forman S, Crofton P, Huang H, et al. The epidemiology of hypernatraemia in hospitalised children in Lothian: A 10-year study showing differences between dehydration, osmoregulatory dysfunction and salt poisoning. *Arch Dis Child*. 2012;97:502.

Hoorn EJ, Betjes MG, Weigel J, et al . Hypernatraemia in critically ill patients: Too little water and too much salt. *Nephrol Dial Transplant*. 2008;23:1562.

Hoorn EJ, Geary D, Robb M, et al. Acute hyponatremia related to intravenous fluid administration in hospitalized children: An observational study. *Pediatrics*. 2004;113:1279.

Knochel JP. The pathophysiology and clinical characteristics of severe hypophosphatemia. *Arch Intern Med*. 1977;137:203.

Lips P. Vitamin D physiology. *Prog Biophys Mol Biol*. 2006;92(1):4-8.

Masilamani K, van der Voort J. The management of acute hyperkalaemia in neonates and children. *Arch Dis Child*. 2012;97:376.

Molla AM, Rahman M, Sarker SA, et al. Stool electrolyte content and purging rates in diarrhea caused by rotavirus, enterotoxigenic *E. coli*, and *V. cholerae* in children. *J Pediatr*. 1981;98:835.

Sterns RH, Hix JK, Silver S. Treatment of hyponatremia. *Curr Opin Nephrol Hypertens*. 2010;19:493.

Weisinger JR, Bellorín-Font E. Magnesium and phosphorus. *Lancet*. 1998;352:391.

DEFINITIONS

URINARY TRACT INFECTION (UTI)

• An infection of the kidney, ureter, bladder, or urethra.

PYELONEPHRITIS

• Inflammatory process of the kidney or upper urinary tract = UTI + systemic symptoms

UROSEPSIS

• UTI/pyelonephritis + systemic inflammatory response syndrome (SIRS) criteria

ETIOLOGY

COMMON ORGANISMS

• Ascending genitourinary (GU) infections: *E. coli*, gram-negative bacteria (*Klebsiella, Proteus, Enterobacter, Pseudomonas*), gram-positive bacteria (enterococci, staphylococci, group B *Streptococcus*)
• Catheter-associated UTI (CAUTI): fungi

PREDISPOSING RISK FACTORS

• Congenital anomalies: hydronephrosis, posterior urethral valves, vesicoureteral reflux
• Neurologic abnormalities: neurogenic bladder, quadriplegia
• Dysfunctional elimination: constipation, voiding dysfunction
• Indwelling catheters
• Sexual activity

CLINICAL MANIFESTATIONS

NEONATES/INFANTS

• Fever of unknown origin
• Jaundice
• Irritability
• Poor feeding or failure to thrive (FTT)

OLDER CHILDREN

• Fever
• UTI symptoms: urinary frequency, urgency, dysuria, enuresis
• Pain: flank, back, abdominal, costovertebral angle (CVA), suprapubic

SYSTEMIC SYMPTOMS IN ANY AGE

• Fever, chills, rigors
• Nausea/vomiting, diarrhea
• Shock

DIAGNOSIS

LABORATORY EVALUATION

• Urinalysis (UA): pyuria + bacteriuria +/- hematuria

○ Routine "test of cure" not necessary
○ Repeat within 48 to 72 hours if clinical response is poor
• Positive urine Gram stain and culture
  ○ Any bacteria from suprapubic tap
  ○ >50k CFU/mL from catheterization specimen
  ○ >100k CFU/mL from "clean catch" (exclude polymicrobial growth)
• Blood culture: to identify concomitant bacteremia

IMAGING

• Recommended for the following patients:
  ○ Children <5 years with febrile UTI
  ○ Females <3 years with first UTI
  ○ Males of any age with first UTI
  ○ Children with recurrent UTI
  ○ Children who do not respond promptly to antimicrobial therapy
• Renal-bladder ultrasound:
  ○ Identifies gross anatomy abnormalities
  ○ Obtain in patients with poor clinical response within 48 hours of antimicrobial therapy
• Voiding cystourethrogram (VCUG):
  ○ Identifies vesicourethral reflux (VUR)
  ○ Perform immediately after therapy
• Technetium 99m-dimercaptosuccinic acid (^{99m}Tc-DMSA) scan:
  ○ Identifies acute pyelonephritis (of limited value) and renal scars (if performed >5 months after infection)

TREATMENT

See *Surviving Sepsis Guidelines* to reverse shock

ANTIMICROBIAL THERAPY

• Empiric IV antibiotics:
  ○ Second- (cefuroxime) or third-generation (cefotaxime, ceftriaxone) cephalosporin
  ○ Ampicillin-sulbactam
  ○ Gentamicin
• Switch to enteral antimicrobial: afebrile and able to tolerate enteral medications
• Narrow antimicrobial therapy: based on culture results
• Duration: 10 to 14 days

COMPLICATIONS

RENAL OR PERINEPHRIC ABSCESS

• Suspect when fever is persistent despite appropriate antimicrobial therapy
• Treatments: drainage + antimicrobial therapy

SUGGESTED READINGS

Kalra OP, Raizada A. Approach to a patient with urosepsis. *J Glob Infect Dis.* 2009;1:57-63.
Roberts KB. Urinary tract infection treatment and evaluation update. *Pediatr Infect Dis J.* 2004;23:1163-1164.
Stucky ER, Kimmons HC. Inpatient management of urinary tract infections in infants and young children. *Hospitalist.* 2005;9(Supplement 2):48-51.

Acute Kidney Injury

The kidneys are responsible for many physiologic functions imperative to homeostasis, including:

• Excretion of organic anions, water-soluble metabolites and drugs
• Regulation of acid–base balance
• Regulation of sodium, chloride, and potassium serum levels
• Regulation of serum osmolality and free water balance
• Production of erythropoietin
• Vitamin D metabolism
• Regulation of systemic vascular resistance through production of renin and angiotensin

The kidneys also receive up to 20% of the cardiac output, making them very sensitive to changes in blood pressure, oxygen delivery, and/or cardiac output.

Acute kidney injury (AKI) is a broad clinical term that includes the subtle signs of renal impairment such as edema or acidosis and extends to complete renal failure and anuria. Staged definitions have been developed to accommodate for the wide clinical variability of patients with a diagnosis of AKI.

CAUSES OF PEDIATRIC AKI

Classically the causes of AKI have been categorized as pre-renal, intrinsic, and post-renal. However, the causes of AKI in critically ill children are more complex and multifactorial than these categories suggest.

Common causes of AKI in the PICU include:

• Hypoxic-ischemic injury
• Sepsis, cytokine, or toxin mediated
• Multiorgan dysfunction syndrome
• Nephrotoxic medications
  ○ *Causes 25% of pediatric AKI*: aminoglycosides, NSAIDs, radiopaque contrast, immuno-suppressive therapy
• Oxidative stress and hypoxia
• Intravascular volume depletion
• Glomerulonephritis
• Interstitial nephritis: idiopathic or drug induced
• Tumor lysis syndrome
• Rhabdomyolysis
• Acute tubular necrosis
• Renal vascular thrombus
• Hemolytic uremic syndrome
• Obstruction of urinary flow from posterior urethral valves, nephrolithiasis, trauma

Children with critical illness are especially vulnerable to AKI as intrinsic renal function does not approach adult levels until over 1 year of age. Neonates and premature infants in normal health have an estimated glomerular filtration rate (GFR) of 50 to 60 mL/min/1.73 m^2 whereas a healthy adult GFR is approximately120 mL/min/1.73 m^2.[1]

DIAGNOSING PEDIATRIC AKI

Approximately 10% of critically ill children will have AKI, most often around the third hospital day.[2] The presence of any signs of renal dysfunction, including fluid overload, systemic hypertension (blood pressure >95th percentile for age and sex), and/or electrolyte derangement should prompt investigation for AKI. The clinical correlate to describe renal function is the GFR, expressed in mL/min/1.73 m^2.

SERUM CREATININE AS A MEASURE OF GFR

The most available serum biomarker of renal function is serum creatinine (SCr). There is a simple bedside calculation to convert SCr levels to an estimated GFR[3]:

$$eGFR = 41.3 \times \left(\frac{Height(m)}{SCr} \right)$$

This equation often overestimates renal function, especially in extremes of age and renal function.

As a by-product of muscle mass with dynamic changes in excretion and renal tubule absorption, SCr has multiple disadvantages as an indicator of renal function in children with critical illness.

The following factors affect SCr levels regardless of actual renal function:

○ Protein malnutrition
○ Age: SCr is very insensitive to small changes in renal function in young children
○ Sex
○ Critical illness
○ Muscle mass
○ Fluid balance: SCr levels should be adjusted for the net fluid balance of a patient to correct for dilution from fluid overload[4]:

$$Adjusted\ SCr = SCr \times \left(1 + \left[\frac{Net\ fluid\ balance(L)}{Wt(kg) \times 0.6} \right] \right)$$

ADULT DEFINITIONS OF AKI

The Kidney Disease: Improving Global Outcomes (KDIGO) international consensus defined AKI in 2012 as an:

• Increase in SCr by ≥0.3 mg/dL within 48 hours; OR
• Increase in SCr to ≥1.5 times baseline, which is known or presumed to have occurred within the 7 days prior; OR
• Urine output < 0.5 mL/kg/hr for 6 hours[5]

PEDIATRIC DEFINITIONS AND STAGING CRITERIA FOR AKI

Consensus definitions or staging criteria have been developed for children; similar to the adult definitions, pediatric definitions for AKI rely primarily on SCr and urine output. The pediatric "Risk" "Injury" "Failure" "Loss" and "End-Stage" (pRIFLE) and Acute Kidney Injury Network (AKIN) are the current definitions and criteria most commonly used by pediatric critical care physicians (Table 51-1)[6].

In a paradigm shift, the Renal Angina Index includes clinical context to describe patients at high risk for AKI in the 2 days after the threshold for "angina" is surpassed (Table 51-2).[7]

TABLE 51-1	The Pediatric-Modified RIFLE and the Acute Kidney Injury Network (AKIN) Criteria Used to Diagnose and Stage Pediatric AKI		
Criteria	**Stage**	**Change in Renal Function**	**Urine Output**
pRIFLE	R–"Risk"	eCrCl* decreases by ≥ 25%	<0.5 mL/kg/hr × 8 hr
	I—"Injury"	eCrCl* decreases by ≥ 50%	<0.5 mL/kg/hr × 16 hr
	F—"Failure"	eCrCl* decreases by ≥ 75% or eCrCl*<35 mL/min/1.73m²	<0.3 mL/kg/hr × 24 hr OR No urine output × 12 hr
	L–"Loss"	Failure >4 weeks	
	E—"End stage"	Failure >3 months	
AKIN	Stage 1	SCr increases by ≥0.3 mg/dL or to 150%–200% above baseline	<0.5 mL/kg/hr × 6 hr
	Stage 2	SCr increases to 200%–300% above baseline	<0.5 mL/kg/hr × 12 hr
	Stage 3	SCr increases to 300% above baseline or >4.0 mg/dL or an acute increase by 0.5 mg/dL	<0.3 mL/kg/hr × 24 hr or no urine output for 12 hr

pRIFLE, pediatric- modified "Risk,""Injury,""Failure,""Loss," and "End-Stage" criteria; *AKIN*, Acute Kidney Injury Network criteria; *eCrCl*, estimated creatinine clearance; *SCr*, serum creatinine.
*Can replace CrCl with SCr if unable to assess creatinine clearance.

TABLE 51-2	Renal Angina Index Used to Describe Thresholds for AKI as Determined by Level of Risk Inherent to Patient Factors
Hazard Tranche	**Renal Angina Threshold**
Moderate-risk patients:	Doubling of SCr or eCrCl decrease >50%; OR
Patients admitted to the PICU	PICU fluid overload >15%
High-risk patients:	SCr increase ≥0.3 mg/dL; OR
Acute decompensated heart failure	eCrCl decrease 25%–50%; OR
Stem cell transplant recipient	PICU fluid overload >10%
Very high-risk patients:	Any SCr increase; OR
Receiving mechanical ventilation and one or more vasoactive medications	eCrCl decrease >25%; OR
	PICU fluid overload >5%

AKI, acute kidney injury; *PICU*, pediatric intensive care unit; *SCr*, serum creatinine; *eCrCl*, estimated creatinine clearance.

DIAGNOSTIC OPTIONS (OTHER THAN SCR) IN PEDIATRIC AKI

It can take up to 2 days and loss of 50% or more of glomerular function for elevations in SCr to occur. Other diagnostic and screening tests used to clinically monitor for and detect AKI include:

• Urinalysis: Casts can indicate tubular damage; microscopic hematuria or proteinuria can indicate glomerular damage
• Renal ultrasound: Rule out vascular thrombi, obstruction
• Renal near infrared regional spectroscopy (NIRS): Monitors for dynamic changes in renal oxygen uptake in patients at high risk of AKI

- Novel biomarkers: Many new serum and urinary tests have been established to replace SCr; none has risen to widespread use. A functional panel of several biomarkers likely holds the most promise for early detection of AKI but is not yet available. The two novel biomarkers most in clinical use in PICUs are:
  - *Cystatin C:* serum or urine, detects earlier and more subtle changes in renal function than SCr
    - AKI threshold >1.0 mg/L
    - Modified Schwartz equation uses serum cystatin C, height (ht), SCr, and blood urea nitrogen (BUN) to estimate GFR with more accuracy that the original Schwartz equation[3]:

$$eGFR = 39.1 \left[\frac{ht(m)}{SCr(mg/dL)} \right]^{0.516} \times \left[\frac{1.8}{cys\,C(mg/L)} \right]^{0.294} \times \left[\frac{30}{BUN(mg/dL)} \right]^{0.169}$$
$$\times \left[\frac{ht(m)}{1.4} \right]^{0.188} \times (1.099 \text{ if male})$$

  - *Neutrophil gelatinase-associated lipocalin (NGAL):* serum or urine, proven to detect changes in renal function in several pediatric populations but is not yet clinically available for use
    - AKI threshold >150 ng/mL in serum and >50 µg/mL in urine

PEDIATRIC AKI MANAGEMENT

No therapies or curative medications exist for pediatric AKI. The key to managing AKI is avoiding further damage through the following tactics:

- Optimize hemodynamics and oxygen delivery
  - *Aim for normotension:* Renal dose dopamine and supraphysiologic blood pressures have shown no benefit in pediatric AKI and may be detrimental.
  - *No role for fenoldopam:* selective dopamine agonist, increases renal blood flow, has shown no improvement in pediatric AKI.
  - *Avoid transfusions if possible:* Transfusing packed red blood cells (pRBCs) likely carries more risk than benefit in augmenting oxygen delivery, depending on the level of anemia. The high potassium load from stored blood products, the extra volume loading, and the potential for transfusion reactions are dangerous side effects of pRBCs that must be considered before administering blood products, especially if the hemoglobin is above 7 mg/dL.
- Optimize nutrition: Use of indirect calorimetry can be helpful to ensure dynamic nutritional needs are met. Renal replacement therapy may be necessary to allow delivery of full nutrition.
- Avoid nephrotoxic medications: Including aminoglycosides, NSAIDs, antifungal agents, calcinuerin inhibitors, and contrast media for computerized tomography (CT) scans.
- Renal replacement therapy (RRT): No standard timing, dosage, or duration has been agreed upon (see Chapter 52 for more details).
- Avoid fluid overload (FO): Increased fluid administration and FO >10% to 20% has been independently associated with mortality in children with AKI and/or requiring renal replacement therapy.[2]
  - *Limit fluid intake to the insensible fluid loss rate* = 300 to 400/m²/day or about one-third of the maintenance IV fluid rate if the body surface area is unknown.

    i. If eating, avoid free water, potassium- or phosphorous-containing food, or a high protein load. Renal formulas such as Suplena are ideal for calorie density and electrolyte composition.

    ii. If on total parenteral nutrition, minimize potassium and limit protein to < 2 grams per day unless on renal replacement therapy.

- *Diuretic therapy*: Diuretics are often used to mitigate further fluid accumulation and improve FO; no prospective pediatric data supports this practice. Electrolyte derangements, hypochloremic alkalosis, and azotemia are expected and manageable side effects from diuretic use (Table 51-3).

TABLE 51-3   Commonly Used Diuretics in Pediatric Critical Care

Class	Diuretics in This Class (Dose Ranges)	Mechanism	Side Effects or Notes
Loop diuretics	Furosemide (0.5–2 mg/kg q6hr), bumetanide (0.02–0.1 mg/kg q6hr) Torsemide (0.25–1 mg/kg q6hr), ethacrynic acid (0.5–1 mg/kg bid)	Inhibit sodium/potassium/chloride transport in the thick ascending loop	Hypercalciuria (potential for stones), ototoxicity, and hypokalemia. Cannot give in sulfa allergy.
Thiazides	Hydrochlorothiazide (0.5–1.5 mg/kg PO bid) Chlorothiazide (10–20 mg/kg PO bid) *Metolazone (0.1–0.2 mg/kg q12–24hr)	Inhibit sodium/chloride cotransport in early distal convoluted tubule	Used for nephrogenic diabetes insipidus and hypercalciuria. Weaker than loops.
Potassium-sparing diuretics	Spironolactone (0.25–0.83 mg/kg q6hr)	Blocks aldosterone action on the cortical collecting ducts	Weak diuretic alone.
Carbonic anhydrase (CA) inhibitors	Acetazolamide (5 mg/kg q8–q24hr)	Inhibit CA in the luminal membrane of the proximal tubule = reduced HCO_3 reabsorption	Also used in glaucoma, altitude sickness, and as adjunctive antiepileptic.
Osmotic diuretics	Mannitol (0.5–1 gm/kg IV) Isosorbide	Expands extracellular fluid and plasma volume to increase renal blood flow, changes concentration gradient in the loop of Henle to avoid water resorption	Works for acute management of elevated intracranial or intra-ocular pressure.
Vasopressin receptor antagonist	Conivaptan (mixed V_2 and V_1 effects, adult dose = 20 mg over 24 hr) Lixivaptan (V_2 only)	With differing selectivity, these drugs block vasopressin receptors in the body, V_2 being local to the kidneys	Cause hypernatremia and free water loss.

*Thiazide-like.

OUTCOMES OF PEDIATRIC AKI

AKI increases mortality in children with multiorgan failure, after organ and stem cell transplantation, on extracorporeal membrane oxygenation (ECMO), with acute respiratory distress syndrome (ARDS), and in septic shock independent of PRISM II scores. In survivors, AKI increases length of mechanical ventilation, inotrope need, and length of stay in the PICU and in the hospital.[2]

LONG-TERM OUTCOMES OF PEDIATRIC AKI

Evidence is growing that a significant amount of previously healthy children after a single episode of AKI during critical illness will have long-term renal impairment. In one study, up to 70% of children with AKI from aminoglycoside therapy had renal impairment 1 year after discharge,[8] and this persists in 40% to 50% of children at 3- and 5-year follow-up.[2]

No consensus guidelines regarding referral to nephrology exist for pediatric AKI after PICU discharge, and current practice is highly variable.[6]

REFERENCES

1. Schwartz GJ, Work DF. Measurement and estimation of GFR in children and adolescents. *Clin J Am Soc Nephrol.* 2009;4(11):1832-1843.
2. Basu RK, Devarajan P, Wong H, et al. An update and review of acute kidney injury in pediatrics. *Pediatr Crit Care Med.* 2011;12(3):339-347.
3. Schwartz GJ, Munoz A, Schneider MF, et al. New equations to estimate GFR in children with CKD. *J Am Soc Nephrol.* 2009;20(3):629-637. PMCID: 2653687.
4. Liu KD, Thompson BT, Ancukiewicz M, et al. Acute kidney injury in patients with acute lung injury: impact of fluid accumulation on classification of acute kidney injury and associated outcomes. *Crit Care Med.* 2011;39(12):2665-2671. PMCID: 3220741.
5. KDIGO Clinical Practice Guideline for Acute Kidney Injury. *Kidney Int Suppl.* 2012;2(1):1-138.
6. Hassinger AB, Garimella S, Wrotniak BH, et al. The current state of the diagnosis and management of acute kidney injury by pediatric critical care physicians. *Pediatr Crit Care Med.* 2016;17(8):e362-e370.
7. Basu RK, Chawla LS, Wheeler DS, et al. Renal angina: An emerging paradigm to identify children at risk for acute kidney injury. *Pediatr Nephrol.* 2012;27(7):1067-1078. PMCID: 3362708.
8. Menon S, Kirkendall ES, Nguyen H, et al. Acute kidney injury associated with high nephrotoxic medication exposure leads to chronic kidney disease after 6 months. *J Pediatr.* 2014;165(3):522-527 e2.

Renal Replacement Therapies 52

THE PHYSIOLOGY OF RENAL REPLACEMENT THERAPY

Renal replacement therapy (RRT), or "dialysis," uses the basic concept of molecular movement across a semipermeable membrane to provide particle and water removal from the blood.[1]

This requires two types of movements:

- Diffusion: Solute exchange across a membrane between two solutions based on concentration gradient (from high to low concentration), permeability of the membrane, and surface area of the membrane
  - Used in HEMODIALYSIS or whenever a dialysate is used
  - Favors small particle movement
  - Faster movement with a large concentration gradient
- Convection: Solute movement or "drag" with filtration across a membrane driven either by hydrostatic or osmotic pressures independent of concentration gradient

  - ULTRAFILTRATION: Water removal across a membrane using a pressure gradient
  - Particles AND water move together; if removing large amounts, will have to provide replacement fluid with electrolytes to compensate for filtration losses
  - Removes small and medium-sized particles; amount depends on amount of filtered water and the sieving coefficient of the membrane
  - Large particles will not be removed if they are larger than the pores of the membrane

RENAL REPLACEMENT THERAPY MODALITIES

PERITONEAL DIALYSIS (PD)

- Description: Uses the peritoneum as the membrane for both convection- and diffusion-based solute clearance. Need a healthy, intact peritoneum (no diaphragmatic hernias, adhesions, or active peritonitis).
- Advantages: Can be run emergently and continuously without vascular access; PD catheters can be placed at the bedside percutaneously by the intensivist or interventional radiologist if pediatric surgeons are unavailable.
- Indications: Efficacious in fluid overload and is less invasive and has little hemodynamic impact, making it safe in neonates and infants.
  - Does not work in hyperammonemia or for drug clearance in toxic exposures
- Complications: Hernias, peritonitis, hyperglycemia, respiratory compromise if giving dwells of more than 60 mL/kg, dialysate leakage, pleural effusions.

INTERMITTENT HEMODIALYSIS (IHD)

- Description: Removes venous blood from the patient into an extracorporeal circuit past a membrane to provide mainly diffusion in a rapid manner via a 3- or 4-hour session
- Advantages: Effective for *small* molecule clearance
- Indications: Good for hyperkalemia, toxic exposures, tumor lysis syndrome
  - Contraindicated in hemodynamic instability, severe uremia (see "Disequilibrium Syndrome" later)

- Considerations: Solute clearance depends on molecular weight, dialysate flow, membrane properties, and blood flow
- Complications: Discussed in detail later

CONTINUOUS RENAL REPLACEMENT THERAPY (CRRT)

- Description: Removes venous blood from the patient into an extracorporeal circuit past a membrane to provide diffusion and/or convention, intended to run 24 hours a day
- Advantages: Provides slow, gentle adjustable removal of fluid and waste over time, more precise in reaching solute clearance and ultrafiltration goals than PD
- Indications: Hemodynamically unstable patients, effective in all indications for RRT
- Complications: Discussed in detail later
- Types of CRRT
  - *SCUF (slow continuous ultra-filtration)*: Free water and some small molecule clearance, no replacement fluid or dialysate is typically used
  - *CVVH (continuous veno-venous hemofiltration)*: Convective-based solute clearance that requires replacement fluids
  - *CVVHD (continuous veno-venous hemodialysis)*: Diffusion-based solute clearance, removes small particles down a concentration gradient; minimal convection
  - *CVVHDF (continuous veno-venous hemodiafiltration)*: Both high-grade convection (replacement fluids) and diffusion (dialysate)

INDICATIONS FOR RENAL REPLACEMENT THERAPY

RRT is indicated emergently for any life-threatening changes in fluid, electrolyte, or acid–base balance.

RECOMMENDED INDICATIONS FOR RRT IN CRITICALLY ILL CHILDREN

- Acute kidney injury with or without oliguria
- Toxic ingestion
  - *RRT modality*: IHD is the preferred modality, may need to augment with CRRT to avoid rebound peak plasma levels in specific situations.
  - *Considerations*: The clearance of a drug depends on a sieving coefficient that is determined by molecular weight, charge, volume of distribution, and stoichiometry. Drugs that have a large volume of distribution, such as vancomycin, will take a long time to clear from the body.

$$\text{Seiving coefficient} = \frac{\text{Drug concentration in the filtrate (Cf)}}{\text{Drug concentration in the plasma (Cp)}}$$

The more protein-bound the drug, the harder it is to remove from the blood because of the molecular size of albumin, a large molecule. Using albumin 2 to 4 mg/dL in the dialysate can improve the efficiency of clearing protein-bound drugs.

- Inborn errors of metabolism with hyperammonemia
  - *RRT modality*: CRRT is preferred because of high efficiency and prevents rebound levels as seen after one session of IHD; NOT CLEARED WITH PD
- Severe electrolyte imbalance refractory to medical therapy (hyperkalemia, hypercalcemia, hyperphosphatemia)

- Symptomatic uremia: No longer using a strict numeric threshold to determine need for RRT for uremia
- Fluid overload >10% to 15%: Equates to a positive fluid balance of >100 to 150 mL/kg; or fluid overload resistant to medical management and leading to systemic hypertension, edema, multiorgan failure, and/or cardiovascular instability

CONTROVERSIAL USES OF RRT

RRT has been used for immunomodulation in multiorgan failure due to septic shock. Studies have shown CRRT can remove some inflammatory mediators nonselectively; however, under closer investigation only a small percentage of cytokines is actually removed from plasma due to molecular size and structure. Despite adjusting modalities and filters, there have not been any reports of sustained or significant decreases in plasma cytokine levels using CRRT alone.[2] There are neither supporting data nor current recommendations to use CRRT in children with septic shock without signs of AKI.

WRITING A PRESCRIPTION FOR CONTINUOUS RENAL REPLACEMENT THERAPY

The subspecialty in charge of ordering CRRT fluids, flow rates, and electrolyte composition is institution dependent. Pediatric intensivists are more commonly taking ownership in place of pediatric nephrologists, especially in hospitals where pediatric nephrologists are not available.

BLOOD FLOW RATES

Small-solute prescription is written in terms of volume of either dialysis fluid (diffusion) and/or replacement fluid (convection) as mL/kg/hr in adults or mL/1.73m^2/hr in children. Typical CRRT flow rate is 2 to 2. 5 L/1.73 m^2/hr divided between dialysate and replacement. This requires a blood flow rate of approximately 3 to 5 mL/kg/min.[3] If using CRRT for hyper-ammonemia, the recommended flow rate is much higher at 8 L/1.73 m^2/hr. Flow rates used in CRRT are slower than IHD but can achieve the same daily clearance over 24 hours with less metabolic variation from a single IHD session.

FLUID REMOVAL RATES

If ordering CRRT, it is important to determine the daily fluid balance goal for your patient. When ordering this, divide the daily goal by 24 to obtain the hourly fluid removal goal. The bedside nurse will use this goal to adjust the amount of fluid removed every hour to adjust for large volume medications or blood products. Current recommendations in hemodynamically unstable children are to set the first 24-hour fluid goal at euvolemia and then begin gentle fluid removal over 48 to 72 hours.

DIALYSATE OR REPLACEMENT FLUID COMPOSITION

The primary electrolytes in standard solutions used for RRT are sodium, potassium, calcium, magnesium, chloride, glucose, and bicarbonate or lactate. There are commercially available solutions that differ in terms of electrolyte composition and the inclusion or exclusion of calcium. Electrolytes can be added to these base solutions to tailor the effects of CRRT to custom patient goals (Table 52-1).

- Specific fluid composition considerations:
  - *Bicarbonate versus lactate:* Bicarbonate-based solutions are used for both diffusion and convection and are recommended over lactate-based solutions for patients with AKI and shock.[4] If a patient is acidotic, the highest bicarbonate concentration is ideal as it will provide a higher serum bicarbonate level to buffer the patient's acidosis.

TABLE 52-1   Electrolyte Composition of Commercially Available Solutions Used in Renal Replacement Therapy

Electrolyte	Dialysate Fluids				Replacement Fluids	
	Normocarb[1] 35HF	PrismaSate[2] BK0/3.5	PrismaSate[2] BK2/0	PrismaSate[2] B22GK4/0	ACCUSOL[2] 35	Duosol[3] solutions
Sodium	140	140	140	140	140	136–140
Calcium	0	3.5	0	0	3.5	0–3
Potassium	0	0	2	4	0–4	0–4
Magnesium	1.5	1	1	1.5	1	1–1.5
Chloride	107	109.5	108	120.5	109	109–117
L-lactate	0	3	3	3	0	0
Bicarbonate	35	32	32	22	35	25–35
Glucose (mg/dL)	0	0	110	110	0–100	100
Osmolarity	**283**	**287**	**292**	**296**	**287**	**278–292**

All electrolytes are displayed in mEq/L unless labeled otherwise. 1. Normocarb, Dialysis Solution, Richmond Hills, Ontario Canada; 2. Baxter Medical, Inc., Bannockburn, Illinois; 3. B Braun Medical, Inc., Bethlehem, Pennsylvania.

- ○ *Calcium:* Calcium-free solutions should be chosen if using citrate regional circuit anti-coagulation. This will allow titratable control over the serum calcium level using the separate calcium infusion.
- ○ *Potassium and phosphorous:* If providing RRT to a patient without AKI, repletion of phosphorous will be necessary, as dialysate and filtration fluids do not typically contain any phosphorous. Use of any dialysate without potassium will quickly remove all potassium from the blood and is not recommended.

ANTICOAGULATION

- Heparin versus citrate: Heparin- and citrate-based protocols exist for anticoagulation to avoid circuit and filter clotting. Heparin requires systemic anticoagulation and can infer bleeding and drug-related risks. The current recommendation is to use citrate regional circuit anticoagulation in CRRT unless a contraindication exists, such as severe liver failure or previous citrate toxicity.
- Citrate anticoagulation: When using citrate, calcium levels in the circuit and patient must be carefully monitored. The calcium bound by citrate in the circuit has to be returned to the patient via a continuous infusion of calcium chloride via an additional access point in the circuit after filtration or, if need be, via an additional central line.
  - ○ *Goal levels of calcium*
    - Circuit: 0.2 to 0.4 mmol/L (0.8–1.6 mg/dL)
    - Patient: 1.1 to 1.3 mmol/L (4.4–5.2 mg/dL)[3]
  - ○ *Ordering citrate and calcium infusions*
    - Typical citrate rates are 1.5 times the blood flow rate.
    - Calcium infusion should run at approximately 0.4 times the citrate rate.
    - Flow rates of citrate should start at approximately 50% lower in neonates because hepatic metabolism of citrate is immature in this age group.

TECHNICAL CONSIDERATIONS

- Obtaining venous access: Both intermittent hemodialysis and CRRT require temporary or permanent venous access (Table 52-2). The right internal jugular vein is the preferred site for placement, followed by the femoral veins. The subclavian should be used in emergency settings only. The catheter should be at least 10 to 14 French to allow adequate blood flow rates[3]; children under 30 kg will require smaller catheters based on weight.
- Priming the circuit: The circuit must be filled with a fluid prior to initiation of CRRT. A typical CRRT circuit can hold approximately 120 to 200 mL of fluid. Normal saline is the fluid of choice if the volume in the circuit is a small percentage of the patient's blood volume. If circuit volume represents more than 10% of the patient's blood volume (which

TABLE 52-2	Temporary Dialysis Catheter Sizes Based on Patient Weight and Preferred Insertion Sites		
Weight	**Catheter Size**	**Preferred Vein for Placement**	**Back-up Insertion Sites**
Neonate	Double lumen 7F	Right internal jugular vein	Femoral, external jugular veins
3–6 kg	Double or triple lumen 7F		
6–15 kg	Double lumen 8F		Femoral, left internal jugular, subclavian veins*
15–30 kg	Double lumen 9F		
>30 kg	Double or triple lumen 10–12F		

Use in an emergency only.

is 60–80 mL/kg), packed red blood cells (RBCs) are a more appropriate priming fluid to prevent hypotension and anemia. Depending on the modality of RRT and the type of circuit used, this could affect any patient less than 15 kg.

○ If blood priming, it is important NOT to reinfuse the blood prime into the patient after RRT is complete, or else it can potentiate volume overload and hypertension.

• Temperature of fluids: Ensure all dialysate and replacement fluids are warmed up to 34.5°C to 37.5°C to avoid hemodynamic instability and hypothermia; higher temperature fluids also provide more efficient solute clearance.

CHOOSING THE TIMING, DOSAGE, AND TYPE OF RENAL REPLACEMENT THERAPY

"EARLY" VERSUS "LATE"

Theoretically, initiating RRT prior to the onset of the damaging effects of metabolic derangements like uremia or fluid overload should provide a survival benefit for children requiring RRT. Retrospective adult data supported the use of early RRT and higher filtration rates in septic shock patients and were validated in two prospective randomized controlled trials (RCTs). However, starting RRT before AKI occurs is not recommended, as prophylactic RRT in adults at risk for AKI without evidence of azotemia provided no survival benefit.[2]

Pediatric data have not been as conclusive about when to start RRT, except in cases of fluid overload (FO). The only consistent independent risk factor for mortality in children requiring RRT remains percent fluid overload at the time of RRT initiation.[5] Estimated glomerular filtration rate (GFR), age, weight, urine output, diuretic use, and severity of illness are all not consistently significantly associated with mortality in pediatric patients with AKI on RRT. Data do agree that having FO greater than 10% to 20% from ICU admission to RRT initiation is an independent risk factor for mortality in several disease states, with an adjusted odds ratio of mortality as high as 8.5.[6] Using CRRT to remove fluid after this threshold is passed does not lessen the mortality risk; only starting RRT before it is met does.[1] Being 20% fluid overloaded equates to having a net fluid balance of 200 mL/kg.

$$\text{Percent FO} = \left[\frac{\text{Fluid intake (L)} - \text{Fluid output (L)}}{\text{Weight}} \right] \times 100\%$$

"HIGH DOSE" VERSUS "LOW DOSE"

Two large randomized, multicenter adult studies—the Randomized Evaluation of Normal versus Augmented Level Renal Replacement Therapy (RENAL) Study and the Veterans Administration/ National Institutes of Health Acute Renal Failure Trial Network (ATN) Study—showed no survival or renal recovery benefit from increasing RRT above 20 to 25 mL/kg/hr of effluent flow.[7] Although no prospective pediatric data exist, retrospective data show no outcome improvement associated with CRRT dose.[8] The most recent Kidney Disease: Improving Global Outcomes (KDIGO) international consensus guidelines recommend delivering an effluent volume of 25 mL/kg/hr, which equates to the standard pediatric CRRT flow rate of 2 to 2.5 L/1.73m²/hr.[4]

IHD VERSUS CRRT

In theory, CRRT should provide more gradual solute and fluid removal leading to fewer episodes of renal and gastrointestinal (GI) ischemia to allow for faster recovery and improved survival than IHD. There are consistent data and strong recommendations for CRRT over

IHD in cases of hemodynamic instability and cerebral edema because of avoidance of blood pressure variability and osmotic cellular shifts.[9] Other indications are less clear.

Prospective randomized adult studies suggest that use of IHD is associated with higher mortality than CRRT in critically ill patients. The RENAL and ATN studies also found that renal recovery and mortality were worse in patients receiving IHD versus CRRT even after adjusting for severity and organ-failure scoring.[7] The conclusion of the adult data is that CRRT is the only appropriate strategy in critically ill patients at risk for hemodynamic instability if renal recovery is to be optimized.

Recent advances in technology have changed the choice of RRT modality by pediatric nephrologists from predominantly PD to now most often CRRT. The Prospective Pediatric CRRT Registry provided data that shows that CRRT is safe and feasible in infants less than 10 kg irrespective of disease severity, contrary to initial beliefs. No prospective randomized pediatric studies exist that compare IHD to CRRT; however, in the critical care unit, CRRT is a safe and feasible option with less hemodynamic and metabolic impact and should be considered first in most circumstances.[1] Choice of modality should also include consideration of the comfort of each institution's staff to administer the therapy. CRRT requires extensive resource utilization, knowledge, and comfort, which could overcome its potential benefit in certain clinical situations.

PICU COMPLICATIONS FROM BLOOD-BASED RENAL REPLACEMENT THERAPY

PEDIATRIC RRT OUTCOMES

- Renal Recovery: Use of RRT does not affect potential for recovery of renal function.
- Mortality: Survival rates for critically ill children with AKI receiving RRT have not changed over the last few decades, persisting around 52%. Survival is lower in those receiving PD (49%–64%) and CRRT (34%–58%) than those receiving IHD (73%–89%).[1]

TIMING OF COMPLICATIONS

The risk of complications is greatest at the initiation of CRRT. It is essential for intensive care physicians to be at the bedside when starting CRRT to provide close monitoring of all vital signs, especially blood pressure, heart rate, oxygen saturation, and neurologic status. Rescue doses of calcium and vasopressors may be necessary depending on the stability of the patient.

LIST OF COMPLICATIONS FROM CRRT OR IHD

- Related to catheter placement or maintenance: Infection, bleeding, thrombosis, pneumothorax, and the other complications associated with placement and maintenance of a large-bore central venous catheter
- Hemodynamic instability: Especially upon initiation of CRRT from fluid shifts and inflammatory response
- Disequilibrium syndrome: Only seen in IHD
  - *Mechanism*: If urea is cleared from blood too quickly, it can cause acute cerebral edema and death
- Hypothermia
- Air embolism
- Anaphylaxis
- Hemorrhage
- Leukopenia
- Electrolyte derangements: Most often sodium, phosphorous, and magnesium

- Metabolic alkalosis: Caused by the normal hepatic metabolism of each citrate molecule into three bicarbonate molecules
- Bradykinin release syndrome: Life-threatening allergic-type reaction causing rapid hypotension, rash, wheezing, and bradycardia
  - *Mechanism:* When acidic whole blood (used to prime a circuit or from the patient) comes in contact with a specific type of dialysis circuit, the AN-69, it can cause a massive bradykinin release. This leads to profound hypotension and an anaphylactic reaction.
  - *Timing:* Immediate, <5 minutes
  - *Management:* Treat like anaphylaxis. May be avoided by rinsing the membrane with bicarbonate, increasing the pH of the blood in circuit or patient, or avoiding use of the AN-69 membrane. The AN-69 membrane is specifically used in small patients and in septic shock as it supposedly provides optimal cytokine removal.
- Citrate toxicity (previously "citrate lock")
  - *Mechanism:* Occurs in patients on CRRT when the citrate infusion is not cleared by normal hepatic metabolism. Citrate then binds to free calcium and forms circulating complexes within the blood, raising the total calcium to very high levels. Ionized calcium should stay the same until more citrate accumulates; then is able to bind and it will start to fall. Tetany can result.
  - *Management:* Once total calcium exceeds 11.5 mg/dL, stop or decrease the citrate infusion and increase circuit clearance by higher dialysate or replacement flow rates.
- Rapid clearance of medications
  - *PICU considerations:* Most notably catecholamine infusions used for blood pressure support can be cleared during CRRT.
  - *Management:* May need higher doses of affected medications while on CRRT.
- To assess if medication doses should be adjusted when on CRRT, go to the Dialysis of Drugs Handbook: http://www.seanmeskill.com/DialysisDrugs2010.pdf

REFERENCES

1. Goldstein SL. Continuous renal replacement therapy: Mechanism of clearance, fluid removal, indications and outcomes. *Curr Opin Pediatr.* 2011;23(2):181-185.
2. John S, Eckardt KU. Renal replacement strategies in the ICU. *Chest.* 2007;132(4):1379-1388.
3. Bunchman TE, Brophy PD, Goldstein SL. Technical considerations for renal replacement therapy in children. *Semin Nephrol.* 2008;28(5):488-492.
4. KDIGO Clinical Practice Guideline for Acute Kidney Injury. *Kidney Int Suppl.* 2012;2(1):1-138.
5. Modem V, Thompson M, Gollhofer D, et al. Timing of continuous renal replacement therapy and mortality in critically ill children. *Crit Care Med.* 2014;42(4):943-953.
6. Sutherland SM, Zappitelli M, Alexander SR, et al. Fluid overload and mortality in children receiving continuous renal replacement therapy: The prospective pediatric continuous renal replacement therapy registry. *Am J Kidney Dis.* 2010;55(2):316-325.
7. Glassford NJ, Bellomo R. Acute kidney injury: How can we facilitate recovery? *Curr Opin Crit Care.* 2011;17(6):562-568.
8. Basu RK, Devarajan P, Wong H, et al. An update and review of acute kidney injury in pediatrics. *Pediatr Crit Care Med.* 2011;12(3):339-347.
9. Khwaja A. KDIGO clinical practice guidelines for acute kidney injury. *Nephron Clin Pract.* 2012;120(4):179-184.

END-STAGE KIDNEY DISEASE (ESKD) IN CHILDREN

Definition: Sustained estimated glomerular filtration rate (eGFR) <15 mL/min/1.73 m^2 (chronic kidney disease or CKD stage 5), requiring either dialysis or kidney transplantation (renal replacement therapy).

Causes: Causes of CKD/ESKD in children differ vastly from those in adults. Hypertension and diabetes mellitus, although common causes of ESKD in adults, are exceedingly rare as causes in children. The most common causes of CKD/ESKD in children are:

- Congenital renal anomalies (57%): Obstructive uropathy (21%), renal aplasia/hypoplasia/dysplasia (18%), reflux nephropathy (8%), polycystic kidney disease (4%)
- Glomerular disease (17%—but 45% of patients >12 yr): Focal segmental glomerulosclerosis (FSGS) most common
- Other (25%): Unknown; hemolytic uremic syndrome (HUS); genetic disorders (cystinosis, oxalosis, Alport's syndrome); interstitial nephritis[1]

Kidney transplantation is preferred over dialysis as treatment for ESKD in children, as the risk for death is more than four times higher on dialysis than after kidney transplantation.[2]

TYPES OF KIDNEY TRANSPLANTATION

Preemptive kidney transplantation: "Preemptive" denotes a kidney transplant performed before a patient requires initiation of dialysis therapy. These transplants result in superior long-term outcomes compared to transplants done after starting dialysis.[3] Preemptive transplants can be done with either living or deceased donor kidney grafts. This approach is not possible or recommended for some conditions (e.g., conditions requiring pretransplant nephrectomies, such as persistent nephrotic syndrome, chronic severe pyelonephritis, and malignant renovascular hypertension).

Note: Patients receiving preemptive kidney transplants, by definition, still have adequate urine output via their native kidneys. This makes using urine output by itself as a marker of transplant graft function postoperatively problematic.

Deceased donor kidney transplantation: The organ is obtained by accruing waiting time on the deceased donor/cadaver kidney list. Highly sensitized patients or those listed for multiple organs are given preference on the list. There is also a pediatric advantage for those listed before turning 18 years old.

Living donor kidney transplantation: Related or unrelated living donors donate one kidney after a thorough medical and psychological evaluation process. Living donor transplants in general demonstrate superior long-term outcomes compared to deceased donor kidney transplantation.

CONTRAINDICATIONS TO KIDNEY TRANSPLANTATION

Contraindications to kidney transplant include sepsis, uncontrolled malignancies, irreversible multisystem organ failure not correctable by transplant, and severe cardiac or pulmonary disease that can't be cured by multiorgan transplant. Active underlying disease (e.g., systemic lupus erythematosus [SLE] or anti-GBM antibody disease) is also a contraindication for transplantation.

IMMUNOSUPPRESSION IN PEDIATRIC KIDNEY TRANSPLANT

INDUCTION THERAPY

- Purpose: To prevent T-cell activation in the perioperative period, when risk of acute rejection is highest.
- *IL-2 receptor antibodies/antagonists (basiliximab): Used for most standard-risk first transplant recipients in our center.
- Alemtuzumab (anti-CD52 monoclonal antibody): Depletes T and B lymphocytes, monocytes, natural killer cells. Used for second transplants, higher immunological risk recipients in our center, but used in standard-risk protocols for induction therapy in many adult centers.
- Antilymphocyte globulin (rATG-thymoglobulin): In our center, used more for cellular rejection treatment than for induction therapy, but widely used in many pediatric centers for induction therapy.
- *IV corticosteroids (methylprednisolone): In our center, standard-risk recipients receive only three daily doses of IV steroids, followed by no maintenance steroid treatment. Steroid use varies widely between pediatric transplant centers.

MAINTENANCE THERAPY

- Oral steroids are not typically used for maintenance immunosuppression for most standard-risk kidney transplant recipients in our center (proven benefits in growth and no increase in risk of rejection).[4] Many pediatric centers do still use corticosteroids as part of their standard maintenance immunosuppression protocols.
- *Tacrolimus (FK-506), calcineurin inhibitor (CNI): Binds to calcineurin (cytosolic receptor) to inhibit transcription of several cytokines by activated T cells. Less rejection and less toxicity than with older CNI (cyclosporine). Side effects include nephrotoxicity, neurotoxicity, hypertension, and diabetes mellitus. Trough levels are followed for medication adjustment given variable metabolism and narrow therapeutic index.
- *Mycophenolate mofetil (MMF), antimetabolite: Inhibitor of inosine 5-phosphate dehydrogenase and guanosine monophosphate synthetase to reduce de novo purine synthesis in T and B lymphocytes (inhibits lymphocyte proliferation and antibody production). MMF has largely replaced azathioprine (less bone marrow toxicity). Side effects are dose related and include diarrhea, leukopenia, and anemia.
- Sirolimus (rapamycin) and other mTOR inhibitors: Block proliferation of lymphocytes in response to IL-2. These medications are not frequently used as part of the protocol at our center due to the potential effect of increasing nephrotoxicity of CNIs, as well as possible side effects of hyperlipidemia, poor wound healing, and proteinuria.

*Denotes standard immunosuppression at our center.

PERIOPERATIVE MANAGEMENT OF KIDNEY TRANSPLANT RECIPIENTS**

**This section is center specific. Protocols may differ significantly between transplant centers.
Each kidney transplant candidate who is either scheduled for living donor kidney transplant or who is active on the deceased donor list has an individualized protocol that will be provided to all managing residents and fellows on admission for kidney transplant.

GENERAL PRINCIPLES

Foley catheter drainage is usually maintained for 3 to 7 days postoperatively (depending on urological history) to keep the bladder decompressed and prevent stress on the bladder-to-transplant ureter anastomosis/potential urine leak. At our center, a ureteral stent is left in place due to concern for postoperative edema/obstruction at this anastomosis. The stent is electively removed 4 to 6 weeks after the transplant.

Initial fluid management is with cc:cc urine output (UOP) replacement to keep overall fluid balance even. If hourly urine output is high, lower dextrose fluid is prescribed. Additional fluid boluses may be given for hypotension/low central venous pressure (CVP) or low UOP. Conversely, overall fluid may be limited if delayed graft function (DGF) is suspected and there are concerns for fluid overload, but these decisions should be made in conjunction with the transplant team.

POST-TRANSPLANT COMPLICATIONS

EARLY/IMMEDIATE

- Delayed Graft Function (DGF): Requirement for dialysis or lack of improvement in baseline degree of native kidney failure in the first week post-transplantation. Grafts with delayed function may have lower long-term graft survival rates. Potential causes of DGF include:
  - *Ischemia-reperfusion injury (acute tubular necrosis or ATN):* Most common cause of DGF
  - *Transplant renal artery or vein thrombosis:* Ultrasound (US) with Doppler and/or nuclear renal scan to diagnose; usually an indication for emergent return to operating room. Higher risk in nephrotic patients, significant hypotensive episodes, multiple arteries/complicated or small vasculature.
  - *Urologic abnormalities:* Urinary leak, hematoma, obstruction. Suspicion usually investigated with US.
  - *Hyperacute or accelerated rejection*
  - *Immediate recurrence of focal segmental glomerulosclerosis (FSGS)*

EARLY/ACUTE (1–12 WEEKS POST-TRANSPLANT)

- Acute rejection: Acute cellular (ACR) or antibody-mediated (AMR) rejection
- Calcineurin inhibitor toxicity
- Urinary obstruction
- Hypovolemia/ATN
- Recurrent disease: FSGS (most frequently recurring glomerular disease), membranoproliferative glomerulonephritis, IgA nephropathy, atypical hemolytic uremic syndrome (aHUS), primary hyperoxaluria, SLE (recurrence rare)

LATE/ACUTE (>3 MONTHS)

- Rejection: ACR and/or AMR
- Calcineurin inhibitor toxicity
- Urinary obstruction
- Hypovolemia/ATN
- Infection/pyelonephritis, BK virus nephropathy
- Recurrent or de novo kidney disease

PROGRESSIVE/CHRONIC (>1 YEAR)

- Chronic allograft nephropathy (CAN): Most likely due to chronic rejection/AMR
- Calcineurin inhibitor toxicity
- Viral infections (e.g., BK virus nephropathy)
- Hypertensive nephrosclerosis
- Recurrent or de novo kidney disease

REJECTION

Kidney graft dysfunction without otherwise apparent cause needs to be investigated by kidney graft biopsy. Type of rejection and grading (usually according to Banff criteria) are necessary to determine appropriate treatment.

ACUTE CELLULAR REJECTION (ACR)

- Borderline or less severe grades of ACR may be treated with IV and/or oral steroid bursts.
- More severe ACR is usually treated with steroids + a course of IV thymoglobulin. Such treatment often requires placement of a central line.

ANTIBODY-MEDIATED REJECTION (AMR)

- When AMR is suspected or seen on biopsy (often with presence of peritubular capillaritis and/or positive C4d staining), the recipient's donor-specific antibody (DSA) levels are measured.
- In addition to IV and/or oral steroids, significant AMR is often treated with multiple plasma exchange/plasmapheresis procedures, with the goal of lowering the recipient's level of circulating DSAs. A hemodialysis catheter is required for this therapy, unless the patient still has a functioning arteriovenous (AV) fistula that may be accessed.
- Intravenous immunoglobulin (IVIG) infusions (promote opsonization and clearance of DSAs) and rituximab (depletes B cells that may contribute to DSA production) are also often used in AMR treatment protocols.
- Resistant cases of AMR may be treated with a trial of bortezomib (a proteasome inhibitor that targets plasma cells) therapy.

INFECTION

Infections are the most common cause of hospitalization during the first 2 years post-transplant (exceed hospitalizations for rejection).[5] Whereas urinary tract infections (UTIs) and pulmonary infections are frequent during the early post-transplant period, viral infections become more important later post-transplant.

- Cytomegalovirus (CMV): CMV may cause disease either from primary infection or from reactivation of primary infection. Infection may be asymptomatic or may manifest as fever, cytopenias, hepatitis, pneumonia, or allograft dysfunction. At our center, all seropositive recipients (and seronegative recipients of seropositive allografts) receive 6 to 12 months of valganciclovir prophylaxis.
- Epstein-Barr virus (EBV): EBV primary infection is usually a severe monolike illness. Reactivation of EBV in a seropositive recipient is usually without symptoms. EBV can induce B-cell proliferation in patients on immunosuppression, leading to post-transplant lymphoproliferative disease (PTLD). PTLD can have a spectrum of severity, ranging from mild/polymorphic proliferation limited to tonsillar/lymphoid tissue (may be self-limited or treated with reduction in immunosuppression) to true monomorphic lymphoma requiring chemotherapy and cessation of immunosuppressive therapy.
- BK virus: This polyoma virus takes up latent residency in uroepithelial cells, where it may become reactivated during states of immunosuppression. It can first be detected in the urine by polymerase chain reaction (PCR) and then in the blood when it gets to high enough levels. Higher levels of this viremia are associated with BK nephropathy and graft dysfunction. Treatment is generally with decrease in immunosuppression +/- antiviral therapy (leflunomide, cidofovir). Cidofovir is often reserved for more severe disease, as the

medication itself is nephrotoxic. Kidney transplant recipients are screened regularly for the presence of BK viruria and/or viremia.

- Varicella: Varicella infection in an immunocompromised host can cause severe disease, including encephalitis, hepatitis, pneumonitis, and death. Nonimmune transplant recipients who have a close contact exposure should receive prophylaxis within 72 hours of exposure. Clinical disease should be treated with IV acyclovir. Varicella vaccine is a live virus vaccine and is usually avoided in patients on chronic immunosuppression.
- Herpes simplex virus (HSV): HSV can also cause either primary or reactivation disease. Acyclovir or valacyclovir can be used to treat infection. Severity of infection dictates whether IV or oral therapy may be appropriate.
- Human papillomavirus (HPV): Warts caused by HPV are common in transplant recipients, and immunosuppressed hosts are also at higher risk for malignancy (e.g., cervical cancer) associated with this virus. Vaccination according to the recommended schedule should be strongly encouraged, as this is a nonlive vaccine.

MALIGNANCY

There is an estimated 2.6% to 6% incidence of malignancy following pediatric kidney transplant. The majority (about 80% of these) are PTLD. The reported incidence of non-PTLD malignancies is approximately sevenfold higher than in the general pediatric population.[6] Skin cancers and native renal cell carcinoma are the most common non-PTLD malignancies in transplant survivors. Routine cancer surveillance should be stressed in long-term primary care follow-up of these individuals.

HYPERTENSION

Hypertension is common after kidney transplantation in children, occurring in up to 80%.[7] Potential causes of hypertension after kidney transplant include fluid overload, steroid treatment, calcineurin inhibitor use or toxicity, rejection, transplant renal artery stenosis, or urinary tract obstruction.

ANEMIA

Anemia is also very common, with an incidence of up to 80% as well.[8] Causes are usually multifactorial: iron deficiency, side effects of immunosuppressive therapy, bone disease, declining graft function/relative erythropoietin deficiency.

POST-TRANSPLANT DIABETES MELLITUS (PTDM)

Treatment with calcineurin inhibitors (especially tacrolimus) and steroids increase risk for developing DM after kidney transplantation. The incidence in pediatric patients is increasing and may be up to 7%.[9]

REFERENCES

1. North American Pediatric Renal Transplant Cooperative Study (NAPRTCS): 2010 Annual report. Rockville, MD. http://www.naprtcs.org. Accessed on August 10, 2016.
2. McDonald SP, Craig JC. Long-term survival of children with end-stage renal disease. *N Engl J Med.* 2004; 350:2654-2662.
3. Jay CL, Dean PG, Helmick RA, et al. Reassessing preemptive kidney transplantation in the United States: Are we making progress? *Transplantation.* 2016;100(5):1120-1127.

4. Sarwal MM, Ettenger RB, Dharnidharka V, et al. Complete steroid avoidance is effective and safe in children with renal transplants: A multicenter randomized trial with three-year follow-up. *Am J Transplant.* 2012;12(10):2719-2729.
5. Dharnidharka VR, Stablein DM, Harmon WE. Post-transplant infections now exceed acute rejection as cause of hospitalization: A report of the NAPRTCS. *Am J Transplant.* 2004;4:384-389.
6. Smith JM, Martz K, McDonald RA, et al. Solid tumors following kidney transplantation in children. *Pediatr Transplant.* 2013;17:726-730.
7. Seeman T. Ambulatory blood pressure monitoring in pediatric renal transplantation. *Curr Hypertens Rep.* 2012;14(6):608-618.
8. Yorgin PD, Belson A, Sanchez J, et al. Unexpectedly high prevalence of posttransplant anemia in pediatric and young adult renal transplant recipients. *Am J Kidney Dis.* 2002;40:1306-1318.
9. Burroughs TE, Swindle JP, Salvalaggio PR, et al. Increasing incidence of new-onset diabetes after transplant among pediatric renal transplant patients. *Transplantation.* 2009;88:367-373.

Hematology/Oncology

Blood Products

The purpose of this chapter is to describe the components of various blood products, indications for transfusions, and complications of transfusion.

TRANSFUSION OF PACKED RED BLOOD CELLS (pRBCs) IN CRITICALLY ILL CHILDREN

OVERVIEW

- pRBCs are red blood cells obtained from donation of whole blood. Most of the plasma and platelets are removed prior to storage, and units of blood are further processed to either reduce or remove leukocytes to decrease the likelihood of leukocyte alloimmunization causing febrile nonhemolytic transfusion reactions (FNHTRs).
- Preservatives, nutrients, and anticoagulants are added to units of pRBCs to ensure a long shelf-life (up to 42–45 days).

TRANSFUSION

- The average pediatric blood volume is estimated to be approximately 80 cc/kg body weight.
- The amount of blood to be given in acute anemia can be calculated using the following formula; for example, assuming that the hematocrit of the unit of pRBCs is 60% or 0.6, the volume to be transfused is:

$$\text{Volume of pRBCs} = \text{Weight(kg)} \times \text{increment desired(g/dL hemoglobin)} \times 3/0.6$$

- In general, transfusion of 1 unit of pRBCs is expected to raise the hemoglobin by approximately 1 g/dL and the hematocrit by 3% in adult patients.
- **Special preparations of pRBCs**
  ○ **Irradiated blood** – to prevent transfusion-associated graft versus host disease (TA-GVHD), a life-threatening condition caused by donor leukocytes. Consider using irradiated blood in immunocompromised states or if directed donor blood (blood donated from relative), such as when transfusing a neonate, in stem cell transplant patients, patients with leukemia, lymphoma, T-cell immunodeficiency, aplastic anemia, or myelodysplastic syndromes. Irradiated blood will have a shorter shelf-life.
  ○ **Washed pRBCs** – use if patient has hyperkalemia or renal failure (to reduce potassium levels) or if known allergic reaction to blood for additional leukocyte and plasma protein reduction (not including febrile reactions to transfusion).
- **Indications for transfusion of pRBCs:**
  ○ Anemia
    ▪ Severe anemia is defined by a hemoglobin less than 5 g/dL even if the patient is asymptomatic and would likely benefit from transfusion.
    ▪ If symptomatic anemia but stable hemodynamics (defined as not having a need for inotropic support, fluid resuscitation, or a mean arterial pressure less than 2 SD below the normal mean for age), consider transfusing prior to reaching a hemoglobin of 5 g/dL. There is no standard threshold at which to transfuse, however one randomized controlled trial performed in 19 tertiary care PICUs, the TRIPICU study, demonstrated that outcomes such as new or progressive organ dysfunction, transfusion reactions, or ICU length of stay were not worse in symptomatic, anemic patients if transfusion was held until the patient had a hemoglobin of 7 g/dL or less.

- If symptomatic anemia and unstable hemodynamics, consider transfusion earlier.
- If transfusing for severe, chronic anemia, consider transfusing in small aliquots (for example, if a hemoglobin of 4 g/dL, some centers transfuse 4 cc/kg of pRBCs over 4 hours followed by a repeat hemoglobin check and additional transfusions) to avoid precipitating heart failure in a patient with a presumed high output state (see Table 54-1).
  - Sepsis
    - Data regarding whether higher hemoglobin thresholds should be targeted in children with sepsis is not definitive. Clinical trials in both children and adults indicate that outcomes were not worse when transfused at a threshold hemoglobin value of 7 g/dL.
  - Cyanotic heart disease
    - No definitive threshold recommended; however, one small randomized controlled trial in single-ventricle patients found no significant difference in mortality or lactate levels if a threshold of 9 g/dL was used compared to those transfused at a higher threshold; however, higher levels of oxygen extraction were found in the restrictive group.

TABLE 54-1 Transfusion Reactions	
Transfusion Reaction	**Clinical Manifestation**
Acute hemolytic transfusion reaction (AHTR)	• Usually from transfusion of antigen-positive RBCs to a recipient with the corresponding antibodies (ex: ABO incompatibility). Hemolysis, activation of inflammatory cascade, DIC occur.
	• Patient may develop hypotension/shock, kidney injury, hypoxia.
Transfusion-related acute lung injury (TRALI)	• New-onset acute lung injury within 6 hours of transfusion with either hypoxemia or PaO_2:FiO_2 <300.
	• Occurs with introduction of human leukocyte antigen (HLA) antibodies or human neutrophil antigens from donor → activation of neutrophils in lung → endothelial damage and pulmonary capillary leak.
Transfusion-associated circulatory overload (TACO)	• New-onset signs and symptoms of acute or worsening respiratory distress or congestive heart failure, including dyspnea, orthopnea, cyanosis, and pulmonary edema manifesting within 6 hours of transfusion.
	• Due to receipt of large volumes of blood in chronically anemic patient or patient with low cardiac reserve.
Febrile nonhemolytic transfusion reaction (FNHTR)	• Fever to 100.4°F or an increase by 1.8°F from start of transfusion.
	• Due to passive transfer of inflammatory mediators like cytokines during transfusion.
	• Less common with leukoreduction.
Transfusion-associated graft versus host disease (TA-GVHD)	• Occurs in patients with transfusion of donor T lymphocytes with HLA that is similar to recipient's (first-degree relative) or if recipient is immunocompromised, allowing proliferation of lymphocytes.
	• Occurs within 2 weeks of transfusion.
	• Symptoms include fever, rash, cholestasis, emesis, pancytopenia.
	• May be prevented through irradiation of blood products for high-risk patients.
	• Mortality rate is high.

TRANSFUSION OF PLATELETS IN CRITICALLY ILL CHILDREN

- Platelets come in two forms: platelet concentrate (PC) and single-donor apheresis platelets. Volumes of platelets range with 1 unit of PC equaling approximately 50 to 70 mL and 1 unit of apheresis platelets equaling approximately 200 to 400 mL.
- Dosing is usually 5 to 10 cc/kg or 1 unit of PC for every 10 kg of body weight.
- Transfusing 5 to 10 cc/kg of platelets in pediatrics is estimated to increase platelet count by 50,000 to 100,000/μL, whereas transfusing 1 unit of apheresis platelets in adults should increase the platelet count by 30,000 to 60,000/μL
- PC is made from 1 unit of whole blood, whereas apheresis platelets are from a single donor.
- Indications for platelet transfusion follow, though are mostly based on adult-related literature.
  - Patients with severe thrombocytopenia are at increased risk of bleeding (platelet count <10,000/μL in most patients; some recommend a threshold of 20,000/μL in neonates, 30,000–50,000 if less than 1 week of age and birth weight <1,000 grams).
  - Many recommend transfusing at platelet counts >10,000/μL if placing a central venous catheter, performing a lumbar puncture, and performing other surgical procedures.
  - Patients in whom to avoid transfusing platelets if possible: those with thrombotic thrombocytopenia purpura (TTP) and heparin-induced thrombocytopenia (HIT), as platelet transfusion may precipitate additional thrombosis.

TRANSFUSION OF FRESH FROZEN PLASMA (FFP) IN CRITICALLY ILL CHILDREN

- Plasma is a component of whole blood that is removed and frozen within 6 to 8 hours of collection for storage. It contains all the coagulation factors as well as additional proteins such as albumin, fibrinogen, immunoglobulins, and transferrin.
- Plasma can be transfused up to 5 weeks after thawing, though labile factors V and VIII activity will be reduced. Transfused plasma must be ABO compatible.
- Dosing is generally based on weight in the pediatric patient (10–15 cc/kg) and is estimated to increase factor levels between 10% and 15%. However, to replace specific factors, dosing is often based on factor levels present and can require much larger than standard volumes of plasma to replenish these.
- Indications for transfusion of plasma:
  - Patients with coagulation disorders, including those with antithrombin III deficiency
  - Patients with factor deficiencies where specific factor concentrates are not available (such as factor V deficiency)
  - Patients with active bleeding
  - Patients with an international normalized ratio (INR) >2 (>1.5 in neurosurgical patients) are often transfused plasma at certain institutions, even if not bleeding
  - Reversal of warfarin therapy only if clinically evident bleeding in order to replace the vitamin K–dependent coagulation factors (factors II, VII, IX, and X)
  - TTP in order to replace the metalloprotease ADAMTS13 that cleaves von Willebrand factor
  - There is little evidence to support the prophylactic transfusion of FFP for invasive procedures in patients with severe liver disease, who may have defects in coagulation factor synthesis

TRANSFUSION OF CRYOPRECIPITATE IN CRITICALLY ILL CHILDREN

- Cryoprecipitate is the precipitate rich in fibrinogen, factor VIII, von Willebrand factor, fibronectin, and factor XIII obtained from the process of fast-freezing plasma. These are all found in greater concentration in cryoprecipitate compared to plasma.

- Cryoprecipitate does not need to be ABO compatible except in the neonatal population.
- Dosing: In adults, 1 unit of cryoprecipitate will increase fibrinogen by approximately 5 to 10 mg/dL, and often adults are given 10 units at a time. In pediatrics, the dose varies, and some centers recommend 5 to 10 cc/kg or 1 to 2 units per 7 to 10 kg of body weight.
- Indications for cryoprecipitate:
  - Fibrinogen replacement that often results from hemorrhage or disseminated intravascular coagulation (DIC).

COMPLICATIONS OF TRANSFUSION

- Transmission of infections. The incidence of this has been greatly reduced with enhanced screening of blood products in the United States prior to transfusion. For example, the risk of acquiring HIV from transfused blood is greater than 1 in 2 million; hepatitis B, approximately 1 in 350,000; and hepatitis C, 1 in approximately 2 million.
- Examples of noninfectious transfusion reactions are in Table 54-1.

INDICATIONS FOR APHERESIS IN CRITICALLY ILL CHILDREN

Apheresis is the process of separating a component of whole blood (such as platelets, plasma, or leukocytes) and retransfusion of the remaining components that were not removed.

INDICATIONS FOR APHERESIS

- **Plasmapheresis**: Because plasma contains immunoglobulins, plasmapheresis is indicated for several antibody-mediated conditions, though most patients will receive plasma exchange therapy by which the patient's plasma with the suspected offending antibodies is removed and the patient receives fresh frozen plasma to replace components lost through the apheresis process.
  - Conditions for therapeutic plasma exchange include (but are not limited to) TTP or atypical hemolytic-uremic syndrome (HUS), myasthenia gravis, Guillain-Barré syndrome, and Goodpasture's syndrome. Also certain types of antibody-mediated rejection of transplanted organs.
- **Red cell apheresis**:
  - Serious events related to sickle cell disease remain the most common disease for which red cell apheresis is performed. Examples include stroke, acute multiorgan failure, acute chest syndrome, acute hepatic sequestration, and progressive intrahepatic cholestasis.
  - Apheresis has some advantages compared to manual exchange transfusions, including speed and prevention of iron overload from chronic transfusions.
  - Some case reports have shown that red cell apheresis in patients with malaria with significant parasite burden may provide benefit.
  - Hyperviscosity syndromes (such as polycythemia vera) to lower hematocrit.
- **Leukapheresis**:
  - Treatment of hyperleukocytosis, such as with certain types of leukemia or myeloproliferative disorders.

SUGGESTED READINGS

Basu D, Kulkarni R. Overview of blood components and their preparation. *Indian J Anaesth.* 2014;58(5):529-537.

Dasararaju R, Marques MB. Adverse effects of transfusion. *Cancer Control.* 2015;22(1):16-25.

Holst LB, Haase N, Wetterslev J, et al. Lower versus higher hemoglobin threshold for transfusion in septic shock. *N Engl J Med.* 2014;371(15):1381-1391.

Karam O, Tucci M, Bateman ST, et al. Association between length of storage of red blood cell units and outcome of critically ill children: A prospective observational study. *Crit Care*. 2010;14(2):R57.

Karam O, Tucci M, Ducruet T, et al. Red blood cell transfusion thresholds in pediatric patients with sepsis. *Pediatr Crit Care Med*. 2011;12(5):512-518.

Kaufman RM, Djulbegovic B, Gernsheimer T, et al. Platelet transfusion: A clinical practice guideline from the AABB. *Ann Intern Med*. 2015;162(3):205-213.

Klein H. G. and Anstee D. J. (eds) (2014) The Transfusion of Platelets, Leucocytes, Haematopoietic Progenitor Cells and Plasma Components, in Mollison's Blood Transfusion in Clinical Medicine, Twelfth Edition, John Wiley & Sons, Ltd, Oxford, UK. doi: 10.1002/9781118689943.ch14.

Lacroix J, Hebert PC, Hutchison JS, et al. Transfusion strategies for patients in pediatric intensive care units. *N Engl J Med*. 2007;356(16):1609-1619.

Szczepiorkowski ZM, Dunbar NM. Transfusion guidelines: When to transfuse. *Hematology Am Soc Hematol Educ Program*. 2013;2013(1):638-644.

Willems A, Harrington K, Lacroix J, et al. Comparison of two red-cell transfusion strategies after pediatric cardiac surgery: A subgroup analysis. *Crit Care Med*. 2010;38(2):649-656.

Yazer MH, Podlosky L, Clarke G, et al. The effect of prestorage WBC reduction on the rates of febrile nonhemolytic transfusion reactions to platelet concentrates and RBC. *Transfusion*. 2004;44(1):10-15.

Coagulation Disorders

55

COAGULATION OVERVIEW

DAMAGE TO VESSEL ENDOTHELIUM ACTIVATES COAGULATION

- Platelets: form the primary platelet plug (primary hemostasis) and help regulate coagulation.
  - *Platelet activation:* initiated by the presence of tissue factor (TF).
    - Platelets adhere to the activated endothelium, aggregate, and provide a surface for clot formation.
- Coagulation cascade: ends with fibrin strand formation, which produces a reinforced cross-linked platelet clot (secondary hemostasis).
  - *Intrinsic pathway:* Activation of factor XII is the first step in the intrinsic pathway.
  - *Extrinsic pathway:* Activation of factor VII, along with presence of TF, is the first step in the extrinsic pathway.
  - *Common pathway:* Activation of factor X then leads to activation of factor II (prothrombin) to factor IIa (thrombin) and finally fibrin formation from fibrinogen. This results in the formation of a cross-linked fibrin clot.

THE MANAGEMENT OF PATIENTS WITH SUSPECTED COAGULATION DISORDERS

DETAILED PATIENT HISTORY

- History of prolonged or excessive bleeding
- History of recurrent or severe thrombosis
  - Deep venous thrombosis (DVT)
  - Pulmonary embolus (PE)
  - Stroke
  - Myocardial infarction (MI)
- History of severe bruising/hematoma formation
- History of hemarthrosis
- History of spontaneous mucous membrane bleeding
- History of prolonged bleeding after surgeries
- History of heavy menses
- Medication history
- Family history of hypercoagulable conditions

PHYSICAL EXAMINATION

- Location of the process: diffuse vs. localized
- Signs of thrombosis: arterial vs. venous
- Depth: superficial (mucocutaneous) vs. deep (intra-articular)
- Presence of splenomegaly: splenic sequestration vs. underlying liver disease vs. marrow infiltration
- Presence of liver disease: varices vs. ascites

LABORATORY TESTS

- Platelet count
- Prothrombin time (PT)

- Activated partial thromboplastin time (aPTT)
- Thrombin time (TT)
- Fibrinogen level
- Fibrin degradation products (FDPs)
- D-dimer
- Platelet and erythrocyte morphology

CONDITIONS ASSOCIATED WITH SERIOUS BLEEDING

DISSEMINATED INTRAVASCULAR COAGULATION (DIC)

- Definition: Imbalance between coagulation and fibrinolysis (either may dominate)
  - Abnormal activation of coagulation (due to TF release)
  - Excessive thrombin generation
  - Excessive fibrin thrombi
  - Eventual consumption of clotting factors and platelets (leads to bleeding)
- Laboratory findings:
  - Prolonged PT, aPTT, TT
  - Decreased fibrinogen and platelets
  - Decreased factors V, VIII, and II (later)
  - Positive D-dimer
- Underlying conditions associated with DIC:
  - Sepsis
  - Multiple organ dysfunction syndrome (MODS)
  - Acute respiratory distress syndrome (ARDS)
  - Liver disease
  - Shock
  - Multiple trauma
  - Penetrating brain injury
  - Necrotizing pneumonitis
  - Tissue necrosis/crush injury
  - Intravascular hemolysis
  - Thermal injury
  - Freshwater drowning
  - Fat embolism syndrome
- Treatment: Treat underlying condition
  - Supportive therapy with blood products to stop bleeding:
    - Packed red blood cells (pRBCs)
      - Dose: 10 to 15 mL/kg
      - Pediatric blood volume is approximately 80 mL/kg
    - Cryoprecipitate: higher fibrinogen content than fresh frozen plasma (FFP) or whole blood; aim to increase fibrinogen level ≥ 100 mg/dL
      - 1 bag of cryoprecipitate per 10 kg body weight, every 8 to 12 hours
    - FFP:
      - Dose: 10 to 15 mL/kg
    - Platelets: maintain platelet counts up to 40,000 to 80,000/mcL of blood
  - Recombinant activated factor VII: indicated during trauma or surgical cases and during severe life-threatening hemorrhage that is refractory to other therapies
    - Increased risk for thrombotic events

LIVER DISEASE

- Etiology: Multifactorial; causes a decrease in synthetic liver function and production of factors II, V, VII, IX, and X
- Early laboratory findings:
  - ○ *Prolonged PT*
  - ○ *Decreased factor VII (occurs first due to its short half-life)*
- Late laboratory findings:
  - ○ Prolonged PT, aPTT
  - ○ Decreased factors II, V, VII, IX, and X
  - ○ Decreased fibrinogen in terminal liver failure
  - ○ Normal platelet count if no splenomegaly/splenic sequestration
  - ○ Normal factor VIII (produced by endothelial cells) and von Willebrand factor (vWF)
- Treatment:
  - ○ No therapy required if patient is not bleeding
  - ○ If bleeding:
    - ▪ Administer vitamin K
    - ▪ Administer FFP until bleeding significantly decreases
      - • Intermittently (10 mL/kg every 6–8 hours)
      - • Continuous infusion (starting at 2–4 mL/kg/hr)
    - ▪ Administer cryoprecipitate to goal fibrinogen levels >100 mg/dL
    - ▪ Transfuse platelets to improve thrombocytopenia (platelets >50,000/mcL of blood)
    - ▪ Consider recombinant activated factor VII if life-threatening hemorrhage
    - ▪ Transfuse pRBCs to maintain hemodynamics and oxygen-carrying capacity
- Other important facts:
  - ○ Portal hypertension–induced esophageal varices puts patients at an increased risk of hemorrhage

VITAMIN K DEFICIENCY

- Etiology:
  - ○ Antibiotics
  - ○ Poor nutrition in the PICU
  - ○ Newborns (failure to receive vitamin K at birth)
  - ○ Medications that interfere with vitamin K activity
  - ○ Fat malabsorption (i.e., cystic fibrosis)
- Pathophysiology: vitamin K needed for γ-carboxylation of factors II, VII, IX, and X
- Laboratory findings:
  - ○ Prolonged PT
  - ○ Normal fibrinogen level, platelet count, and factor V
- Treatment:
  - ○ Administration of vitamin K: 1 to 5 mg (subcutaneous or intravenous)
  - ○ If patient actively bleeding, administration of FFP (10–15 mL/kg)

HEPARIN OVERDOSE

- Forms:
  - ○ Unfractionated heparin (UH): interacts with antithrombin III (AT-III) to decrease clot formation by inactivating thrombin
    - ▪ Works immediately
    - ▪ Monitor effects by following aPTT

- Low-molecular-weight heparin (LMWH): inhibition of activated factor Xa
  - Longer half-life (3–5 hours) than UH
  - Monitor effects by following anti-Xa assay
- Laboratory findings:
  - Prolonged aPTT, TT
  - +/− Prolonged PT
- Management:
  - No intervention if patient doesn't have significant bleeding
  - Significant bleeding:
    - Protamine sulfate: 1 mg neutralizes ~100 units of UH; given IV *slowly* over 8 to 10 minutes

WARFARIN OVERDOSE

- Etiology:
  - Medications that enhance warfarin's effects: antibiotics, azole antifungals, metronidazole, trimethoprim-sulfamethoxazole, steroids, phenytoin, thyroxine
  - Hepatic dysfunction: warfarin is metabolized by the liver
- Pathophysiology:
  - Warfarin causes competitive inhibition of vitamin K epoxide reductase (necessary to regenerate the reduced form of vitamin K)
  - Causes depletion of vitamin K–dependent factors
- Laboratory findings:
  - Prolonged PT, INR
  - +/− Prolonged aPTT if severe enough
  - Vitamin K–dependent factors (II, VII, IX, X) decreased
  - Factors V, VIII normal
  - Normal TT, fibrinogen, and platelets
- Management:
  - Administration of vitamin K
  - If patient actively bleeding, administration of FFP (10–15 mL/kg) or recombinant activated factor VII for life-threatening hemorrhage

MASSIVE TRANSFUSION SYNDROME

- Etiology:
  - Administration of multiple blood transfusions (pRBC only) without also giving FFP and platelets
  - Leads to dilution of plasma coagulation proteins and platelets
  - Causes a "washout syndrome" and coagulopathy
- Laboratory findings:
  - Prolonged PT, aPTT, and TT
  - Decreased fibrinogen and platelets
- Management:
  - Supportive: correct electrolyte abnormalities (hypocalcemia, hyperkalemia/hypokalemia, acidosis) and hypothermia
  - Identify high-risk patients early: transfuse platelets and FFP prior to progression of coagulopathy in an appropriate ratio to pRBCs given

PLATELET DISORDERS

- Quantitative platelet disorders (thrombocytopenia): decreased number of platelets due to either increased destruction in the peripheral blood or decreased production by the bone marrow.

- ○ Sepsis
- ○ Immune thrombocytopenia (ITP):
  - ▪ Antibodies against platelet antigens
  - ▪ Treat with corticosteroids and IVIG
- ○ TTP/HUS: See later
- ○ Drugs: heparin, sulfonamides, vancomycin, cephalosporins, valproic acid, chemotherapy, thiazide diuretics (usually reversible after drug is discontinued)
- ○ Mechanical destruction: cardiopulmonary bypass (CPB)
- ○ Viral illnesses: cytomegalovirus (CMV), Epstein-Barr virus (EBV), herpes simplex, parvovirus, etc.
- ○ Splenic sequestration
- ○ DIC
- ○ Dilution
- • Qualitative platelet disorders: impaired platelet function
  - ○ Anti-inflammatory agents:
    - ▪ Aspirin (irreversible)
    - ▪ Nonsteroidal anti-inflammatory drugs (NSAIDS) (reversible within 24 hours)
    - ▪ Corticosteroids
  - ○ Antibiotics: especially β-lactam antibiotics (reversible)
  - ○ Phosphodiesterase inhibitors: (methylxanthines – theophylline), dipyridamole
  - ○ Furosemide
  - ○ Heparin
  - ○ α-blockers: phentolamine
  - ○ β-blockers: propranolol
  - ○ Tricyclic antidepressants
  - ○ Nitrates: sodium nitroprusside, nitroglycerin
  - ○ Stored whole blood
  - ○ DIC
  - ○ Hypothyroidism
  - ○ Uremia: usually reversible
- • Management:
  - ○ Removal or substitution of offending medication, if possible
  - ○ Platelet transfusion usually not recommended

MICROANGIOPATHIES WITH MICROVASCULAR THROMBOSIS

HEMOLYTIC UREMIC SYNDROME (HUS)

- • Definition: a multisystem disease; classic triad of symptoms, including
  - ○ GI dysfunction: diarrhea (often bloody) +/− colitis, intussusception, bowel perforation/acute abdomen AND
  - ○ Hemolytic anemia
  - ○ Thrombocytopenia
  - ○ Acute renal injury/oliguria
- • Etiology: often caused by strains of *Escherichia coli* (O157:H7) or *Shigella* (shigatoxin induced)
- • Laboratory tests:
  - ○ Hemolytic anemia with microangiopathy
  - ○ +/− Thrombocytopenia
  - ○ Usually normal PT, aPTT
  - ○ Renal insufficiency

- Treatment:
  - Supportive
  - +/− Renal replacement therapy (RRT)

THROMBOTIC THROMBOCYTOPENIC PURPURA (TTP)

- Definition:
  - Hemolytic anemia with microangiopathy
  - Thrombocytopenia
  - Fever
  - Renal dysfunction
  - Neurological symptoms
- Etiology: absence or deficiency of the von Willebrand factor–cleaving protease ADAMTS-13 (normally cleaves vWF).
  - Inherited
  - Acquired: inhibitory autoantibodies against ADAMTS-13
- Laboratory tests:
  - Thrombocytopenia
  - Mild anemia with microangiopathy
  - ADAMTS-13 deficiency
  - Normal/slightly abnormal PT, aPTT, fibrinogen
- Treatment: plasma exchange by apheresis
  - Replaces plasma ADAMTS-13 and removes inhibitory antibodies from circulation
  - +/− steroids
  - Platelet administration not advised due to increased risk of thrombosis

THROMBOCYTOPENIA-ASSOCIATED MULTIPLE ORGAN FAILURE (TAMOF)

- Etiology: decrease in ADAMTS-13 in patients with sepsis; similar clinical picture to TTP
- Treatment: plasma exchange by apheresis

THROMBOTIC SYNDROMES

INHERITED CONDITIONS

- Protein C deficiency:
  - Vitamin K–dependent protein
  - Protein C normally cleaves activated factors V and VIII
- Protein S deficiency:
  - Vitamin K–dependent cofactor for protein C
  - Normally cleaves activated factors V and VIII
- Antithrombin III (AT-III) deficiency:
  - Inherited
  - Acquired: hepatic failure, nephrotic syndrome, shock, DIC, ECMO
  - Normally AT-III activity is enhanced by heparin
- Factor V Leiden mutation: activated protein C (APC) resistance
- Congenital heart disease:
  - Polycythemia, sluggish blood flow, and qualitative platelet defect

ACQUIRED CONDITIONS/RISK FACTORS

- Central venous line (CVL)–associated thrombosis/deep venous thrombosis
  - Indwelling catheter: most common acquired risk factor for thrombotic events

- Pulmonary embolism (PE)
- Coronary thrombosis/acute myocardial infarction
- Cerebral venous thrombosis/stroke
  - Dehydration is primary cause
- Congenital heart disease
- Atrial fibrillation
- Autoimmune disease
- Nephrotic syndrome
  - Due to factor IX and AT- III deficiency
- Leukemia and chemotherapy
  - Hyperviscosity, hyperleukocytosis, inflammation, infection
  - Decreased AT-III level by L-asparaginase
- Hemoglobinopathies
- Trauma
- Shock
  - Hypovolemia, dehydration
- Prolonged immobilization (>5 days)
- Morbid obesity
- TTP/HUS
- Heparin-induced thrombocytopenia (HIT)

MANAGEMENT

- Anticoagulation: initiation of UH or LMWH therapy
  - Thrombolytic therapy: not recommended as first-line treatment in uncomplicated venous thrombosis; consult hematology/oncology prior to initiation
- Monitoring: follow aPTT or anti-Xa level, respectively
- Thromboprophylaxis: no consensus for thromboprophylaxis in children
  - Pneumatic compression devices: postpubertal PICU patients with >1 to 2 days of immobility
  - LMWH: routine use not recommended

SELECTED DISORDERS

- Systemic diseases associated with factor deficiencies
  - Hemophilia A: factor VIII deficiency
  - Hemophilia B: factor IX deficiency

SUGGESTED READINGS

McCrory MC, Brady KM, Takemoto CM, Easley RB. Hematologic emergencies. In David G. Nichols and Donald H. Shaffner: *Rogers' Textbook of Pediatric Intensive Care*. 5th ed., Kindle ed., Philadelphia, PA: Lippincott Williams & Wilkins, a Wolters Kluwer business; 2016.

Parker RI, Nichols DG. Coagulation issues in the PICU. In David G. Nichols and Donald H. Shaffner: *Rogers' Textbook of Pediatric Intensive Care*. 5th ed. Kindle ed., Philadelphia, PA: Lippincott Williams & Wilkins, a Wolters Kluwer business; 2016.

56   Sickle Cell Anemia

MOLECULAR DESCRIPTION

NORMAL ADULT HEMOGLOBIN STRUCTURE

- Hemoglobin A (Hb A): A protein tetramer composed of two α and two β chains. Each chain contains:
  - *An iron-containing heme group* = binds oxygen
    - Identical in each chain
  - *A globin chain* = amino acid sequence
    - Variable in each chain

SICKLE CELL HEMOGLOBIN STRUCTURE

- Hemoglobin S (Hb S): Mutation in the adult β-globin chain allele, which replaces valine (hydrophobic) for glutamine/glutamic acid (hydrophilic) at the position of the sixth amino acid.
- Sickle cell anemia (SCA): Patients possess two abnormal β-globin chain alleles (homozygous) of the hemoglobin molecule (Hb SS).
- Sickle cell trait (SCT): Patients possess one normal and one abnormal β-globin chain allele (heterozygous) of the hemoglobin molecule (Hb AS).

INHERITANCE PATTERN

- Autosomal recessive

SICKLE CELL DISEASE (SCD) PHENOTYPE

PRODUCTION OF SICKLED ERYTHROCYTES

- Hemoglobin deoxygenation and polymerization:
  - Exposure to deoxyhemoglobin increases Hb S polymerization and causes it to take on the classic sickle shape.
  - Increased Hb S polymerization the longer the erythrocyte is exposed to a deoxygenated, cold, and acidic environment.
  - Irreversible polymerization leads to decreased erythrocyte flexibility.

EFFECTS OF SICKLED ERYTHROCYTES ON THE BODY

- The increased Hb S polymerization and sickle cell formation leads to:
  - Chronic hemolysis
  - Recurrent vascular occlusions
  - Painful crises
  - Ischemic end-organ injury (chronic)
  - Acute life-threatening manifestations of the disease
  - Chronic organ dysfunction

PATHOPHYSIOLOGY OF SICKLE CELL COMPLICATIONS

INTERACTION BETWEEN ABNORMAL HEMOGLOBIN AND THE CIRCULATORY SYSTEM

- Erythrocytes:
  - *The abnormal β-globin allele causes:*
    - Accelerated breakdown of oxygenated hemoglobin

- Decreased solubility of deoxygenated hemoglobin
  - *Accumulation of Hb S causes:*
    - Polymerization of Hb S
    - Precipitation of deoxygenated Hb S
    - Formation of an erythrocyte-deforming gel
  - *Erythrocyte cell membrane damage causes:*
    - Loss of membrane flexibility
    - Inability of erythrocyte to traverse capillary beds
    - Ischemic injury
  - *Depletion of erythrocyte glutathione can lead to:*
    - Increase in erythrocyte hemolysis
    - Increased risk of developing pulmonary hypertension.
- Hemoglobin:
  - *Accelerated destruction of the globin chain causes:*
    - Increased oxidation of iron to the ferric state
    - Increased generation of superoxide, hydrogen peroxide, and hydroxyl radical, increasing oxidative injury
    - Disruption of normal phospholipid membrane structure
    - Increased mean corpuscular hemoglobin concentration (MCHC)
- Endothelium:
  - There is an amplified expression of cell surface adhesion molecules that increase vascular inflammation, including vascular cell adhesion molecule-1 (VCAM-1), intercellular adhesion molecule-1 (ICAM-1), E-selectin, and P-selectin
  - Activated endothelial cells promote thrombosis and vasculopathy via increased affinity for interactions with abnormal erythrocytes, activated leukocytes, hemostatic pathway, and activated platelets
- Leukocytes:
  - Vascular injury in SCD due to leukocyte adhering to endothelial cells and causing release of destructive proteolytic enzymes
- Platelets:
  - Platelet activation is prominent.
  - Platelets are in a chronic state of heightened activity.
  - Platelets have a shortened life span due to rapid destruction and increased turnover.
- Coagulation cascade:
  - *Increased risk of vascular thrombosis due to:*
    - Inhibition of VWF protease ADAMTS-13
    - Enhanced thrombin generation
    - Reduced protein C + S activity
    - Decreased factor V
    - Increased factor VIII
    - Decreased plasminogen levels
    - Shorter thrombin times
    - Higher serum fibrinogen degradation products (FDPs)
- Nitric oxide (NO) scavenging:
  - *There is decreased availability of NO:*
    - Interaction between free hemoglobin released from erythrocytes and NO, producing nitrate.
    - Causes diminished NO-mediated vasodilation of tissue beds, stimulating vasoconstriction, ischemia, and further erythrocyte sickling

COMMON ACUTE COMPLICATIONS OF SICKLE CELL ANEMIA

VASO-OCCLUSIVE CRISIS

- Definition: Intermittent episodes of vascular occlusion leading to tissue ischemia, reperfusion injury, and variable degrees of hemolysis leading to multiorgan dysfunction.
  - Most common reason for hospital admission
  - Usually does not require PICU admission
- Treatment: Supportive
  - Aggressive hydration
    - 1.5 times maintenance rate
  - Pain management/control
    - Acetaminophen
    - Nonsteroidal anti-inflammatory drugs (NSAIDS)
      - Ibuprofen
      - Ketorolac
    - Opioid medications
      - Intermittent dosing
      - Patient-controlled analgesia
    - Regional anesthesia techniques
  - Supplemental oxygen
  - Treat underlying cause
    - Pain
    - Infection (antibiotics)
  - Incentive spirometer
    - Encourage every 2 hours while awake

ACUTE CHEST SYNDROME

- Definition: Clinical syndrome characterized by
  - Fever
  - Cough
  - Pleuritic chest pain
  - Hypoxemia
  - Tachypnea
  - A new or rapidly progressive pulmonary infiltrate on chest radiograph
- Risk factors:
  - Younger age
  - Higher steady-state hemoglobin level
  - Lower fetal hemoglobin percentage
  - Increased neutrophil count
  - History of asthma in patient
  - Active smoking
  - Environmental smoke exposure
- Etiology:
  - Infection (pulmonary or systemic)
  - Fat embolism
  - Pulmonary infarction
- Laboratory studies:
  - A decrease in hemoglobin concentration
  - A decrease in platelet count
  - An increase in LDH (due to intravascular hemolysis and thrombosis)

- Initial management:
  - Analgesia
    - Acetaminophen
    - NSAIDS
    - Opioids
  - Corticosteroids if patient has history of asthma
  - IV fluids
  - Oxygen supplementation
    - $PaO_2 \geq$ to 80 to 100
    - $SaO_2 > 95\%$
  - *Empiric antibiotics*
    - Third-generation cephalosporin
    - Macrolide
    - ± Vancomycin
  - Ambulation in milder disease
  - Incentive spirometer
  - Transthoracic echocardiogram: Evaluate tricuspid valve jet velocity, right and left ventricular function, and estimated pulmonary artery pressure
- Transfusion indications: To dilute the Hb S–containing erythrocytes with Hb A–containing ones, with the hope that the microvascular occlusion of the pulmonary circulation is removed and systemic oxygen delivery increased
  - Multilobar involvement in the setting of anemia or thrombocytopenia
  - Rapidly progressive disease
  - Underlying cardiac disease
  - Respiratory failure
  - Mild to moderate disease: Simple transfusion to increase the hemoglobin concentration to 10 g/dL
  - Severe/rapidly progressive disease: Exchange transfusions can be used for patients who are not significantly more anemic than baseline but who have a high concentration of Hb SS (usual goal <30)
- Sequelae: Can rapidly progress to acute respiratory failure resembling acute respiratory distress syndrome (ARDS)
- Management of severe acute lung injury or ARDS

  - Noninvasive mechanical ventilation
  - Invasive mechanical ventilation strategies:
    - Minimize plateau pressure and tidal volume
    - Optimize positive end-expiratory pressure (PEEP) and lung compliance
  - Administration of inhaled nitric oxide (iNO)
  - Extracorporeal membrane oxygenation (ECMO) to support pulmonary and cardiovascular function.

ACUTE SPLENIC SEQUESTRATION CRISIS

- Presentation: Usually presents in infants and toddlers with
  - Sudden drop in hemoglobin concentration (anemia)
  - Pallor
  - Splenomegaly (often tender)
  - Reticulocytosis
  - Intravascular volume depletion
  - Shock

- Treatment:
  - ○ Restoration of circulating blood volume
    - ▪ Crystalloid infusion
    - ▪ Simple transfusion with packed red blood cells
- Rapid exchange transfusion in setting of heart failure or shock
- Splenectomy in patients who do not respond to aggressive medical therapy

APLASTIC CRISIS

- Definition: Acute suppression of bone marrow function
- Most common cause: Viral infection (especially parvovirus B19)
- Treatment: Supportive with simple PRBC transfusion until marrow function recovers and reticulocytosis resumes (goal hemoglobin 7–9 g/dL)

SEPSIS

- Increased risk for serious bacterial infections: Especially encapsulated organisms such as
  - ○ *Streptococcus pneumoniae*
  - ○ *Neisseria meningititidis*
- Treatment: Early with broad-spectrum antibiotics (ceftriaxone)

STROKE/CEREBROVASCULAR EVENTS

- Background information:
  - ○ Important to have a high index of suspicion for stroke in patients with SCA and altered mental status.
  - ○ High incidence of both ischemic and hemorrhagic stroke
    - ▪ Silent infarctions are the most common form of central nervous system (CNS) injury
  - ○ Highest risk during first decade of life with an incidence of 1% per year between the ages of 2 and 5 years.
- Presentation:
  - ○ Usual clinical signs and symptoms of cerebral vascular accident (CVA) (hemiplegia, aphasia, etc.)
  - ○ Altered or depressed mental status
  - ○ Seizures (generalized or focal)
- Management:
  - ○ Computerized tomography (CT) brain (acute bleed)
  - ○ Magnetic resonance imaging (MRI) brain (early detection of ischemic parenchymal changes)
  - ○ MR angiography
  - ○ If CVA present, immediate exchange transfusion to reverse or prevent progression of ischemic CNS injury
  - ○ Exchange transfusion: To decrease Hb S percentage <30% while hemoglobin concentration is maintained at 10 g/dL
  - ○ Airway protection
  - ○ Suppression of seizure activity
  - ○ Preservation of hemodynamic and respiratory function
  - ○ Monitor for intracranial hypertension

PERIOPERATIVE CONSIDERATIONS IN SCD

OXYGENATION

- Oxygenation to the body in SCD is ensured by:
  - ○ Increasing cardiac output
  - ○ Increasing 2,3-diphosphoglycerate (2,3 DPG) concentrations

- Preservation of arterial oxygenation (PaO_2), oxygen-carrying capacity, and cardiac output is crucial to minimize prolonged hemoglobin desaturation
- Essential to closely monitor PaO_2 with initiation of supplemental oxygen to keep PaO_2 in normal range

HYDRATION

- Transit time through circulation is adversely affected by:
  - Dehydration
  - Systemic hypotension
  - Tourniquet use can be occlusive
  - Physiology or pharmacologically induced vasoconstriction
- Presence of intracellular erythrocyte dehydration can induce
  - Hemoglobin polymerization and gel formation
- Provide generous IV hydration and maintain euvolemia

TEMPERATURE

- Preserve normothermia
- Hypothermia:
  - Limits the unloading of oxygen off hemoglobin
  - Stimulates cutaneous vasoconstriction
  - Increases erythrocyte tissue–lung transit time
  - May induce erythrocyte sickling
- Hyperthermia:
  - Due to:
    - Infection
    - Atelectasis
    - Systemic inflammation
  - Shifts the hemoglobin-oxygen dissociation curve to the right: increases the unloading of oxygen to the tissues and hemoglobin desaturation

ACID–BASE STATUS

- Maintain pH in reasonable physiologic range

SUGGESTED READINGS

Bender MA, Nielsen KR. Hemoglobinopathies. In: *Furhman,& Zimmerman's Pediatric Critical Care*. 4th ed. Kindle ed.,Philadelphia, PA: Elsevier Mosby; 2011.

Sullivan KJ, Coletti E, Goodwin SR, Gauger C, Kissoon N. Sickle cell disease. In David G. Nichols and Donald H. Shaffner: *Rogers' Textbook of Pediatric Intensive Care*. 5th ed. Kindle ed., Philadelphia, PA: Lippincott Williams & Wilkins, a Wolters Kluwer business; 2016.

Piccini JP, Nilsson KR. *The Osler Medical Handbook*. 2nd ed. Elsevier Health Sciences; 2006.

57 Hematologic and Oncologic Emergencies

TUMOR LYSIS SYNDROME[1,2]

- Definition: Potentially life-threatening clinical syndrome that results in electrolyte derangements secondary to significant tumor cell death and impairment in the kidney's ability to maintain homeostasis
  - Most commonly occurs in patients with tumors with high cell turnover (acute leukemia, Burkitt's lymphoma) with initiation of therapy, but can occur in any malignancy, even without chemotherapy
  - Can lead to renal failure
- Common electrolyte derangements include:
  - Hyperkalemia (typically the first to develop and most life threatening)
  - Hyperuricemia
  - Hypocalcemia
  - Hyperphosphatemia
- Therapy:
  - *Aggressive hydration:* 1.5 to 2 times maintenance IV fluids (without potassium or phosphorus)
  - *Prevention of hyperuricemia:* allopurinol (first-line), rasburicase
  - *Dialysis:* Reserved for severe kidney injury with electrolyte disturbances and/or fluid overload

HYPERLEUKOCYTOSIS AND LEUKOSTASIS[3]

- Definition: Hyperleukocytosis is defined as a white blood cell (WBC) count $>100,000/\mu L$, most commonly seen in children with acute lymphocytic leukemia (ALL). As WBC count increases, the viscosity of blood is increased, which can lead to aggregation of leukocytes and obstruction of blood vessels. Leukostasis causes local hypoxia and invasion of the blood vessels by leukemic cells.
  - Children with hyperleukocytosis have higher rates of morbidity and mortality:
    - Neurologic complications: Intracranial hemorrhage, ischemia (can present with headache, mental status changes, seizures, or visual disturbances)
    - Pulmonary leukostasis: Presenting with respiratory distress, hypoxemia
    - Tumor lysis syndrome
- Therapeutic approach: Supportive care
  - Avoid diuretics and blood transfusions (may increase blood viscosity further)
  - Prevent bleeding complications by correcting coagulopathy
  - Treat/prevent tumor lysis syndrome
  - Consider exchange transfusion or leukapheresis-limited evidence of efficacy

MEDIASTINAL MASS[4]

- Definition: Presence of a mass in the mediastinum can be seen in benign or malignant disease and should be considered when widened mediastinum is seen on chest radiograph.
  - Most commonly occurs in patients with lymphoma or neuroblastoma
  - Patients may report respiratory distress or orthopnea

- Therapeutic considerations:
  - Masses in anterosuperior or middle mediastinum can compress the tracheobronchial tree, heart, and great vessels with a high risk of airway or vascular compromise, especially when lying flat
  - Sedation/anesthesia is high risk; complications vary from hypotension to complete cardiopulmonary collapse and occur in 9% to 20% of patients with mediastinal mass undergoing anesthesia

FEVER AND NEUTROPENIA[5]

- Definition: Temperature of >38.5°C (or multiple temperatures >38°C) in a patient with an absolute neutrophil count (ANC) of <1,000
  - ANC = WBC count * % neutrophils * 1000
- Workup:
  - Complete blood count (CBC) to confirm neutropenia and assess for anemia, thrombocytopenia
  - Blood (central and peripheral) and urine (noncatheterized) cultures
  - Remainder of workup depends on symptoms
    - Consider chest x-ray (CXR), respiratory polymerase chain reaction (PCR) if respiratory symptoms
    - Stool studies if gastrointestinal (GI) complaints
    - Cerebrospinal fluid (CSF) studies/central nervous system (CNS) imaging if neurologic changes
- Therapeutic approach:
  - Follow sepsis guidelines: Fluid resuscitation, inotropic support, steroids if evidence of adrenal insufficiency, increased oxygen delivery, and decreased oxygen demand
- Antibiotic therapy:
  - Gram-negative coverage: Including *Pseudomonas* (ceftazidime, cefepime, piperacillin-tazobactam)
  - Additional gram-positive coverage (especially in the setting of a central line or AML: higher risk for *Streptococcus mitis* infection)
  - Empiric antifungal coverage is not recommended in the absence of specific risk factors

DISSEMINATED INTRAVASCULAR COAGULATION (DIC)[6]

- Definition: Condition characterized by widespread activation of coagulation, resulting in intravascular fibrin formation and occlusion of small and medium-sized vessels, concurrent with depletion of platelets and coagulation proteins resulting in severe bleeding. Commonly seen in the setting of sepsis (especially with gram-negative organisms, trauma, and cancer).
- Workup:
  - Clinical evaluation: Underlying disease process known to be associated with DIC
  - Coagulation studies:
    - Prolonged/elevated prothrombin time (PT)
    - Prolonged activated partial thromboplastin time (aPTT)
    - Low antithrombin III (AT III) levels
    - Elevated fibrin degradation products (D-dimer)
    - Low or normal fibrinogen (acute-phase reactant, may be artificially normal)
  - Complete blood count: low (<100,000) platelet count or decreasing platelet count

- Therapeutic approach:
  - Treat the underlying disease process
  - Replacement of platelets and plasma only if bleeding is severe or patient is having invasive procedure; there is no role for prophylactic platelet or fresh frozen plasma (FFP) administration
  - Variable evidence for heparin, coagulation factor replacement, and fibrinolysis, but not common practice

REFERENCES

1. Burns RA, Topoz I, Reynolds SL. Tumor lysis syndrome risk factors, diagnosis and management. *Pediatr Emerg Care.* 2014;30(8):571-576.
2. Henry M, Sung L. Supportive care in pediatric oncology oncologic emergencies and management of fever and neutropenia. *Pediatr Clin North Am.* 2015;62(1):27-46.
3. Aspesberro FP, Roberts JS, Brogan TV. Hematology and oncology problems in the intensive care unit. *Pediatric Critical Care.* 4th ed. 2011;1157-1158.
4. Pearson JK, Tan GM. Pediatric anterior mediastinal mass: A review article. *Semin Cardiothorac Vasc Anesth.* 2016;19(3):248-254.
5. Downes KJ, Zaoutis TE, Shah SS. Guidelines for management of children with fever and neutropenia. *J Pediatric Infect Dis Soc.* 2013;2(3):281-285.
6. Levi M, ten Cate H. Disseminated intravascular coagulation. *N Engl J Med.* 1999; 341:586-592.

Complications of Stem Cell Transplant

58 CHAPTER

ACUTE GRAFT VS. HOST DISEASE (GVHD)[1,2]

- Definition: Pro-inflammatory syndrome affecting the skin, liver, and gastrointestinal (GI) tract, typically within 100 days of hematopoietic stem cell transplant; immunocompetent transplanted cells mount an inflammatory response to cells in an immunosuppressed host.
  - Skin: Most commonly affected organ, commonly maculopapular eruption, can progress to bulla formation and epidermal necrosis
  - Gastrointestinal: Symptoms include watery diarrhea, severe abdominal pain, GI bleeding or ileus (endoscopy and biopsy are recommended for diagnosis when possible)
  - Hepatic: Cholestatic jaundice most common, but can progress to hepatic failure
  - See Table 58-1 for staging and grading of GVHD
- Therapy:
  - First-line therapy is corticosteroids (decrease inflammatory cytokines that propagate acute GVHD)
    - *Skin GVHD typically responds most quickly to steroid therapy*
  - Variety of second-line therapies include polyclonal (ATG) and monoclonal antibodies, TNF-blockade (infliximab, etanercept), and calcineurin inhibitors
  - Supportive care: Organ specific, including wound care, antimotility agents, bowel rest, ursodeoxycholic acid, and antimicrobial prophylaxis

TABLE 58-1	Staging and Grading of Graft vs. Host Disease (GVHD)		
	Skin	**Gastrointestinal (GI)**	**Liver**
Stage			
1	<25% skin surface	Diarrhea 10–19.9 mL/kg/day or persistent nausea, vomiting or anorexia, with a positive upper GI biopsy	Bilirubin 2–3 mg/dL
2	25%–50% skin surface	Diarrhea 20–30 mL/kg/day	Bilirubin 3.1–6 mg/dL
3	>50% skin surface	Diarrhea >30 mL/kg/day	Bilirubin 6.1–15 mg/dL
4	Generalized erythroderma with bullae formation	Severe abdominal pain with or without ileus	Bilirubin >15 mg/dL
Grade			
I	Stages 1–2	None	None
II	Stage 3 or	Stage 1 or	Stage 1
III	-	Stages 2–4 or	Stages 2–3
IV	Stage 4	-	Stage 4

Grade II requires Stage 3 Skin or Stage 1 GI or Stage 1 Liver
Grade III requires Stage 2–4 GI or Stage 2–3 Liver

VASOOCCLUSIVE DISEASE (VOD)/SINUSOIDAL OBSTRUCTION SYNDROME (SOS)[1-3]

- Definition: Clinical syndrome of tender hepatomegaly, fluid retention, weight gain, and elevated serum bilirubin
  - Reported incidence varies from 5% to 60% of pediatric patients undergoing stem cell transplant
  - Poor prognosis with mortality rates as high at 90% in severe disease
- Diagnosis: Clinical diagnosis based on physical exam and laboratory findings. Liver ultrasound with Doppler is an adjunctive test but may be normal.
- Treatment:
  - Supportive care: Focus on fluid balance and preservation of renal blood flow, using fluid restriction, diuretics, dialysis
  - Defibrotide: Polydisperse mixture of single-stranded oligonucleotide with antithrombotic and fibrinolytic effects on microvascular endothelium
    - *Bleeding is serious complication and requires frequent monitoring of platelet count and markers of coagulation*

IDIOPATHIC PNEUMONIA SYNDROME[1,2]

- Definition: Widespread alveolar injury following hematopoietic stem cell transplant in the absence of an active lower respiratory tract infection or cardiogenic causes
  - Spectrum of disease that includes interstitial pneumonitis, diffuse alveolar hemorrhage, periengraftment respiratory distress syndrome, and bronchiolitis obliterans organizing pneumonia
    - *Widespread alveolar injury: Multifocal infiltrates, signs/symptoms of pneumonia, and impaired pulmonary physiology (widened alveolar-arterial gradient, abnormal or worsening pulmonary function tests)*
    - *Absence of infection (including bacterial, viral, and fungal studies)*
    - *Absence of cardiac dysfunction, renal failure ,or iatrogenic fluid overload*
- Incidence and risk factors: Reported in 5% to 15% of pediatric allogeneic stem cell transplant patients, with increased incidence in patients with acute GVHD, those who received unrelated-donor transplant or pretransplant total-body irradiation
- Treatment:
  - Supportive care, including mechanical ventilation, conservative fluid management
  - Broad-spectrum antimicrobials
  - Corticosteroids, etanercept

REFERENCES

1. Forman SJ, Negrin RS, Blume KG. *Thomas' Hematopoietic Cell Transplantation: Stem Cell Transplantation.* 4th ed. Blackwell Publishing, Hoboken, NJ; 2009.
2. Chima RS, Abulebda K, Jodele S. Advances in critical care of the pediatric hematopoietic stem cell transplant patient. *Pediatr Clin North Am.* 2013;60(3):687-707.
3. Corbacioglu S, Kernan N, Lehmann L, et al. Defibrotide for the treatment of hepatic veno-occlusive disease in children after hematopoietic stem cell transplantation. *Expert Rev Hematol.* 2012;5(3):291-302.

Endocrine

59 Diabetic Ketoacidosis

DEFINITION AND DIAGNOSIS

Diabetic ketoacidosis (DKA) mainly affects children with type 1 diabetes mellitus (T1DM) and is caused by a deficiency in circulating insulin levels and elevations in other hormones like glucagon and cortisol. This, in turn, leads to:

- Impaired glucose consumption by the peripheral tissues with elevations in plasma glucose levels
- Increased glucose production by the liver through gluconeogenesis and glycogenolysis
- Increased serum osmolality
- Increased lipolysis with production of ketone bodies (ß-hydroxybutyrate) and resultant ketonemia
- Profound anion gap metabolic acidosis

The hyperglycemia and acidosis associated with DKA result in a profound osmotic diuresis, significant dehydration, glycosuria, ketonuria, ketonemia, and electrolyte disturbances.

SIGNS AND SYMPTOMS OF ACUTE DKA CAN INCLUDE:

- Polyuria/increased urination
- Polydipsia/increased thirst
- Vomiting and dehydration
- Abdominal pain
- Irregular respirations (Kussmaul breathing: large, deep, gasping breaths)
- Weakness and lethargy
- Altered mental status and confusion
- Loss of consciousness or coma

THE DIAGNOSTIC CRITERIA FOR DKA INCLUDE:

- Hyperglycemia (serum glucose >250–300 mg/dL)
- Significant venous acidosis (pH <7.3)
- Serum bicarbonate levels ≤15 mmol/L

DKA IS GENERALLY CATEGORIZED ACCORDING TO THESE pH AND BICARBONATE VALUES (TABLE 59-1).

TABLE 59-1	Classification of DKA severity	
Severity of DKA	**Venous Blood pH**	**Serum Bicarbonate Level (mmol/L)**
Mild	<7.30	<15
Moderate	<7.20	<10
Severe	<7.10	<5

INCIDENCE OF DKA

- As mentioned, DKA occurs more commonly in patients with T1DM but has been seen in older children with type 2 diabetes mellitus. DKA at the onset of T1DM occurs more frequently in:
  - Young children (age <4 years)
  - Children of lower socioeconomic status
  - Children without a significant family history of diabetes
- Children with known relatives with T1DM are more frequently evaluated by clinicians and are less likely to present in DKA.
- Children with known T1DM have a 1% to 10% risk of having an episode of DKA/year
- Children at higher risk for DKA after the diagnosis of T1DM are:
  - Peripubertal/adolescent girls
  - Children from lower-income households
  - Children with mood or eating disorders
  - Children with poor self or parental compliance to medical therapy
- DKA can often be precipitated by:
  - An intercurrent illness (e.g., viral or bacterial infection)
  - Inadequate insulin administration
  - Corticosteroid or diuretic use
  - Exacerbation of another underlying disease that puts the body under a stress state (e.g., pancreatitis, trauma, heart disease)

MANAGING DKA

In known T1DM patients with evidence of urinary ketones or elevated glucose without significant acidosis, care can be managed at home in close contact with a pediatric endocrinologist.

Children with new-onset T1DM or moderate to severe DKA should be considered for inpatient or pediatric intensive care admission.

INITIAL STABILIZATION OF PATIENTS IN DKA IN AN ACUTE CARE SETTING SHOULD INCLUDE:

1. Establishing a protocolized monitoring system:
   - Hourly vital sign monitoring of heart rate, blood pressure, respiratory rate, and fluid intake
   - Hourly blood sugar assessments through point-of-care capillary glucose
   - Frequent electrolyte assessments (~ every 2 hours) for alterations in sodium, phosphate, urea, potassium, and laboratory glucose values
   - Frequent blood gases (~ every 2 hours) to monitor for improvement in pH
   - Frequent neurologic checks to monitor for signs of cerebral edema
2. Proper fluid resuscitation and management of sodium:
   - High levels of circulating osmolytes create a significant depletion in intracellular fluid volume and are further exacerbated by extracellular volume contraction and diuresis
   - Small-volume boluses of isotonic fluids like normal saline (0.9) or lactated Ringer's in 5 to 10 mL/kg doses should be given slowly over 1 to 2 hours to restore circulating volume and improve kidney glomerular filtration rates and restore normal electrolytes
   - Serum sodium levels are often falsely low due to the pseudo-hyponatremic effect of increased glucose and do not adequately reflect the degree of extracellular volume contraction

- Fluid goals for children usually range between 3600 and 4000 mL/m²/day, or approximately 1.5 to 2 times the usual daily requirement of sodium-containing fluids after accounting for the initial fluid resuscitation
- Urine output should not be replaced or utilized in calculating daily fluid volume
3. Insulin therapy
    - Correction of the patient's underlying insulin deficiency should begin immediately at 0.1 U/kg/hour IV and should remain at this rate until resolution of the patient's ketoacidosis (improved pH >7.3, bicarbonate >15 mmol/L, and correction of the anion gap)
    - IV insulin boluses are not indicated for the treatment of DKA in children
    - Glucose should be added to fluids once serum glucose levels have reached ~250 mg/dL to prevent hypoglycemia in the face of insulin therapy
    - Transition to a more stable insulin regimen will begin once a child is out of DKA
4. Potassium supplementation
    - Children may present with low, normal, or elevated potassium levels, so serum potassium levels should be followed closely
    - In general, once insulin therapy has begun, potassium will be driven intracellularly, so supplementation may be necessary shortly after to prevent hypokalemia
    - Potassium should not be supplemented until the child has demonstrated the ability to produce urine
5. Recognizing phosphate depletion:
    - Like potassium, phosphate enters the cell with insulin therapy, but may take much longer to respond to supplementation
    - The addition of potassium phosphate to IV fluids should be considered for low phosphate levels; however, electrolytes should be closely monitored because phosphate supplementation can lower serum calcium levels
6. Monitoring bicarbonate levels and acidosis without direct treatment:
    - While incredibly low on presentation, IV bolus doses of bicarbonate or continuous bicarbonate infusions are not recommended for pediatric DKA because data shows no clinical benefit from treatment with these measures
    - Although not well studied, there remains concern that bicarbonate treatment causes paradoxical central nervous system (CNS) acidosis and can drastically alter CNS sodium load and predispose patients to cerebral edema
7. Referral and early consultation with a pediatric endocrinologist
    - Allows for proper transition of care from the acute care to outpatient setting for both short- and long-term therapy
    - Helps determine the best treatment course during hospitalization and after discharge
    - Introduces parents and patients to diabetic educators who teach about diabetes, the natural treatment course, and concerning signs and symptoms of DKA
    - Diabetic dietitians may often aid patients in learning how to properly count carbohydrate loads and institute sliding-scale insulin regimens

DKA AND THE ASSOCIATION WITH CEREBRAL EDEMA

Children are at greater risk for cerebral edema than adults and should be monitored closely for mental status changes.

THE PATHOPHYSIOLOGY OF CEREBRAL EDEMA IN DKA IS NOT FULLY UNDERSTOOD BUT MAY BE RELATED TO:

- Changes in cerebral blood flow
- Alterations in cerebral ion transport and aquaporin channel permeability

- Production of pro-inflammatory mediators that disrupt the blood–brain barrier
- Generation of intracellular osmolytes that create a gradient, promoting cerebral swelling

SYMPTOMS OF CEREBRAL EDEMA INCLUDE:

- Acute or subacute onset of a dull aching headache
- Graduate changes in mental status or alterations in consciousness
- Elevations in blood pressure due to the impact on cerebral autoregulation
- Bradycardia with changes in distal peripheral pulses

CHILDREN WITH GREATER RISK FOR CEREBRAL EDEMA INCLUDE:

- Patients presenting with T1DM for the first time in DKA
- Patients meeting criteria for severe DKA
- Younger children (age <5 years)
- Patients who have had many days of unrecognized symptoms

EVALUATION AND MANAGEMENT OF CHILDREN WITH SUSPECTED CEREBRAL EDEMA SHOULD INCLUDE:

- Emergent treatment with IV mannitol (1 g/kg) or hypertonic (3%) saline (5 to 10 mL/kg) over 30 minutes; repeat as clinically indicated
- Endotracheal intubation and mechanical ventilation if the Glasgow Coma Scale <9 or if the patient is unable to maintain an adequate airway while awake
- Avoidance of prolonged hyperventilation
- Head imaging by computerized tomography (CT) or quick magnetic resonance imaging is not required but may aid in prognosis in severe cases

PREVENTING DKA

Clinicians should continue to educate the general public on the signs and symptoms of early-onset diabetes in children. Increasing awareness of these symptoms should lead to more frequent diagnoses and reduced occurrences of DKA.

SUGGESTED READINGS

Dunger D, Sperling M, Acerini C, et al. European Society for Paeduatric Endocrinology/ Lawson Wilkins Pediatric Endocrine Society Consensus Statement on Diabetic Ketoacidosis in Children and Adolescents. *Pediatrics.* 2004;113(2):133-142.

Nichols DG; section editors, Alice D. Ackerman, Andrew C. Argent, *Rogers Textbook of Pediatric Intensive Care.* 4th ed. Philadelphia, PA: Lippincott Williams & Wilkins; 2008.

60 Adrenal Insufficiency

ADRENAL INSUFFICIENCY AND CRITICAL ILLNESS

BACKGROUND

- An acquired, reversible adrenal insufficiency can occur in any critically ill patient, but occurs most commonly in the context of sepsis and septic shock. Common etiologies of adrenal insufficiency in critical illness are listed in Table 60-1.
- Many of the patients who are admitted to the ICU have been/are on chronic steroid therapy and may lack an intact hypothalamic–pituitary axis (HPA), leading to refractory hypotension.
- The incidence of adrenal insufficiency ranges widely (17%–52%) in children with septic shock. This variability is partly due to the lack of consensus in terms of diagnostic strategies.[1-4]

DIAGNOSIS

- A diagnosis of adrenal insufficiency may be made by checking a cortisol level (morning or random), but may need to be verified with an adrenocorticotropic hormone (ACTH) stimulation test.
- There is variability in corticotropin stimulation testing dosing, using basal cortisol values vs. threshold values after corticotropin stimulation, and controversy over whether to use total vs. free cortisol levels. Table 60-2 reveals the variability in diagnostic criteria.

TABLE 60-1	Common Etiologies of Adrenal Insufficiency	
Location	**Etiology**	**Pathophysiology**
Central	Hypothalamic or pituitary disease	
	Brain injury/brain death	
	Recent or chronic steroid use	
Peripheral	Preexisting adrenal failure	Addison's disease, congenital adrenal hyperplasia (CAH)
	Acute adrenal destruction	Adrenal hemorrhage, autoimmune adrenalitis
	P450 enzyme dysfunction	Etomidate, antifungals (azoles), sepsis, prematurity
	Increased clearance	Occurs with phenytoin, phenobarbital, rifampin
	End-organ/tissue/cellular unresponsiveness	Cytokines and inflammatory mediators can alter glucocorticoid receptor sensitivity
Other	Sepsis/inflammation	HPA axis suppression secondary to CIRCI

HPA, hypothalamic pituitary axis; *CIRCI*, critical illness related corticosteroid insufficiency.

TABLE 60-2	Diagnostic Criteria, Dose of ACTH Used for Adrenal Stimulation, and Incidence of Adrenal Insufficiency in Children with Septic Shock		
Authors	**Diagnostic Criteria**	**ACTH Dose Used**	**Incidence of AI**
Hatherill et al.	Peak cortisol increase <7 μg/dL	145 μg/m²	52%
Bone et al.	A.M. basal cortisol <5 μg/dL;	0.5 μg/m²	17%
	Peak cortisol <18 μg/dL		
Pizarro et al.	Peak control increase <9 μg/dL	250 μg	44%
Menon et al.	Basal cortisol <7 μg/dL	125 μg (<10 kg)	31%
	Peak cortisol <18 μg/dL	250 μg (>10 kg)	

ACTH, adrenocorticotropin hormone. *AI,* adrenal insufficiency. Peak cortisol is cortisol level after administration of ACTH.

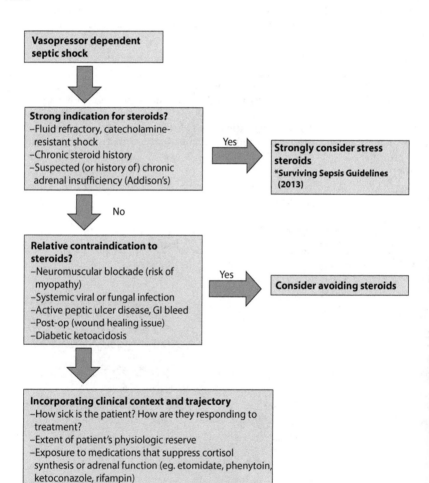

FIGURE 60-1 **Approach to steroids in septic shock.**

TREATMENT

- In cases of adrenal insufficiency, hydrocortisone is generally started at 50 mg/m^2/day divided every 6 hours.
  - Dosing should be verified to ensure that the patient is actually on "stress dose" steroids in relation to their previous dose of steroid.
- In sepsis, hydrocortisone is given as a daily stress dose of 50 mg/m^2 or divided over 24 hours as currently recommended by the Surviving Sepsis Guidelines.[5]
- Steroids are generally weaned over several days according to physician preference and patient status.

See Chapter 13 for a list of systemic steroids and a glucocorticoid equivalency table.

CURRENT THOUGHTS

- Total cortisol and ACTH stimulation are inadequate markers for identifying critical illness related corticosteroid insufficiency (CIRCI), as much of the altered regulation associated with critical illness and the steroid response occurs at the cellular level.
- To date there is no clinically relative, time-sensitive test capable of assessing intracellular glucocorticoid regulation/dysfunction.
- Figure 60-1 reveals a pragmatic approach for the use of steroids in septic shock.

REFERENCES

1. Hatherill M, Tibby SM, Hilliard T, et al. Adrenal insufficiency in septic shock. *Arch Dis Child.* 1999;80:51-55.
2. Bone M, Diver M, Selby A, et al. Assessment of adrenal function in the initial phase of meningococcal disease. *Pediatrics.* 2002;110:563-569.
3. Pizarro CF, Troster EJ, Damiani D, et al. Absolute and relative adrenal insufficiency in children with septic shock. *Crit Care Med.* 2005;33:855-859.
4. Menon K, Clarson C. Adrenal function in pediatric critical illness. *Pediatr Crit Care Med.* 2002;3:112-116.
5. Dellinger RP, Levy MM, Rhodes A, et al. Surviving sepsis campaign: International guidelines for management of severe sepsis and septic shock. *Crit Care Med.* 2013;41:580-637.

Diabetes Insipidus & Syndrome of Inappropriate Antidiuretic Hormone

DIABETES INSIPIDUS (DI)

- Uncontrolled free water losses lead to severe hypernatremia and significant dehydration

NORMAL WATER HOMEOSTASIS

- Normal plasma osmolality: 275 to 295 mOsm/L
- Controlled via thirst and arginine vasopressin
- Arginine vasopressin (AVP): Produced in supraoptic and paraventricular nuclei of hypothalamus, released in posterior pituitary
  - Vasopressin receptors
    - V1: liver, vasculature – contributes to vasoconstriction, hepatic gluconeogenesis
    - V2: kidney – functions to increase renal tubule water permeability
  - AVP mechanism
    - **Binds V2 in renal collecting ducts**: increases permeability via aquaporin-2 channels – allows diffusion of water from tubules to plasma
    - Release regulated by osmoreceptors near anterior hypothalamus
    - Nonosmotic factors affecting AVP release: volume depletion, hypotension, pain, nausea, medications
    - Desmopressin (DDAVP) – lacks smooth muscle contraction effects; more specific for V2 receptor

PATHOPHYSIOLOGIC MECHANISMS

- Central DI: defect in secretion or synthesis of vasopressin → decreased free water reabsorption in renal collecting tubules
  - Genetic
  - Injury/damage to pituitary gland and/or hypothalamus
    - Post–hypothalamic-pituitary surgery; may be transient (permanent if transection of pituitary stalk)
    - Central nervous system (CNS) infections
    - CNS tumors (e.g., craniopharyngioma)
    - Traumatic brain injury
    - Hypoxic ischemic injury
    - Brain death
- Nephrogenic DI: impaired ability to concentrate urine
  - Genetic
  - Drugs: lithium, amphotericin B, rifampin
  - Neoplasm
  - Sickle cell
  - Metabolic derangements
  - Obstructive uropathy

DIAGNOSIS

- Hallmarks:
  - Polyuria and polydipsia
  - Urine specific gravity <1.005

- ○ Urine output (UOP) >4 mL/kg/hr
- ○ Serum Na >145 mEq/L
- ○ Serum osmolality >285 mOsm/L
- ○ Urine osmolality <100 to 200 mOsm/L
- Serum sodium and osmolality depend on hydration status

CLINICAL MANIFESTATIONS

- Thirst, polyuria, dilute urine, hypovolemia, tachycardia, poor perfusion, shock
- CNS abnormalities – lethargy, irritability, seizure, coma
- Hyperosmolar state – risk of venous sinus thrombosis

TREATMENT

- Fluid resuscitation to reverse hypovolemic shock if necessary
- Then hypotonic fluid to replace urine losses in addition to maintenance requirements
- Avoid hyperglycemia if giving large volumes of dextrose-containing fluids – risk of osmotic diuresis worsening dehydration
- If vasopressin sensitive (central DI), initiation of vasopressin administration
- Avoid rapid correction of hypernatremia – correct over 48 to 72 hours to avoid cerebral edema

SYNDROME OF INAPPROPRIATE ANTIDIURECTIC HORMONE SECRETION (SIADH)

- Relative hypersthenuria (increased urine osmolality) and hyponatremia

PATHOPHYSIOLOGIC MECHANISMS

- Pituitary hypersecretion of vasopressin → excess of water in extracellular and intracellular compartments → renin/aldosterone activity reduced → increased natriuresis due to expansion of extracellular volume
- Causes of SIADH
  - ○ CNS: brain injury, tumors, infections
  - ○ Adrenal insufficiency
  - ○ Drugs: vincristine, cyclophosphamide, carbamazepine, barbiturates
  - ○ Malignancy
  - ○ Hypothyroidism
  - ○ Guillan-Barre
  - ○ Infant botulism
  - ○ Pulmonary diseases: tuberculosis, cystic fibrosis
  - ○ Positive end-expiratory pressure (PEEP)

DIAGNOSIS

- Hypotonic hyponatremia
- Serum sodium <125 mEq/L
- Serum osmolality <260 mOsm/L
- Urine sodium >18 mEq/L
- Inappropriate urine concentration at some level of serum hypo-osmolality
- Elevated urinary sodium excretion with normal salt and water intake
- *Signs of hypovolemia or hypervolemia should raise concern for other causes of hypo-osmolality*

TABLE 61-1	Diabetes Insipidus vs. SIADH	
	DI	**SIADH**
Disorder	ADH deficit	ADH excess
	Decreased water reabsorption in distal tubules	Increased renal distal tubule permeability and increased water reabsorption
Volume status	Decreased	Increased or euvolemic
Salt balance	Variable	Variable
Serum sodium	Increased >150 mEq/L	Decreased <130 mEq/L
Urine sodium	Decreased <40 mEq/L or normal	Increased >60 mEq/L
Serum osmolality	Increased >305 mOsm/L	Decreased <275 mOsm/L
Urine osmolality	Decreased <250 mOsm/L	Increased >500 mOsm/L
Urine specific gravity	Decreased <1.005	Increased >1.025

CLINICAL MANIFESTATIONS

- Nausea, vomiting, weakness, mental status changes, irritability, headache, seizures
- May be more pronounced if hypo-osmolality develops acutely
- Rate of decrease in sodium correlates more strongly with morbidity and mortality than extent of decline (less time for regulation – cerebral edema intensified)

TREATMENT

- Eliminate underlying disorder
- Restrict fluid intake
- In acutely symptomatic patient with severe hyponatremia, hypertonic saline (3%) to restore serum sodium >125 mEq/L
- Goal to raise serum sodium slowly, goal increase <1 mEq/h, to avoid central pontine myelinolysis
  ○ *Sodium deficit*

COMPARISON OF DIABETES INSIPIDUS AND SIADH

- There are several features and laboratory values that differentiate DI from SIADH. See Table 61-1.

SUGGESTED READINGS

Lynch R, Wood E. Fluid and electrolyte issues in pediatric critical illness in pediatric critical care. In: Fuhrman B, Zimmerman J, et al. eds. *Pediatric Critical Care* Philadelphia, OA: Elsevier; 2011:944.

Roberston GL. Regulation of arginine vasopressin in the syndrome of inappropriate anitdiuresis. *Am J Med.* 2006;119:S36.

Sterns RH. Disorders of plasma sodium – causes, consequences, and correction. *NEJM.* 2015;372:55.

Gastroenterology/Nutrition/Hepatology

62 Critical Care Nutrition

Nutrition support intervention varies depending on which phase of illness a patient may be in. Three phases of critical illness are highlighted.[1–3]

FIRST PHASE OF ILLNESS: ACUTE PHASE

- **Duration:** 6 to 8 hours after onset of illness or trauma
- **Characteristics:** Fever, tachycardia, hypoglycemia
- **Nutrition intervention:** Usually NPO during resuscitation with fluids, inotropes, pressors, and/or blood products

Please note, though, that growth is inhibited at this time. Energy metabolism is diverted toward the stress or injury.

SECOND PHASE OF ILLNESS: EBB PHASE

- **Duration:** Varies
- **Characteristics:**
  ○ INCREASED: Catecholamines, counterregulatory hormones (glucagon, cortisol) → hyperglycemia, growth hormone, cytokine production, free fatty acids → possible hypertriglyceridemia, antidiuretic hormone (ADH), gluconeogenesis
  ○ DECREASED: Insulin level, insulin growth factor-1, acute decrease in metabolic rate
- **Nutrition intervention:** These metabolic and hormonal changes are not reversed or impaired by providing an increased amount of calories. Calories should be limited because providing an excess amount of nutrients could be deleterious.

Weights most likely will reflect increased fluid status due to increased ADH and not reflect the true somatic status of the patient.

THIRD PHASE OF ILLNESS: FLOW PHASE

TWO SUBCATEGORIES: CATABOLIC AND ANABOLIC

Catabolic Flow Phase

- **Duration:** Varies
- **Characteristics:** Hypermetabolism due to endogenous catabolism of fat, carbohydrate, and protein stores; active inflammatory processes; hyperglycemia; glucose intolerance; lipolysis; and negative nitrogen balance
- **Nutrition intervention:** Until the metabolic and hormonal alterations subside, nutrient provision should remain toward basal metabolic needs with the exception of providing an increased amount of protein as permissible per renal and liver status. Amino acids are pulled from muscle, connective tissue, and the gut (if inactive) to promote gluconeogenesis and production of acute-phase proteins, such as C-reactive protein (CRP).

There will be a decrease in synthesis of visceral protein stores of albumin and prealbumin.

Anabolic Flow Phase

- **Duration:** Varies
- **Characteristics:** Restoration of tissue composition, depleted energy reserves, and positive nitrogen balance

- **Nutrition intervention:** Nutrient provision should now be increased to promote nutrition repletion. Patient is now approaching convalescence and growth will resume; thus, more calories will be needed.

COMPONENTS OF ENERGY EXPENDITURE

Total energy expenditure = Basal metabolic rate + Energy from thermogenesis + Energy for activity* + Energy for growth* + Energy for healing process[4]

*Please note patients in the PICU are usually not active nor are they growing, so these components are excluded in determining energy needs.[5]

CONSIDERATIONS FOR DETERMINING ENERGY NEEDS

1. Phase of illness
2. Severity and duration of illness
3. Respiratory status: intubated vs. O_2 (mask ventilation/nasal cannula) vs. room air
4. Sedation status
5. Muscle relaxed or pentobarbital coma
6. Injury or stress factors, such as fever, sepsis, wounds, burns, cardiac failure, status post surgery
7. Baseline calorie needs (especially if chronically ill)

CALCULATING CALORIE PROVISIONS

There are many predictive equations, of which none are based on the critically ill pediatric population except for the *White equation.* This equation includes many patient variables (based on age, weight, weight for age Z score, body temperature, number of days after intensive care admission, and primary reason for admission) and is not easy to calculate.[6] Table 62-1 provides a basic approach to calculating calorie needs.

The gold standard for determining calorie needs is to measure the patient's calorie needs by indirect calorimetry, otherwise known as a metabolic cart study, which is reviewed in Chapter 9.[7] A metabolic cart may be available in the PICU and be conducted by the appropriate trained personnel.

See Table 62-1 for the predictive equation to use to estimate resting energy expenditure (REE = Basal metabolic needs X Factor for thermogenesis) needs during the acute and ebb phases of illness[8]:

TABLE 62-1 Resting Energy Expenditure	
Age	**REE (kcals/kg/d)**
2–6 mo	54
7–12 mo	51
13–35 mo	56
3 yr (boys/girls)	57/55
4–8 yr (boys/girls)	48/45
9–13 yr (boys/girls)	36/32
14–18 yr (boys/girls)	28/26
>18 yr (boys/girls)	28/23

As the patient's acute illness status improves, the energy needs may increase, with the goal of moving toward the patient's usual baseline calorie needs.[9]

PROTEIN NEEDS

• Protein needs during acute illness are usually more than when healthy (Table 62-2)
• Increased protein provision can help promote a positive nitrogen balance (16% of protein molecule is nitrogen)

NUTRITION SUPPORT

Enteral mode: Use of the gut is always preferred.

Contraindications: Gastrointestinal surgery, prolonged ileus, severe emesis, and/or diarrhea.

Formula selection: Formulas available vary per institution. Selection of the type of formula is based on the patient's acute clinical/medical status to discern the use of a standard intact, semi-elemental, or elemental formula.

Please note the use of fiber-containing formula may be prudent, as constipation may be an issue due to use of sedation agents in the PICU (formulas for children >1 year old contain fiber).

Mode of delivery: Continuous versus bolus

Continuous feeds are recommended if the patient is sedated and/or muscle relaxed or if concern for aspiration/reflux.

Bolus feeds can be started if the patient is more alert and concern for reflux/aspiration is absent. Bolus feeds mimic a more physiologic feeding pattern.

NJ versus NG is a debated issue. If there is increased concern for reflux or aspiration post-pylorus (transpyloric tube—ND or NJ), it may help to reduce occurrence of reflux/aspiration.[6] Transpyloric tubes need to be placed by a trained health care provider or interventional radiologist.

NG feeds reflect more normal feeding route and are easily placed by bedside nurse.

Note: Cannot provide bolus feeds via an NJ tube.

Total parenteral nutrition (TPN) mode: Less physiologic, more expensive, and increased risk of complications, including infection and line placement problems.[10]

TPN is individually tailored to the patient by determining the amount of macronutrients and micronutrients to provide.

Dextrose: 3.4 kcals/gm (gm = % dextrose × volume)

Amino acids: 4 kcals/gm

Fat (20% IV fat solution): 10 kcals/gm or 2 kcals/mL

Recommended ratio of calories = 50% to 60% carbohydrate, 10% to 20% protein, 30% to 55% fat[10]

Indications for use are the contraindications for enteral mode.

TABLE 62-2	Protein Recommendations During Critical Illness[5]
Age	**Protein in g/kg/day**
0–2 yr	2–3
2–13 yr	1.5–2
13–18 yr	1.5

LABORATORY VALUES

During critical illness, shifts in fluid and electrolyte status can occur. Monitoring electrolytes (sodium, potassium, chloride, bicarbonate, glucose, blood urea nitrogen [BUN], creatinine, and calcium) is helpful to assess changes and possible need for electrolyte supplementation or adjustments.[1-3]

TPN labs (electrolytes, ionized calcium, magnesium, phosphorus, and triglyceride) should be checked with every change in TPN concentration.[10]

C-reactive protein (CRP) levels can help indicate current acute illness status of patient, and obtaining serial measurements can better guide patient's nutrient provision.[11]

Prealbumin level is a marker of visceral protein stores. During acute illness, prealbumin levels decline. Prealbumin synthesis may resume when the first few phases of illness subside. Serial measurements can indicate the trend of the illness and better guide how much protein to provide (given that CRP levels are within normal limits at the time).[11]

FORMULA LIST

Premature Infant Formulas
Preterm formulas
Preterm post-discharge formulas
Full-Term Infant Formulas
Infant standard intact formulas
Infant cow's milk protein–based, lactose-free formulas
Infant soy-based formulas
Infant cow's milk–based with thickening agent formula
Infant cow's milk–based with low mineral content formula
Infant impaired long chain fat digestion/absorption formulas
Infant casein hydrolysate formulas
Infant elemental protein formula
Children formulas (1–10 years of age)
Children standard intact formulas (milk protein based)
Children standard intact formulas (soy protein based)
Children semi-elemental protein formulas
Children elemental protein formulas
Children calorie-dense formulas
Children semi-elemental protein, calorie-dense formulas
Children impaired long chain fat digestion/absorption formulas
Adolescent and Adult Formulas (>10 years old)
Adolescent and adult standard intact formulas
Adolescent and adult calorie-dense formulas
Adolescent and adult semi-elemental protein formulas
Adolescent and adult elemental protein formulas
Adolescent and adult renal formulas
Oral Supplements for Children (1–10 years) and Adolescents/Adults (>10 years)
Ketogenic formulas
Metabolic formulas

REFERENCES

1. Kallas HJ, Dimand R. Metabolic and nutritional support of the critically ill child. In: Reifen R, Lerner A, Branski D, et al., eds. *Pediatric Nutrition. Pediatric Adolescent Medicine*. Vol 8. Basel, Switzerland: Karger; 1998:154-181. doi: 10.1159/000061914.

2. De Carvalho WB, Leite HP. Nutritional support in the critically ill child. In: Nichols DG, ed. *Roger's Textbook of Pediatric Intensive Care*. 4th ed. Philadelphia, PA: Wolters-Kluwer/Lippincott Williams & Wilkins; 2008:1500-1515.

3. Chwals RJ. Energy metabolism and appropriate energy repletion in children. In: Baker SS, Baker RD, Davis AM, eds. *Pediatric Nutrition Support*. Boston, MA: Jones and Bartlett Publishers; 2007:65-82.

4. Shulman RJ, Phillips S. Parenteral nutrition in infants and children. *J Pediatr Gastroenterol Nutr* 2003;36(5):587-607.

5. Mehta NM, Compher C, A.S.P.E.N. Board of Directors, et al. A.S.P.E.N. Clinical guidelines: Nutrition support of the critically ill child. *J Parenter Enteral Nutr*. 2009;33(3):260-278.

6. White MS, Sheperd RW, McEniery JA. Energy expenditure in 100 ventilated, critically ill children: Improving the accuracy of predictive equations. *Crit Care Med*. 2000;28:2307-2312.

7. Skillman HE, Wischmeyer P. Nutrition therapy in critically ill infants and children. *J Parenter Enteral Nutr*. 2008;32:520-534. doi:10.1177/0148607108322398.

8. Bunting KD, Mills J, Ramsey E, et al., eds. *Pediatric Nutrition Reference Guide*. 10th ed. Houston: Texas Children's Hospital; 2013.

9. Steinhorn DM, Russo LT. Nutrition issues in critically ill children. In: Fink MP, Abraham E, Vincent JL, et al, eds. *Textbook of Critical Care*. 5th ed. Philadelphia, PA: Elsevier Saunders, 2005:951-959.

10. Leonberg B, ed. *Pediatric Nutrition Practice Group. Pediatric Nutrition Care Manual*. Academy of Nutrition and Dietetics: Chicago; 2012.

11. Beck FK, Rosenthal TC. Prealbumin: A marker for nutritional evaluation. *Am Fam Physician*. 2002;65(8):1575-1579.

Gastrointestinal Bleeding

Gastrointestinal (GI) bleeding is categorized into upper GI bleed (UGIB), bleeding from a source proximal to the ligament of Treitz, and lower GI bleed (LGIB) occurring distal to this duodenojejunal junction point.

TYPICAL CLINICAL PRESENTATIONS

- Upper GI bleed: hematemesis (bright red blood or coffee ground) and/or melena
- Lower GI bleed: hematochezia (bright red blood per rectum)

ETIOLOGY

- Likelihood of various etiologies depends on age and geography.
- Upper GI causes include coagulopathy, gastric or duodenal ulcer, gastritis, Mallory-Weiss tear, varices, esophagitis, and foreign body.
- Lower GI causes include anal fissure, milk protein colitis, coagulopathy, vascular malformations, necrotizing enterocolitis, malrotation with midgut volvulus, intussusception, infectious colitis, Meckel's diverticulum, inflammatory bowel disease, hemolytic uremic syndrome (HUS), Henoch-Schonlein purpura (HSP), lymphonodular hyperplasia, and graft-versus-host disease.

DIAGNOSTIC EVALUATION

- Physical exam: Look for evidence of shock in vital signs, pulses, and perfusion. Evaluate for abdominal distension or tenderness, ascites, jaundice. Examine the anus for fissures.
- History: Ask about Timing/frequency, abdominal pain, severity/amount of blood loss, comorbid conditions, medication exposure, and associated symptoms.
- Serum labs: Coagulation factors, complete metabolic panel, amylase, lipase, complete blood count
- Stool guaiac in lower GI bleed
- Stool for testing for infectious etiology if indicated by the history and symptoms

MANAGEMENT

- Initial evaluation should focus on assessment and treatment of shock in cases of severe and/or brisk bleeding.
- If patient is hemodynamically unstable, follow resuscitation pathway for hemorrhagic shock.
  - Establish IV access, preferably two large-bore IVs.
  - Initial labs should include type and cross-match of blood. If patient has significant hemodynamic instability, obtain universal donor blood products quickly.
  - Resuscitation of hemodynamics should focus on giving blood products. Guidelines for traumatic hemorrhagic shock resuscitation recommend high ratio of plasma:packed red blood cells. Ratio of 1:1 or 1:2 (plasma:PRBC) is appropriate.
- Gastric lavage via nasogastric tube to evaluate for presence of ongoing gastric bleeding is an option, though negative lavage does not entirely rule out bleeding.
- Initiate proton pump inhibitor, which may help to reduce UGIB.
- Consider prophylactic antibiotics in patients with UGIB from esophageal varices.

- In ongoing UGIB, octreotide or somatostatin may be helpful to diminish bleeding, especially in variceal bleeding.
- Endoscopy/colonoscopy is often indicated for diagnosis and/or therapy to stop bleeding.
- Endoscopy is ideally performed once patient has been resuscitated and bleeding is better controlled. In cases of ongoing severe bleeding, endoscopy may be indicated for acute therapeutic interventions.
- If source of bleeding is not identified via endoscopy, other diagnostic modality options include angiography, tagged red cell scan, or video capsule endoscopy.

SUGGESTED READINGS

Chang R, Holcomb JB. Optimal fluid therapy for traumatic hemorrhagic shock. *Crit Care Clin*. 2017;33:15-36.

Richard L. Management of upper gastrointestinal bleeding in children: Variceal and nonvariceal. *Gastrointest Endosc Clin N Am*. 2016;26:63-73.

Sahn B, Bitton S. Lower gastrointestinal bleeding in children. *Clin N Am*. 2016;26:75-98.

GENERAL PERIOPERATIVE CONSIDERATIONS

Gastrointestinal emergencies are a frequent cause of hospitalization in children, and despite a wide range of etiologies, many of the principles in management are the same. Initial therapy should always include adequate resuscitation with establishment of stable IV access, IV fluid administration with isotonic solution such as Ringer's lactate, correction of electrolyte abnormalities, and consideration of a Foley catheter for careful monitoring of fluid shifts. Patients should be made NPO, and insertion of a nasogastric tube may be considered in cases of refractory vomiting or concern for an obstructive or ischemic process. Additionally, prompt administration of broad-spectrum IV antibiotics is often indicated when underlying infection or sepsis is suspected.

NECROTIZING ENTEROCOLITIS (NEC)

BACKGROUND

Necrotizing enterocolitis affects 5% to 10% of all infants admitted to the neonatal intensive care unit. Ninety percent of patients with NEC are also premature. Although the exact etiology is unknown, the hypothesized mechanisms include the presence of bacteria in an immature gut, inflammatory response, failure of the intestinal immunologic barrier, and resultant coagulation necrosis. Well-established risk factors include prematurity and low birth weight.

FINDINGS

Signs and symptoms may range from mild and nonspecific to an acute abdomen with evidence of intestinal perforation.

1. Symptoms: Abdominal distention, gastric residuals, bloody stools, abdominal wall erythema, apnea, hemodynamic instability.
2. Labs: Leukocytosis or leukopenia, thrombocytopenia, elevated C-reactive protein (CRP), metabolic acidosis
3. Imaging (plain radiographs): Ileus gas pattern, pneumatosis, portal venous gas, pneumoperitoneum (Figure 64-1)

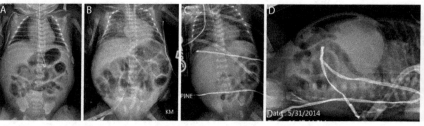

FIGURE 64-1 **(a) Pneumatosis, (b) portal venous gas, (c and d) free air.**

STAGING: MODIFIED BELL'S STAGING CRITERIA (TABLE 64-1)

Differential diagnosis – sepsis, medical ileus

TABLE 64-1	Modified Bell's Staging Criteria			
Stage	Classification	Clinical Findings	Radiographic Findings	Gastrointestinal Symptoms
Ia	Suspected	Apnea, bradycardia, temperature instability	Mild ileus	Increased gastric residuals, mild distention, fecal occult blood
Ib	Suspected	Same as above	Same as above	Grossly bloody stools
IIa	Definite, mild	Same as above	Ileus, intestinal dilation, focal pneumatosis	Prominent distention, absent bowel sounds, grossly bloody stools
IIb	Definite, moderate	Thrombocytopenia, early metabolic acidosis	Diffuse pneumatosis, ascites, portal vein gas	Abdominal tenderness, abdominal wall edema
IIIa	Advanced, severe	Acidosis, oliguria, hypotension, coagulopathy	Same as above, prominent bowel loops	Worsening edema, erythema, palpable loops
IIIb	Advanced, perforated bowel	Shock, decompensation	Pneumoperitoneum	Bowel perforation

MANAGEMENT

1. Medical management (stage I–II): Bowel rest, gastric decompression, IV fluids and resuscitation, broad-spectrum antibiotics. Obtain blood and urine cultures prior to initiation of antibiotics. Follow with serial abdominal exams and radiographs. Clinical deterioration or failure to improve are indications for surgical management.
2. Surgical management (stage III): Laparotomy, resection of necrotic bowel, second-look laparotomy for areas of questionable ischemia, ostomy creation. Primary anastomosis performed selectively. Placement of a Penrose drain alone, without laparotomy, used as definitive management in some neonates <1 kg.

PEARLS

1. Focal intestinal perforation (FIP)
   a. Spontaneous, isolated perforation occurring primarily in extremely premature neonates
   b. May be managed with peritoneal drainage alone in some cases
2. Complications
   a. Short gut syndrome – NEC is leading cause of short gut syndrome, accounting for >50% of cases
   b. Stricture – feeding intolerance after medical management should prompt contrast studies (contrast enema followed by upper GI series) to assess for strictures. Strictures occur most frequently in the colon and distal ileum.

3. Future directions
   a. A Cochrane review found that probiotic administration in premature neonates may reduce the incidence of necrotizing enterocolitis.[1] Clinical trials are underway to further delineate this relationship.

MALROTATION/VOLVULUS

BACKGROUND

Normal intestinal rotation during gestation is 270 degrees in the counterclockwise direction. Failure of normal rotation results in Ladd's band (adhesions crossing from the abdominal wall to the cecum, which may compress the duodenum) and a narrow-based mesentery, which is prone to midgut volvulus.

FINDINGS

1. Signs and symptoms:
   a. Acute presentation: Acute-onset bilious emesis is assumed to be malrotation with midgut volvulus until proven otherwise. Abdomen can be distended or scaphoid and is tender to palpation. Prompt surgical intervention is required to avoid bowel ischemia, peritonitis, shock, and potential loss of the entire small bowel.
   b. Chronic: Malrotation without volvulus can present with feeding intolerance, failure to thrive, and intermittent abdominal pain. Symptoms are due to duodenal obstruction by Ladd's bands and/or intermittent partial volvulus.
2. Labs: Leukocytosis and metabolic acidosis (seen variably)
3. Imaging:
   a. No imaging indicated if clinical presentation concerning for midgut volvulus with bowel ischemia. Proceed immediately with operation.
   b. Abdominal radiograph (two-view) – gastric distention, gasless abdomen, "double bubble" sign of duodenal obstruction. Radiographic findings are variable.
   c. Upper GI – This is the definitive study for malrotation. The ligament of Treitz fails to cross to the left of midline and return to the level of the pylorus in the cranial-caudal axis. Corkscrew sign or "beaking" concerning for volvulus (Figure 64-2).
   d. Ultrasound – "whirlpool sign" of superior mesenteric vein (SMV) around superior mesenteric artery (SMA).

MANAGEMENT

1. Acute presentation (concern for volvulus): Fluid resuscitation, NG decompression, broad-spectrum IV antibiotics, immediate laparotomy for reduction of volvulus, resection of necrotic bowel, and Ladd procedure.
2. Chronic presentation (malrotation without volvulus): Elective Ladd procedure (laparoscopic or open). Components of Ladd procedure include (1) division of Ladd's bands to relieve duodenal obstruction, (2) appendectomy, (3) broadening of mesentery, and (4) positioning the small bowel in the right and large bowel in the left hemi-abdomen.

SMALL BOWEL OBSTRUCTION

BACKGROUND

Common causes in pediatric population include adhesive disease, internal hernia, incarcerated inguinal hernias, intussusception, volvulus, omphalomesenteric band, and intestinal stricture.

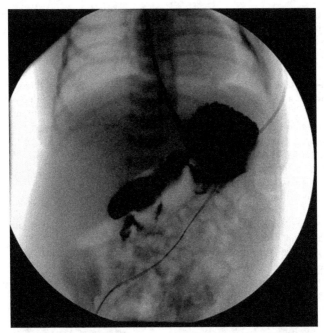

FIGURE 64-2 UGI showing malrotation with midgut volvulus resulting in "corkscrew" appearance.

FINDINGS

1. Signs and symptoms: Crampy abdominal pain, bilious emesis, abdominal distention, obstipation
2. Labs: May be normal or show signs of dehydration, metabolic acidosis, leukocytosis
3. Imaging:
   a. Abdominal radiograph – distended loops of intestine, paucity of gas in rectum, air fluid levels
   b. Computerized tomography – useful for identifying transition point, distinguishing between complete and partial small bowel obstruction (SBO), and identifying emergent findings such as internal hernia.

MANAGEMENT

1. Nonoperative: IV hydration and NG decompression indicated for patients without peritonitis or other signs of bowel ischemia, especially in the setting of partial obstruction attributable to adhesions.
2. Operative: Laparoscopy or laparotomy indicated for any signs of peritonitis, any obstruction without explanation (e.g., no prior abdominal operations), and/or failure to improve with nonoperative management (typically within 48–72 hours).

PEARLS

1. Intussusception
   a. Primary intussusception may occur after gastroenteritis or respiratory viral infection. Secondary intussusception occurs due to a lead point (e.g., Meckel's).

    b. Most common between ages 3 months and 3 years old. Atypical cases include older children and teenagers where other etiologies and lead points such as tumors should be considered.

    c. Although a "target sign" is sometimes visible on plain radiograph, diagnosis is typically made by ultrasound.

    d. First-line treatment in typical patients is with air or water-soluble contrast enema reduction and is successful in up to 85% of patients. Delayed reduction enema can be utilized if the initial reduction is partially successful, and repeat reduction may be attempted for recurrences. Recent studies do not demonstrate an increased incidence of complication with repeat enemas.[2]

2. Meckel's band

    a. Consider omphalomesenteric band if patient has obstruction without previous abdominal surgeries or other known etiology.

    b. Diverticulum may also serve as lead point in intussusception.

3. Hernias

    a. Incarcerated inguinal hernia is a common cause of intestinal obstruction, especially in babies.

    b. A complete physical exam is crucial in patients with obstruction.

4. Stricture

    a. Important consideration in patients with previous necrotizing enterocolitis (NEC) or bowel ischemia

    b. Diagnosed with upper and lower contrast studies

ACUTE APPENDICITIS

BACKGROUND

Appendicitis occurs due to obstruction of the appendiceal lumen resulting in inflammation, ischemia, necrosis, and eventually perforation. Obstruction may be due to a variety of causes, including fecal material (fecalith), hyperplasia of lymphoid tissue, or foreign bodies. Infection is usually polymicrobial, and enteric organisms are most commonly seen.

FINDINGS

Presentation is widely variable and may not follow the classic pattern of diffuse periumbilical pain followed by localized right lower quadrant (RLQ) tenderness, particularly in young children. Common signs and symptoms include abdominal pain, fever, nausea/vomiting, and tachycardia. Exam is often notable for focal peritonitic pain in the RLQ. Laboratory findings are also variable, but a leukocytosis with left shift is common. Diagnosis can be confirmed by imaging. Ultrasound (US) is typically the first-line imaging in children, with computerized tomography (CT) or magnetic resonance imaging (MRI) reserved for those with nondiagnostic ultrasound.

MANAGEMENT

Children with acute, nonperforated appendicitis are managed with appendectomy and can be discharged home within 24 hours of operation, often on the same day. Non-operative management of acute appendicitis is currently under investigation in a number of clinical trials, but is still considered experimental. Those with complicated (perforated) appendicitis have more complex management challenges, which may occasionally necessitate ICU care.

1. Initial management

    a. Most children presenting with clinical and imaging findings concerning for perforation still benefit from up-front appendectomy. Early appendectomy is associated with lower costs and fewer readmissions compared to those who undergo initial nonoperative management.

b. In rare cases, perforated appendicitis can involve the base of the appendix at the cecum, necessitating ileocecectomy.

c. Those presenting with a well-defined abscess may benefit from initial image-guided drainage and antibiotic therapy tailored to the culture results.

d. For those who undergo initial nonoperative management, delayed "interval appendectomy," typically after 6 to 12 weeks, is recommended by some surgeons to avoid recurrence.

2. Routine postoperative management of perforated appendicitis

a. Patients who undergo appendectomy for perforated appendicitis require fluid resuscitation, careful monitoring of intake and output, and a prolonged course of antibiotic therapy.

b. Most surgeons keep these children on broad-spectrum IV antibiotics (piperacillin-tazobactam or ceftriaxone/metronidazole) until they are afebrile, tolerating a general diet, and pain free.

c. Some check a complete blood count (CBC) and/or C-reactive protein (CRP) prior to discharge.

d. Patients can then be discharged home to complete a course of oral antibiotics.

3. Postoperative abscess

a. Postoperative abscess occurs in 20% to 25% of patients who undergo appendectomy for perforated appendicitis.

b. Patients with fever, pain, and/or feeding intolerance persisting beyond 5 to 7 days should undergo CT scan to assess for abscess.

c. Postoperative abscess is managed by image-guided drainage (or, rarely, by operative drainage) followed by prolonged antibiotic therapy (typically 10–14 days) tailored to the culture results. Patients with smaller, undrainable collections may be managed by antibiotics alone.

COLITIS

BACKGROUND

Variety of etiologies, including infectious and inflammatory causes.

CLINICAL FINDINGS

Fever, abdominal distention, diarrhea, leukocytosis.

MANAGEMENT

Although management is dependent on the etiology of colitis, initial management is usually nonoperative except in cases of perforation or septic shock.

ETIOLOGIES

1. Ulcerative colitis with toxic megacolon

a. Emergent surgical intervention may be required for those presenting with fulminating disease with abdominal distention, bloody diarrhea, severe cramping, fever, tachycardia, and sepsis.

b. Abdominal radiograph demonstrates massively dilated colon.

c. Surgical management of patients presenting acutely is typically with a three-stage procedure: (1) acute intervention with total colectomy with end ileostomy; (2) subsequent completion proctectomy, ileoanal pouch creation, and loop ileostomy; and (3) final ileostomy closure.

2. *Clostridium difficile*
   a. Septic shock from fulminant colitis is a rare but serious complication of *C. difficile* infection.
   b. Bacteria release exotoxins, which cause mucosal injury and inflammation of the colon, leading to pseudomembrane formation, ulceration, and systemic toxicity.
   c. Toxic megacolon is a clinical diagnosis based upon radiographic evidence of extreme colonic dilation in the setting of severe sepsis.
   d. Failure to improve with resuscitation and appropriate antimicrobial therapy is an indication for emergent colectomy.
3. Hirschprung-associated enterocolitis (HAC)
   a. HAC is a potentially life-threatening complication of Hirschsprung's disease (HD). It may be the initial presenting finding in children with undiagnosed HD, or it may occur after definitive pull-through procedure.
   b. The etiology is bacterial overgrowth in the setting of distal obstruction due to aganglionosis of the bowel and internal sphincter.
   c. Initial management is with fluid resuscitation, broad-spectrum antibiotics, and prompt rectal irrigations.
4. Neutropenic enterocolitis
   a. A necrotizing infection of the intestine occurring in patients with neutropenia, usually as a result of cytotoxic chemotherapy. The etiology is not fully understood but is likely due to mucosal injury and loss of host defenses secondary to chemotherapy, often seen in patients with hematologic malignancies. It was first described in the pediatric population with acute leukemia undergoing induction therapy.
   b. Historically referred to as "typhlitis," it most commonly occurs in the ileocecal region. However, it may be found anywhere in the small bowel or colon. Usually a polymicrobial infection.
   c. Important to consider for a child with fever and abdominal pain in the setting of severe neutropenia (absolute neutrophil count <500 cells/μL); CT is diagnostic imaging of choice.
   d. Optimal medical management includes bowel rest, gastric decompression, IV fluids, correction of coagulopathy, and broad-spectrum IV antibiotics. Surgical intervention is rarely required and reserved for frank perforation, clinical deterioration, or persistent GI bleed.

FOREIGN BODIES/INGESTIONS

BACKGROUND

The most frequently swallowed items include coins, toys, and batteries. The most common area of impaction is the esophagus below the cricopharyngeus muscle. The majority of foreign bodies that pass into the stomach will pass through the remainder of the GI tract uneventfully. Plain radiograph is usually sufficient to demonstrate the object.

ESOPHAGEAL FOREIGN BODIES

1. Clinical findings include drooling, poor feeding, neck or throat pain
2. Three main areas of impaction: the upper esophageal sphincter, level of the aortic arch, and lower esophageal sphincter.
3. Items impacted in upper and mid-esophagus usually require retrieval by rigid or flexible endoscopy or Foley balloon extraction under fluoroscopy.
4. Protect the airway and avoid inadvertently dropping the object into the airway during extraction from the esophagus.

GASTROINTESTINAL FOREIGN BODIES

1. Once an object reaches the stomach, removal is rarely indicated (see later for exceptions)
2. Potential areas of impaction include the pylorus and the ileocecal valve
3. Acute onset of pain warrants a two-view radiograph to exclude free air

SPECIFIC INGESTIONS

1. Batteries
   a. May release low-voltage current or leak alkali solution – causes liquefaction necrosis.
   b. Look for double contour rim on x-ray (Figure 64-3).
   c. Injury may occur in as little as 60 minutes; needs **immediate removal** when in esophagus.
   d. Complications include perforation, stricture, tracheoesophageal fistula (TEF).
2. Alkali ingestion (lye)
   a. More dangerous with greater extent of injury than acidic ingestions, causes liquefactive necrosis with penetration into deeper tissues.
   b. High risk of esophageal perforation during reparative phase of healing (5–10 days).
   c. Scar formation results in high risk of stricture.
   d. Management includes resuscitation and supportive care.
   e. Endoscopy should be performed on all symptomatic patients between 24 and 48 hours after injury to evaluate extent of injury (see Table 64-2).
   f. Contrast esophagram utilized as clinically indicated to assess for stricture.

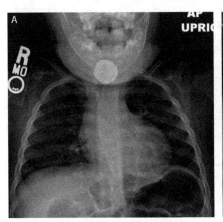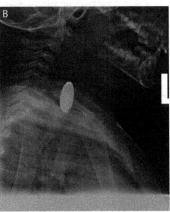

FIGURE 64-3 **Button battery in esophagus.**

TABLE 64-2	Grading of Caustic Esophageal Injury
Grade	**Endoscopic Findings**
0	Normal mucosa
1	Mucosal edema, erythema
2a	Friable mucosa, blisters, hemorrhage, erosions, white exudate
2b	Same as 2a with deep or circumferential ulcerations
3a	Scattered, small areas of necrosis
3b	Extensive necrosis

3. Magnets
   a. Problematic when (1) multiple and (2) separated along the length of the gastrointes-
      tinal system. May attach across intestinal wall in two separate areas of lumen causing
      perforation, obstruction, or fistula formation.
   b. Managed with close observation and serial exams
4. Sharp objects
   a. Low risk of perforation; however, close observation is warranted until the object
      passes into the colon.
   b. May flush GI tract with polyethylene glycol to assist with clearance.

SPECIAL CONSIDERATIONS

ESOPHAGEAL PERFORATION

Background

The majority of esophageal perforations are due to iatrogenic injuries; causes include
endotracheal intubation, NG tube placement, or stricture dilations. Other common causes
include foreign body ingestion, caustic ingestions, or trauma. The most common location for
perforation is in the thoracic esophagus.

Clinical Findings

1. Dysphagia, respiratory distress, fever, chest pain, subcutaneous emphysema
2. Chest x-ray may demonstrate pneumothorax, pleural effusion, pneumomediastinum,
   pneumopericardium, or subcutaneous emphysema.
3. Contrast esophagram with evidence of leak is diagnostic study of choice. Water-soluble
   contrast is used initially, but may be followed by barium if no leak identified.

Management

1. Initiation of broad-spectrum antibiotics
2. If identified early (<24 hr), may undergo primary surgical repair. If there is a delay in
   diagnosis, diversion with drainage of leak is preferred.
3. The majority will heal spontaneously with appropriate diversion.

DUODENAL PERFORATION

Background

Etiologies for perforation include trauma, obstruction (atresia), ulcers (rare), Crohn's disease, or iatrogenic injury. Signs and symptoms are similar to other intestinal perforations
and include abdominal pain, distention, nausea and vomiting, leukocytosis, sepsis, and free
air on imaging. Management is made more difficult by the inability to resect the affected
portion of bowel and the high risk of leak with primary repair.

Management

1. Principles of operative management rely on wide drainage of the injury in addition to
   repair.
2. Pyloric exclusion may be performed (suturing closed the pylorus) with gastrojejunos-
   tomy for complete but temporary diversion of gastric secretions from repaired area. This
   reduces the incidence of duodenal fistula.
3. Feeding jejunostomy should be considered for enteral access and nutrition.

ABDOMINAL COMPARTMENT SYNDROME

Background

Sustained intra-abdominal hypertension that is associated with new-onset organ dysfunction or failure. Increased pressure on capillary beds leads to decreased perfusion of abdominal viscera, resulting in ischemia, acidosis, and eventual cardiopulmonary collapse. Causes include trauma, sepsis, and massive fluid resuscitation.

Clinical Findings

1. Firm, distended abdomen, oliguria, decreased tidal volumes with increased peak, and plateau pressures on ventilator
2. Elevated intra-abdominal pressure >20 mmHg

Management

1. Measure serial bladder pressures. Should be measured with child paralyzed in supine position.
2. Decrease abdominal wall compliance with sedation and paralysis. Optimize fluid balance.
3. Decompressive laparotomy and diuresis until decrease in edema allows for tension-free closure.

REFERENCES

1. AlFaleh K, Anabrees J. Probiotics for prevention of necrotizing enterocolitis in preterm infants. *Cochrane Database Syst Rev.* 2014;4:CD005496.
2. Fisher JG, Sparks EA, Turner CG, et al. Operative indications in recurrent ileocolic intussusception. *J Ped Surg.* 2015;50(1):126-130.

DEFINITIONS

Inflammation of the peritoneal lining of the abdominal cavity

- Primary: without an intra-abdominal source
- Secondary: caused by viscus rupture/perforation, bowel necrosis, or extension of an intra-peritoneal organ infection or abscess

ETIOLOGY

Most commonly associated with nephrotic syndrome, liver failure, acute abdominal infections (i.e., appendicitis)

COMMON ORGANISMS

- Pneumococci
- Group A streptococci
- Gram-negative enteric organisms: *Escherichia. coli, Klebsiella*
- Staphylococci
- Enterococci
- Candida
- *Pasteurella multocida*
- *Mycobacteria tuberculosis*

CAUSES OF SECONDARY PERITONITIS

- Ruptured appendicitis
- Incarcerated hernia
- Midgut volvulus
- Meckel's diverticulum
- Intussusception
- Necrotizing enterocolitis (NEC)
- Hemolytic uremic syndrome (HUS)
- Ruptured peptic ulcer
- Trauma
- Genital tract infections and pelvic inflammatory disease (PID): mixed flora, *Neisseria, Chlamydia*, anaerobes
- Foreign bodies: ventriculoperitoneal (VP) shunts, peritoneal dialysis (PD) catheters
- Autoimmune disorders: systemic lupus erythematosus (SLE)

CLINICAL MANIFESTATIONS

- Fever, abdominal pain, anorexia, vomiting, diarrhea, acute abdomen, mental status changes, toxic appearance, shock.
- Clinical signs may be unreliable; therefore, have a low threshold for diagnostic paracentesis.

DIAGNOSIS

LABORATORY EVALUATION

- Complete blood count (CBC): increased white blood cells (WBCs) with neutrophil predominance
- Urinalysis (UA): proteinuria
- Ascitic fluid: >250 polys/mm^2, increased lactate, decreased pH (<7.35), Gram stain with organisms

IMAGING

- Upright abdominal x-ray: may show free air in patients with ruptured viscus

TREATMENT

See *Surviving Sepsis Guidelines* to reverse shock.

ANTIMICROBIAL THERAPY

- Empiric IV antibiotics:
  - Ampicillin or ceftriaxone + an aminoglycoside
  - Anaerobic coverage (metronidazole or clindamycin) if secondary peritonitis suspected
- Switch to enteral antimicrobial: afebrile and able to tolerate enteral medications
- Narrow antimicrobial therapy: based on culture results
- Duration: 10 to 14 days

SURGICAL INTERVENTION

- Drainage of abscess
- Repair of perforated viscus
- Excision of necrotic bowel
- Removal of foreign body

SUGGESTED READINGS

Rangel SJ, Moss RL. Chapter 69: Peritonitis. In: Long SS, Pickering LK, Prober CG, eds. *Principles and Practice of Pediatric Infectious Diseases*. 3rd ed. Churchill Livingstone–An Imprint of Elsevier Science; 2009:420.

Solomkin JS, Mazuski JE, Bradley JS, et al. Diagnosis and management of complicated intra-abdominal infection in adults and children: Guidelines by the Surgical Infection Society and the Infectious Diseases Society of America. *Clin Infect Dis*. 2010;50:133-164.

Acute Liver Failure

CLINICAL PRESENTATION

- Symptoms may include nausea, vomiting, itching, fever.
- Signs may include encephalopathy, ascites, scleral icterus/jaundice.
- Though there are no strict diagnostic criteria, consider acute liver failure if all of these are present:
  - Hepatic failure within 8 weeks of onset of hepatic disease
  - Elevated serum AST, ALT, and/or bilirubin
  - Coagulopathy (PT >15, INR >1.5) does not correct with vitamin K
  - No prior history of chronic liver disease
  - Encephalopathy (confirmatory, not required)

ETIOLOGY

- Likelihood of various etiologies depends on age and geography
- Causes can be classified into the following categories:
  - Infectious
  - Metabolic
  - Autoimmune
  - Toxin or drug mediated
  - Indeterminate
  - Other

DIAGNOSTIC EVALUATION

- Physical exam: look for jaundice, encephalopathy, Kayser-Fleischer rings.
- History: ask about timing of symptom onset, family history, medications or recreational drugs, and fever.
- Serum labs: coagulation factors, complete metabolic panel, amylase, lipase, complete blood count, acetaminophen level, ammonia, lactate
- Secondary testing once diagnosis of acute liver failure is confirmed:
  - If cytopenia is present in two cell lines perform hemophagocytic lymphohistiocytosis (HLH) testing with ferritin, triglyceride, and fibrinogen.
  - If older than 5 years perform Wilson's disease testing with serum ceruloplasmin.
  - Viral hepatitis serology, viral PCR (herpes simplex virus [HSV], Epstein-Barr virus [EBV], cytomegalovirus [CMV], adenovirus, parvovirus, enterovirus)
  - Perform tests for specific genetic etiologies based on age of patient and newborn screening results.
- Liver biopsy may be indicated if etiology remains unknown.

MANAGEMENT

- Acute liver failure may lead to rapid systemic decompensation, so PICU admission is often appropriate.
- Frequently monitor for hyponatremia, hypoglycemia, hypokalemia, and hypophosphatemia.
- Manage fluids to avoid fluid overload. Consider continuous renal replacement therapy early in the treatment course.

- Routine monitoring of coagulation factors:
  - Give vitamin K one time to assess response in coagulopathy.
  - Empiric correction of coagulopathy with plasma infusion is not indicated, unless done prior to an invasive procedure.
- Respiratory support: respiratory failure requiring mechanical ventilation is common due to fluid overload, pulmonary edema or hemorrhage, encephalopathy, or sepsis.
- Frequently reassess the clinical exam, including assessment of encephalopathy staging. See table 66-1.
- Neurologic care in early stages of hepatic encephalopathy (grades 0–II):
  - Head of bed elevated 30 degrees
  - Oxygen saturation >96%
  - Temperature control to maintain normothermia
  - Maintain adequate blood pressures to ensure good cerebral perfusion pressure (CPP)
  - Target serum sodium 145 to 150 mEq/L and serum osmolarity 300 to 320 mOsm/L with hypertonic saline
  - Baseline EEG
  - Obtain baseline head imaging to evaluate for cerebral edema (MR ventricle with diffusion weighted imaging [DWI]).
- Neurologic care when worsening clinical exam and/or hepatic encephalopathy grades III and IV:
  - Invasive intracranial pressure (ICP) monitoring can be considered, but there is risk of bleeding and lack of evidence it improves survival.
    - Mannitol and/or hypertonic saline may be used for acutely elevated ICP
    - CPP goal range 40 to 60 mmHg depending on age
  - Target $PaCO_2$ 35 to 40 mmHg using mechanical ventilation.
  - Active cooling to keep temperature <37.5°
- Monitor for infections. If antibiotics are indicated, consider using ceftriaxone due to its ability to protect astrocyte glutamate transporters.

TABLE 66-1	Stages of Pediatric Hepatic Encephalopathy	
Grade	**Neurologic Behaviors**	**Deep Tendon Reflexes**
Grade 0	Normal	Normal
Grade I	Confused, inconsolable crying, irritable, mood changes; not acting like usual self	Normal or hyperreflexic
Grade II	Drowsy, inappropriate behavior, inconsolable crying; not acting like usual self	Normal or hyperreflexic
Grade III	Stupor, somnolence, combativeness, may obey simple commands	Hyperreflexic, + Babinski's
Grade IV	Comatose, arouses with painful stimuli or no responses to painful stimuli	Absent

- Therapies for specific etiologies:
  - Acetaminophen toxicity: N-acetyl cysteine
  - Autoimmune causes: steroids
  - Herpes simplex virus: acyclovir
  - Hepatitis B: lamivudine
  - Wilson's disease: chelation, plasmapheresis
  - HLH: steroids, chemotherapy

- ○ Gestational alloimmune liver disease/neonatal hemochromatosis: IVIG, exchange transfusion
- ○ Tyrosinemia type 1: nitisinone (NTBC)
- • Liver transplant
  - ○ Treatment with liver transplant is a multidisciplinary decision. There are no existing standardized indications for liver transplant for pediatric acute liver failure (see Chapter 67).

SUGGESTED READINGS

Hussain E, Grimason M, Goldstein J, et al. EEG abnormalities are associated with increased risk of transplant or poor outcome in children with acute liver failure. *J Pediatr Gastroenterol Nutr.* 2014;58(4):449-456.

Lutfi R, Abulebda K, Nitu ME, et al. Intensive care management of pediatric acute liver failure. *J Pediatr Gastroenterol Nutr.* 2017;64(5):660-670.

Squires RH, Shneider BL, Bucuvalas J, et al. Acute liver failure in children: The first 348 patients in the pediatric acute liver failure study group. *J Pediatr.* 2006;148(5):652-658.

67 Liver Transplantation

INDICATIONS FOR LIVER TRANSPLANT

- Biliary atresia often following the Kasai procedure
- Metabolic diseases
  - Alpha-1-antitrypsin deficiency
  - Tyrosinemia
  - Wilson's disease
  - Urea cycle defects
  - Hemochromatosis
  - Glycogen storage disease
- Fulminant hepatic failure (see Chapter 66)
  - Infection
  - Toxin
  - Drug ingestion
- Hepatic malignancy
- Chronic liver disease
- End-stage liver disease

CONTRAINDICATIONS FOR LIVER TRANSPLANT

- Absolute contraindications
  - Unresectable hepatic malignant tumor
  - Uncontrollable extrahepatic sepsis
  - Neurologic devastation (arrived by consensus, as stage IV hepatic encephalopathy can mask brain death)
- Relative contraindications
  - Acceptable alternative medical therapy
  - Expected suboptimal outcome
  - Impairment of other organ systems that would compromise function of the graft
  - Major systemic infection
  - Cancer with a high postsurgical recurrence rate

OPERATIVE TECHNIQUE

- Recipient hepatectomy phase
- Anhepatic phase
- Reperfusion phase
  - Arterial anastomoses
  - Biliary reconstruction
  - Hemostasis

TYPES OF TRANSPLANTS

- Reduced size graft
- Split liver graft
- Living related donor transplantation

POSTOPERATIVE MANAGEMENT

RESPIRATORY MANAGEMENT

- Most pediatric patients will return from the operating room intubated and mechanically ventilated.
- The goal should be to extubate as quickly as medically possible, generally within 48 hours.
- Factors that determine extubation readiness for all patients include ventilatory parameters, sedation and analgesia requirements, and hemodynamics.
- Extubation is often delayed until the 12-hour assessment of graft function.
- Prolonged ventilation increases the risk of nosocomial infection and ventilator-associated pneumonia.
- Age and nutritional status play a role in extubation readiness, as does the transplant type.
- Pleural effusion is common, and the right side is more frequently affected. These effusions can generally be managed with diuretics and fluid restriction and rarely require pleurocentesis and drainage.
- Atelectasis is a common problem, especially in young children, and contributes to respiratory distress and difficulty weaning from mechanical ventilation.
- Diaphragmatic dysfunction is associated with prolonged ventilatory requirement and prolonged PICU stay and may require diaphragmatic plication.
- Monitoring includes oxygen saturation, capnography, and arterial blood gas analysis (Table 67-1).

CARDIOVASCULAR MANAGEMENT

- Patients should be monitored with invasive and noninvasive blood pressure monitoring and central venous pressure monitoring, as well as heart rate monitoring (Table 67-1).
- Hemodynamic instability in the early postoperative period is contributed to by acid–base status, fluid status, and bleeding issues.
- A small percentage of patients will have evidence of bacterial translocation intraoperatively (taking down an old Roux-en-Y, manipulating bowel) and present with a sepsis-like picture.
- Maintaining good flow to the liver is paramount, and hypotension must be avoided at all costs.
- Following liver transplantation, children frequently have hypertension requiring medical control.
- Hypertension results from pain, side effects of immunosuppression (steroids), or volume overload.

TABLE 67-1	Postoperative Liver Transplant Monitoring
System	**Monitoring**
Respiratory	ABG, pulse oximetry, capnography, serial CXR
Cardiovascular	Invasive and noninvasive BP monitoring, CVP monitoring, cardiac monitor
Renal	Urine output
Fluids and electrolytes	Serial BMP, iCa, Mg, Phos, CVP monitoring
Hematology	Serial CBC, PT/PTT, INR
Liver function	Serial LFTs, liver ultrasound with Doppler
Neurologic function	Frequent neuro exam, imaging as needed, EEG as needed

- Hypertension can be particularly dangerous in post-transplant patients due to coagulopathy and thrombocytopenia, and vigilance for hemorrhagic stroke is indicated.
- Calcium channel blockers such as nicardipine and amlodipine are often considered first-line agents in the treatment of acute hypertension in the immediate post-transplant period.

FLUID, ELECTROLYTE, AND ACID–BASE STATUS

- It is important to follow fluid status and electrolytes closely in the postoperative period. Key electrolytes and metabolites to follow post-transplant are serum glucose, pH, and serum phosphorous (Table 67-1).
- Postoperatively, patients are often fluid overloaded due to intraoperative fluid administration. Monitoring should include urine output as well as total fluids in and total fluids out.
- In the child with significant ascites and increased Jackson-Pratt (JP) drainage post-transplant, there may be an associated decrease in urine output.
- Maintaining euvolemia is best accomplished by fluid replacement strategies matching JP drainage with cc/cc fluid replacement intravenously.
- Drainage from the abdominal drains should be measured hourly. This can be an early indicator of intra-abdominal bleeding, coagulopathy, or issues with vascular anastomoses.

GASTROINTESTINAL ASSESSMENT OF GRAFT FUNCTION

- It is imperative to monitor and assess graft quality and function.
- Follow laboratory markers, including pH, glucose, coagulation studies, phosphorous, bilirubin, and transaminases (Table 67-1).
- Issues with graft function are often related to the degree of ischemia-reperfusion during the transplant procedure and blood flow in general postoperatively.
- Ultrasound with Doppler is generally performed in the first 12 hours post-transplant.
- Biliary complications are the most common technical complication after liver transplantation and range from early anastomotic leaks to late obstruction.
- The serum biochemical abnormalities associated with biliary system complications include an elevated bilirubin level and changes in canalicular enzyme levels of alkaline phosphatase and γ-glutamyl transferase (GGT).
- Ultrasonography is not as reliable in assessing biliary pathology.
- Follow coagulation studies closely and replace JP abdominal fluid drainage with fresh frozen plasma if the international normalized ratio (INR) is >1.7. With an INR of <1.7, replacement can be with 5% albumin or lactated Ringer's (LR) depending on the acid–base status of the patient.
- An elevated INR is indicative of poor graft function or an ongoing consumptive process, is consistent with bleeding, and is the first clue that the patient may require re-exploration.
- In these cases, stop all anticoagulation interventions and support with blood products until a surgical problem is clearly defined.

NEUROLOGIC MANAGEMENT

- It is important to assess and reassess neurologic function in the postoperative period.
- Drugs with prolonged half-lives, hepatic metabolism, or a propensity for delirium should be used cautiously. Benzodiazepine administration is avoided.
- Most neurologic complications are related to (1) the degree of pretransplantation encephalopathy or (2) the post-transplant metabolic abnormalities caused by immunosuppressive agents, most notably the calcineurin inhibitors (CNIs).
- Neurologic complications following pediatric liver transplant include seizures, encephalopathy, posterior reversible encephalopathy syndrome (PRES), and headache.

- Seizures are the most common neurologic complication and occur in up to 30% of children following transplant. Causes of seizures include hypoglycemia, electrolyte abnormalities, and high levels of CNI, as well as ischemic or hemorrhagic stroke and infection.
- Neuroimaging should be obtained to rule out intracerebral hemorrhage in any patient with a new-onset seizure or altered mental status.
- CNI-related neurotoxicity occurs in approximately 25% of liver transplant recipients. Many are dose related, and treatment includes reducing or completely discontinuing the suspected offending agent. In some cases, substitution of one CNI by another is all that is needed.
- Primary graft nonfunction causes cerebral edema and increased intracranial pressure, often requiring intracranial pressure monitoring to manage and maintain cerebral perfusion pressure. The treatment is to replace the nonfunctioning liver.
- Electroencephalogram and transcutaneous Doppler studies are valuable to differentiate cerebral edema from encephalopathy from drug effect, especially when prognosis is a factor in determining retransplant candidacy.
- If there are concerns for brain death, a nuclear medicine scan for brain perfusion may be the only study to differentiate hepatic encephalopathy (+ flow) from brain death (− flow).

IMMUNOSUPPRESSION

- The immune system recognizes the graft as foreign and begins a destructive immune response mediated principally by T lymphocytes.
- In order to avoid graft destruction, immunosuppressive drugs must be administered.
- Most patients, regardless of age, will begin maintenance immunosuppressive therapy with a triple drug regimen consisting of a CNI, an antiproliferative agent, and steroids (Table 67-2).

TABLE 67-2 Postoperative Liver Transplant Medications

Medication Class	Medication Types	Specific Medications
Immunosuppression	Calcineurin inhibitors	Tacrolimus Cyclosporine
	Antiproliferative agents	Mycophenolate mofetil
	Corticosteroids	Methylprednisolone Prednisone Prednisolone
	Antimetabolites	Azathioprine
	Monoclonal antibody	Basiliximab
Anticoagulation	Bleeding prevention	Vitamin K
	Clot prevention	Heparin infusion
	Antiplatelet, clot prevention	Aspirin
	Platelet aggregation inhibition Decrease reperfusion injury	Alprostadil
Infection prevention	Perioperative antibiotics	Ampicillin Cefotaxime
	Prophylactic antimicrobials	Sulfamethoxazole/trimethoprim Nystatin Ganciclovir

- The goal is to minimize CNI exposure and facilitate early steroid withdrawal, thereby preventing the long-term toxicities: abnormal growth development, steroid-induced osteoporosis and post-transplant lymphoproliferative disease.

ANTICOAGULATION (TABLE 67-2)

- All patients receive one dose of vitamin K immediately upon arrival to the PICU post-transplant.
- All patients are candidates for low-dose heparin infusion. This is viewed as prophylactic dosing, and patients are started on a 10 units heparin/hour regardless of weight. The goal of this therapy is *not* to alter the partial thromboplastin time (PTT), but rather to prevent small clot formation in critical vessels.
- Patients who are identified by transplant surgery as being at high risk for vascular thrombosis will receive treatment-dose heparin infusion. In these patients the therapeutic goal will be to increase the PTT by 1.5 to 2.0 times normal.
- Prior to the initiation of the heparin drip, the following criteria must be met: prothrombin time <25 seconds (INR = 2.1), no obvious evidence of bleeding, and platelet count must be >20,000/mm^3.
- Heparin therapy should be discontinued 24 hours after antiplatelet therapy with aspirin has begun *and* with approval from transplant surgery.
- Aspirin is started on postoperative day #3 as long as the following criteria are met: platelet count ≥20,000, no anticipated procedures requiring adequate platelet function, approval from the transplant team. The duration of aspirin therapy is intended to be 6 months.
- The transplant team may request that the patient be placed on a prostaglandin drip (alprostadil) to reduce vascular resistance and improve blood flow to the liver graft.
- Patients receiving a split liver graft from a deceased donor, patients receiving grafts from marginal donors, patients with rapidly climbing liver enzymes, or patients with a suboptimal intraoperative course (i.e., prolonged ischemia time, poor perfusion) are candidates for alprostadil therapy.
- Alprostadil has potent vasodilatory and antiplatelet effects in addition to its cytoprotective and immunomodulatory properties. These beneficial qualities modulate ischemic reperfusion injury and minimize the risk of primary nonfunction of the graft in the early post-transplant period.
- The duration of therapy is intended to be 3 to 5 days or until AST/ALT normalize.

INFECTION PREVENTION (TABLE 67-2)

- All patients are placed on empiric antibiotics for at least 48 hours after transplantation.
- Ampicillin and cefotaxime are the standard antibiotics for patients with normal renal function.
- All patients receive *Pneumocystis jiroveci* pneumonia (PCP) prophylaxis with sulfamethoxazole-trimethoprim for 1 year post-transplant unless contraindicated.
- All patients receive *Candida* prophylaxis for prevention of oral thrush with nystatin for 3 months post-transplant.
- Select patients will receive antiviral prophylaxis for cytomegalovirus (CMV) with ganciclovir based on the transplant recipient's age, CMV serologic status at the time of transplant, and the donor's CMV serologic status.
- Patients who are retransplanted and those who have been treated with antithymocyte globulin are considered high risk for acquiring CMV disease and should be treated with antivirals for a total of 3 months.

NUTRITION

- Nutrition in the post-transplant patient is critically important.
- For the child who is well nourished preoperatively, the transition is easier. Frequently the patient's preoperative profile includes malnutrition, preexisting ascites, and edema.
- For the first 3 to 5 days postoperatively, the patient is treated like a surgical abdomen patient.
- Enteral calories begin once there are bowel sounds, flatus, and no evidence of ileus.
- In a liver transplant, a choledochojejunostomy is performed to allow for bile drainage. In a patient who has had a previous Kasai procedure, they will already have had a choledocho-jejunostomy with a Roux-en-Y loop, so this does not need to be created.
- A child with an existing choledochojejunostomy with a Roux-en-Y loop can be fed when they meet postsurgical criteria on postoperative day #3, whereas a fresh choledochojeju-nostomy with a new Roux-en-Y loop cannot be fed until postoperative day #5 as per the surgical team.
- The liver is essential for the digestion and absorption of protein, fat, and carbohydrate as well as the fat-soluble vitamins (A, D, E, and K). The transplant child also needs supple-mentation with iron, zinc, calcium, and magnesium.

POST-TRANSPLANT COMPLICATIONS

- Postoperative complications usually present with a nonspecific combination of cholestasis, rising hepatocellular enzyme levels, fever, lethargy, and anorexia.
- Early complications include
  - Primary nonfunction
  - "Small for size" syndrome
  - Technical complications
  - Vascular thrombosis
  - Biliary leak
  - Rejection
  - Infection
- Late complications include
  - Infection
  - Rejection
  - Hypertension
  - Renal dysfunction
  - Lymphoproliferative disease

PRIMARY NONFUNCTION

- The lack of graft functional recovery can be seen in the first hours following transplanta-tion, with high lactate levels, increasing prothrombin time and partial thromboplastin time, rapidly rising liver enzyme levels, bleeding, vasoplegia, progressive renal and multi-system failure, and encephalopathy.
- It is the most common cause of early graft loss. Biopsy reveals histologic evidence of hepa-tocyte necrosis in the absence of any vascular compromise.
- The only treatment is emergent retransplantation.
- A possible cause is hyperacute rejection.
- With improved donor selection and management, operative techniques, reducing cold ischemia times, and newer preservative solutions, the risk of primary nonfunction has decreased but remains around 5%.

- Patients with initial dysfunction, also known as primary graft dysfunction, might recover with support, but those who progress to show evidence of extrahepatic complications as listed earlier must be considered as having primary nonfunction and listed for retransplantation.

VASCULAR COMPLICATIONS

- Hepatic artery thrombosis is the most common vascular complication. The incidence in children ranges between 5% and 20%.
- It may present as acute liver failure, biliary fistula, or enzyme elevation.
- Hepatic artery thrombosis is associated with small-size donors and presents with massive graft necrosis and graft loss.
- Hepatic artery thrombosis occurs in children three to four times more frequently than in adult transplant patients and usually within the first 30 days after transplantation.
- Late thromboses can manifest with biliary complications.
- Hepatic artery thrombosis and biliary complications are correlated because the blood supply of the biliary tract is exclusively arterial. Diagnosis is made based on an absence of flow using Doppler ultrasound.
- Surgical exploration and thrombectomy may be required.
- Anticoagulation or antiplatelet agents are often used to help.
- Portal vein thrombosis is less frequent than hepatic artery thrombosis, occurring in 4% to 15% of recipients and is more frequent in children transplanted for biliary atresia.
- The incidence of vascular thrombosis is related to vessel size
- Presentation includes elevation in liver enzymes, portal hypertension, and encephalopathy.
- Diagnosis is also made by Doppler ultrasound.
- Thrombectomy is often required.
- Prevention includes anticoagulation and avoidance of hemoconcentration.

BILIARY COMPLICATIONS

- Biliary complications occur in approximately 8% to 30% of pediatric liver transplant recipients.
- In the early postoperative period, the presence of bile-like fluid in the abdominal drains is strongly suggestive of a bile leak.
- Ultrasound evidence of intrahepatic biliary ducts dilatation, elevated alkaline phosphatase, and gamma-glutamyl transferase (GGT) suggest biliary stricture. Patients may require dilation and internal stenting.

REJECTION

- Acute cellular rejection is very common, and about 20% to 50% of patients develop at least one episode of acute rejection in the first few weeks after liver transplant, with about 45% of patients developing at least one episode of rejection within 6 months of transplant.
- Clinical signs include fever, irritability, malaise, and leukocytosis.
- Increases in GGT, bilirubin, and/or transaminases after transplant in a stable patient may be the first sign of rejection.
- Histologic biopsy evaluation of the liver is essential for making the diagnosis of rejection.
- Treatment involves pulse steroids and adjustment in immunosuppression.
- Based on the severity of the rejection, the patient receives additional treatments, which could range from an increase in the baseline immunosuppressive regimen to the administration of steroid boluses and the addition of other drugs to the maintenance therapy, or the administration of antilymphocyte antibodies in case of resistance to the primary line of therapy.

INFECTION

- Infectious complications now represent the most common source of morbidity and mortality following transplantation. This includes sepsis, nosocomial infection, and opportunistic infection.
- About 38% of patients develop serious bacterial or fungal infections <30 days and 14% have serious viral infections <15 months after liver transplant.
- The risk of infection in liver transplant recipients is determined by the intensity of exposure to infectious agents (hospital or community sources) and the overall immunosuppression level.
- In the first few weeks, bacterial pathogens are more common offending organisms with gram negative bacteria, enterococci or staphylococci.
- Fungal infections are also frequent, with the most common agent being *Candida albicans*.
- Fungal infection most often occurs in high-risk patients, requiring multiple operative procedures, retransplantation, hemodialysis, or multiple antibiotic courses.
- Viral infections occur later, with cytomegalovirus (CMV) being the most common viral infectious agent. Epstein-Barr virus (EBV) infection occurs in the first year after transplant.
- The risk of developing either CMV or EBV infection is influenced by the preoperative serologic status of the transplant donor and recipient.
- Most young children are EBV seronegative at the time of transplant, and during primary exposure to EBV, significant immunosuppression increases the risk of post-transplant lymphoproliferative disease (PTLD).
- Risk factors for PTLD include young age at transplant (less than 2), primary EBV infection, and at least one episode of rejection.
- The incidence of PTLD is decreasing in pediatric liver transplant recipients due to improved immunosuppression regimens.

SUGGESTED READINGS

Fullington NM, Cauley RP, Potanos KM, et al. Immediate extubation after pediatric liver transplantation: A single-center experience. *Liver Transpl.* 2015;21:57-62.

Ganschow R, Nolkemper D, Helmke K, et al. Intensive care management after pediatric liver transplantation: A single-center experience. *Pediatr Transpl.* 2000;4:273-279.

Ghosh PS, Hupertz V, Ghosh D. Neurological complications following pediatric liver transplant. *J Pediatr Gastroenterol Nutr.* 2012;54:540-546.

Gungor S, Kilic B, Arslan M, et al. Early and late neurological complications of liver transplantation in pediatric patients. *Pediatr Transpl.* 2017;21(3):e12872.

Kerkar N, Danialifar T. Changing definitions of successful outcomes in pediatric liver transplantation. *Curr Opin Organ Transplant.* 2014;19:480-485.

Kukreti V, Daoud H, Bola SS, et al. Early critical care course in children after liver transplant. *Crit Care Res Practice.* 2014;2014:725748.

Manczur TI, Greenough A, Rafferty GF, et al. Diaphragmatic dysfunction after pediatric orthotopic liver transplantation. *Transplantation.* 2002;73:228-232.

Miloh T. Medical management of children after liver transplantation. *Curr Opin Organ Transplant.* 2014;19:474-479.

Miloh T, Barton A, Wheeler J, et al. Immunosuppression in pediatric liver transplant recipients: Unique aspects. *Liver Transpl.* 2017;23:244-256.

Murase K, Chihara Y, Takahashi K, et al. Use of noninvasive ventilation for pediatric patients after liver transplantation: Decrease in the need for reintubation. *Liver Transpl.* 2012;18:1217-1225.

Narkewicz MR, Green M, Dunn S, et al. Decreasing incidence of symptomatic Epstein-Barr virus disease and posttransplant lymphoproliferative disorder in pediatric liver transplant recipients: Report of the studies of pediatric liver transplantation experience. *Liver Transpl.* 2013;19:730-740.

Shepherd RW, Turmelle Y, Nadler M, et al. Risk factors for rejection and infection in pediatric liver transplantation. *Am J Transpl.* 2008;8:396-403.

Spada M, Riva S, Maggiore G, et al. Pediatric liver transplantation. *World J Gastroenterol.* 2009;15:648-674.

Tannuri U, Tannuri AC. Postoperative care in pediatric liver transplantation. *Clinics.* 2014;69(S1):42-46.

8 Environmental/Toxicology Emergencies

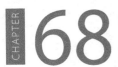
BACKGROUND

- In 2014, over 2 million calls were made to poison control centers across the United States. It is the leading cause of injury-related death in the United States. Of these calls 64% were exposures of children between ages 0 and 19; 50% of total exposures were children younger than 6 years old.[1]
- The top four pediatric exposures were cosmetics/personal care products (15%), household cleaning substances (11%), analgesics (10%), and foreign bodies (7%).[1]

GENERAL PRINCIPLES

- First things first! Your initial assessment should, as always, focus on imminently life-threatening problems. Mind your ABCs prior to additional assessment. Specifically:
  - **Airway**: Toxic exposures can cause tongue/airway edema, flaccid airway structures, and depressed mental status. All these things can necessitate support (oral/nasal airway, suctioning, or an endotracheal tube). When in doubt, secure the airway.
  - **Breathing**: Toxic ingestions can depress respiratory effort or cause inflammation anywhere from the trachea (stridor), airways (wheeze), or alveoli (crackles).
    - If respiratory effort is depressed, bag mask ventilation should be instituted without delay. Naloxone should be administered for a suspected opiate ingestion, but intubation and mechanical ventilation may be necessary if the desired effect is not achieved expediently.
    - In a spontaneously breathing patient, you can consider supplemental oxygen for hypoxia and/or bronchodilators (albuterol/racemic epinephrine) for wheezing.
    - If there is stridor, strongly consider intubation for airway protection.
  - **Circulation**: Ensure adequate circulation. Mind your heart rate and blood pressure. Volume resuscitation, vasopressors, and inotropes might be necessary (review section on shock for guidance in fluid/inotrope/vasopressor management).
- Use your resources! In the event of a known or unknown ingestion, the toxicologists at poison control can help you identify potential toxins and/or ensure appropriate surveillance and management for your patient (U.S. telephone number: 800-222-1222).
- In the event of an unknown ingestion, a prudent history and physical are paramount to making the diagnosis. Interview anyone who might have information about the circumstances of the ingestion. Ask about available substances in the household, routes of administration, behavioral changes/trajectory of illness, etc. In older patients, assess for suicidal intentions.
- If available, review the product/medication containers rather than solely relying on the narrative history.

PHYSICAL EXAM

- Careful physical examination can provide crucial information in identifying an unknown toxidrome or the extent of physiologic derangement in the event of a known ingestion.
- Your initial assessment, beyond the ABCs noted earlier, should be comprehensive but efficient. First attention should be paid to potential threats to life. Vital signs, mental status, and pupillary exam will often provide your first clues to the responsible toxin (see Table 68-1).
- Though "toxidromes" are extremely helpful in identifying and treating a toxic ingestion, know that not every patient will fit cleanly into a known toxidrome.

TABLE 68-1	Clinical Toxidromes	
Toxidrome	**Signs/Symptoms**	**Drug/Toxin**
Anticholinergic	Tachycardia, hypertension, hyperthermia, altered mental status, mydriasis, seizure, flushing, urinary retention, dry mucous membranes	Antihistamines, scopolamine, atropine, tricyclic antidepressants (TCAs), phenothiazines
Sympathomimetic	Tachycardia, hypertension, tachypnea, hyperthermia, mydriasis, hyperactivity, agitation, seizures, diaphoresis	Amphetamines, methamphetamines, cocaine, ephedrine
Cholinergic	Bradycardia, miosis, salivation, lacrimation, bladder/bowel incontinence, bronchorrhea, emesis, bronchospasm, agitation, confusion, weakness, seizures	Organophosphates, insecticides
Opiate	Bradycardia, hypotension, respiratory depression/arrest, miosis, confusion, lethargy, ataxia, coma	Morphine, heroin, oxycodone, codeine, hydrocodone, fentanyl, methadone
Sedative-hypnotic	Bradycardia, hypotension, hypothermia, respiratory depression/arrest, confusion, stupor, coma	Barbiturates, benzodiazapines, alcohol (methanol, ethanol)
Serotonergic	Tachycardia, hypertension, tachypnea, hyperthermia, mydriasis, trismus, diaphoresis, hypertonicity/myoclonus, agitation, confusion, seizures, coma	Selective serotonin reuptake inhibitors (SSRIs), methamphetamines, dextromethorphan, TCAs, monoamine oxidase (MAO) inhibitors, lithium, MDMA ("ecstasy," "Molly"), PCP

DIAGNOSTIC TESTING

- Laboratory data and point-of-care testing can help to clarify diagnosis and direct therapy in a poisoned patient. Nearly every patient should have glucose, electrolytes ($+/-$ liver function testing), serum osmolality, drug screen (urine and serum), and ECG.
- Depending on the clinical circumstances, consideration should be given to checking an arterial blood gas, coagulation panel, head imaging (CT or MRI), abdominal x-ray or CT scan, and blood levels for suspected ingestions or possible co-ingestions. If there is any doubt about the toxidrome or possibility of co-ingestions, levels for acetaminophen, salicylates, and ethanol should be tested.
- Anion gap should always be calculated in the poisoned patient with metabolic acidosis: $(Na^+ + K^+) - (Cl^- + HCO_3^-)$. Normal values are 8 to 16. Causes of anion-gap acidosis is remembered by the mnemonic MUDPILES (methanol, uremia, diabetic ketoacidosis, propylene glycol, isoniazid/iron, lactic acidosis, ethylene glycol, salicylates).
- Osmolal gap should also be calculated for all unknown ingestions. It is calculated by the formula as the difference between the *measured* serum osmolality and the *calculated* osmolarity. Osmolarity is calculated by the formula: $(2 \times Na^+) + (BUN/2.8) + (Glucose \times 18)$. Elevated osmolal gap >10 suggests osmotically active, unmeasured solutes in the bloodstream. Common osmotically active compounds include ethanol, methanol, isopropyl alcohol, acetone, propylene glycol, and mannitol.

OPTIONS FOR DECONTAMINATION

- Often decontamination occurs prior to the PICU in the emergency department or other care site where the child first presents.
- **Surface decontamination:** In the event of a topical toxin exposure, clothing should be removed and the affected area should be liberally irrigated with large volumes of water. After this is done, the area should be cleansed with soap and water. Consideration should be given to consultation with colleagues in dermatology and/or plastic surgery depending on the extent and nature of the injury.
- **Ocular decontamination:** Caustic exposures to the eyes represent an emergency, as the cornea is very easily damaged by caustic agents. Irrigation should be immediate and copious—generally no less than 1 liter of normal saline per eye. pH should be checked following irrigation, and irrigation continued until pH is normal (7.5–8). Contact lenses should be removed, and fluorescein testing should be performed for corneal injury. If there is any evidence of corneal injury, alteration of vision, or other concerns, ophthalmology should be consulted to better assess.
- **Gastric decontamination:** In the pediatric patient, gastric decontamination is most commonly performed by using activated charcoal (AC). Other methods such as syrup of ipecac and gastric lavage have fallen out of favor due to side effects and technical difficulty in the pediatric patient.
  - Even AC is becoming less common due to the lack of evidence for effect on clinical outcomes.
  - AC should be considered within 60 minutes of a potentially toxic ingestion.
  - AC is distributed as an aqueous preparation and should be administered at a dose of 1 g/kg (max 100 g) orally or via NG tube. It is recommended that NG position be confirmed prior to administration. Repeated doses may be considered in consultation with poison control.
- **Forced diuresis:** For primarily renally cleared toxins, historically, providers have utilized a combination of IV volume repletion and osmotic or loop diuretics to force urinary throughput. However, there is no evidence of efficacy of this practice; therefore, it is not recommended.
- **Urine alkalinization:** For many toxins, increasing the pH of the urine will cause the toxin to exist predominantly in the ionized form in the urinary collecting system. In this form, it is less likely to diffuse back into the blood and thus is functionally "trapped."
  - *Methotrexate* and *salicylate*s are two toxins for which urinary alkalization is recommended to promote clearance
  - Alkalinization can be achieved by administration of bicarbonate solutions, acetazolamide, or a combination.
  - Urine alkalinization should be done with serial monitoring of both urine pH and serum electrolytes, as this can cause systemic alkalosis, as well as hypokalemia.
- **Hemodialysis**
  - Small, water-soluble, unbound toxins can often be removed by hemodialysis.
  - Given the invasiveness and potential morbidities of this, it is generally reserved for potentially life-threatening ingestions.
  - Some commonly dialyzed toxins include carbamazepine, ethylene glycol, lithium, methanol, phenobarbital, salicylate, theophylline, and valproic acid.
  - This should generally be done with the consultation of a toxicology expert.

MANAGEMENT OF SPECIFIC TOXINS

ACETAMINOPHEN

- Most common intentional overdose

- **Mechanism**:
  - Major clearance mechanism is by conjugation or sulfation followed by urinary excretion.
  - A less common pathway, an enzyme CYP2E1 can convert acetaminophen to N-acetyl-p-benzoquinone-imine (NAPQI), a potent hepatotoxin.
  - Ordinarily, this by-product is detoxified by glutathione; however, with overdose, NAPQI can accumulate in excess of what glutathione stores can detoxify and cause liver injury.
- **Presentation**:
  - Can present with nausea/vomiting/abdominal pain.
  - Often asymptomatic on presentation.
  - Occasionally will have altered mental status, but this is often not present at time of initial presentation.
- **Course:** Usually, laboratory evidence of liver injury will manifest at ~24 hours and peak in 2 to 3 days. Patients will either gradually recover function or progress to fulminant hepatic failure and thus need to be considered for liver transplantation.
- **Treatment:**
  - N-acetylcysteine (NAC)
    - Works by multiple mechanisms, including increasing glutathione production.
    - It is extraordinarily effective in decreasing risk of liver failure and death after toxic acetaminophen ingestions and should be given as early as possible.
    - The Rumack-Matthew nomogram (Figure 68-1) can help to determine whether or not to treat with NAC based on acetaminophen level. Anything above the broken line in the figure should be treated.
    - Any patients with evidence of acidosis, altered mental status, or hepatic toxicity should also be treated, regardless of level. Erring on the side of administration for any border-line case is recommended, as the drug is extraordinarily well tolerated and the consequences of not treating are high.

SALICYLATES

- By far the most common is acetylsalicylic acid, or aspirin.
- Other salicylates are found in over-the-counter antidiarrheal products, analgesics, cold/cough combination products, antihistamines, and wintergreen oil (methyl salicylate).
- Toxicity is generally seen with ingestions >60 mg/kg.
- **Presentation:**
  - Early signs include tachypnea, nausea, emesis, and tinnitus.
  - Laboratory data early in the course can show a metabolic acidosis and a respiratory alkalosis. Salicylate levels are also available at most laboratories to confirm ingestion, with >35 mg/dL predicting minor symptoms and >45 mg/dL showing more significant toxicity.
  - Rarely salicylate ingestion can cause cerebral or pulmonary edema.
- **Treatment:**
  - As discussed earlier, urine should be alkalinized to enhance toxin clearance. This is generally done by continuous infusion of sodium bicarbonate to target urine pH >7.5
  - Electrolytes , glucose, and systemic acid–base status should be closely monitored.
  - If intubation is required, respiratory alkalosis must be maintained to prevent decompensation via worsening acidosis causing increased CNS salicylate concentration.
  - Hemodialysis should be considered for renal failure if levels are extraordinarily high, if clinical toxidrome is imminently life-threatening or not responding to therapy, if mental status is altered, if there is concern for cerebral edema, or if electrolyte/volume/acid–base status is otherwise untenable.

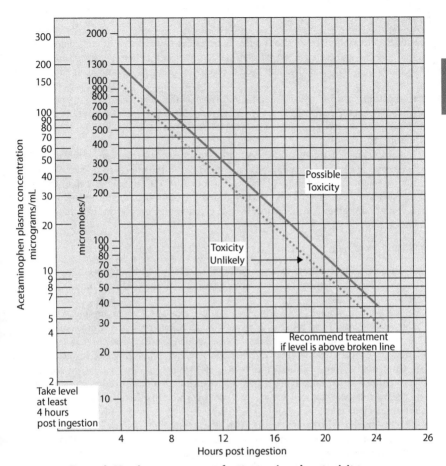

FIGURE 68-1 Rumack-Matthew nomogram for acetaminophen toxicity.
Reproduced with permission from Hung OL, Nelson LS. Acetaminophen. In: Tintinalli JE, et al, eds. *Tintinalli's Emergency Medicine: A Comprehensive Study Guide,* 8e New York, NY: McGraw-Hill; 2016.

BENZODIAZEPINES

- **Mechanism:** Exert action via GABA receptors in the CNS which causes hyperpolarization via chloride influx.
- **Presentation:** Can include bradycardia, hypotension, respiratory depression, stupor, confusion, and coma.
- **Treatment:**
  - Initial treatment is supportive with attention to airway, breathing, and circulation.
  - Can use crystalloid fluid boluses for hypotension; may require endotracheal intubation for respiratory depression.
  - Flumazenil is a competitive GABA antagonist that can reverse the effects of benzodiazepines, but can also precipitate seizures and cardiac dysrhythmias.

OPIATES

- Includes prescription medications such as oxycodone, hydrocodone, morphine, methadone, codeine, and fentanyl, as well as drugs of abuse such as heroin and opium.
- **Mechanism:** Works as agonist to μ- and κ-receptors, which cause both analgesia and toxic side effects.
- **Presentation:** Consists of depressed mental status/coma, depressed respirations, and miosis. Can also entail bradycardia and hypotension. Often causes shallow, rather than slow, respirations so hypercapnea may present before hypopnea.
- **Treatment:**
  - Initial treatment is supportive with attention to airway, breathing, and circulation.
  - Naloxone is a μ- and κ- antagonist and can reverse the effects of opiates. Dose for a life-threatening ingestion is 0.1 mg/kg, but doses of 1/10 or even 1/100 of that starting dose can be effective for partial reversal of less hyperacute ingestions. Doses are generally given IV, but can also be given intramuscularly, subcutaneously, or endotracheally.

RECREATIONAL DRUGS

- Recreational drugs continue to be a source of morbidity and mortality among teenagers. The list of potential toxins is vast and ever growing due to a continual influx of new synthetic drugs of abuse.
- Cocaine is a commonly abused stimulant and presents as a sympathomimetic toxidrome (Table 68-1). Toxicity can result from hypertension, coronary ischemia/myocardial infarction, rhabdomyolysis, cardiac dysrhythmias, sudden cardiac death, renal failure, and pulmonary edema. Treatment is largely supportive, but a high index of suspicion should be maintained for myocardial infarction, and cardiac enzymes should be monitored. Hypertension should initially be treated with benzodiazepines to address toxidrome, but can also be treated with other agents. However, beta blockers should be avoided due to the unopposed alpha effect.
- 3,4-Methylenedioxymethamphetamine (MDMA), commonly sold as "ecstasy" or "Molly," causes release and inhibits reuptake of serotonin, dopamine, and norepinephrine. Its effects include euphoria, changes in perception, mydriasis, tachycardia, and hypertension. MDMA can cause heat stroke, rhabdomyolysis, renal failure, liver damage, disseminated intravascular coagulation (DIC), seizure, and cerebral edema. Treatment is primarily supportive. There is some evidence that dantrolene can be used to treat hyperpyrexia from MDMA.[2]
- Ethanol is an extraordinarily common toxic ingestion among teenagers. Its ingestion can cause altered mental status, coma, emesis, hypothermia, metabolic acidosis, and multiple electrolyte derangements. Activated charcoal is not of benefit in the absence of co-ingestions. Management is supportive, with emphasis on volume repletion and maintaining airway, breathing, and circulation.

OTHER TOXINS

Given the breadth of potential toxins, this chapter does not contain all possible ingestions. In all cases, we recommend consulting with your local Poison Control Center as early as possible for expert guidance. See Table 68-2 for a list of antidotes for common toxins.

TABLE 68-2	Antidotes for Common Toxins
Toxin	**Antidote**
Acetaminophen	N-Acetylcysteine (NAC)
Anticholinergics	Physostigmine
Benzodiazepines	Flumazenil (use with caution for seizures)
Beta-blockers	Glucagon
Botulism (infantile)	Botulism immune globulin
Calcium channel blockers	Calcium chloride, glucagon, dextrose + insulin
Carbon monoxide (CO)	Oxygen, hyperbaric oxygen
Cyanide	Hydroxocobalamin, amyl nitrate, or sodium thiosulfate
Digoxin	Digoxin immune fab
Ethylene glycol	Fomepizole or ethanol
Flouride	Calcium chloride
Heparin	Protamine
Iron	Desferoxamine
Isoniazid, hydralazine	Pyridoxine
Lead	Dimercaprol, calcium disodium EDTA, succimer
Mercury	Dimercaprol
Methanol	Fomepizole or ethanol
Methemoglobinemia (nitrates/nitrites)	Methylene blue
Opiates	Naloxone
Organophosphates/insecticides	Atropine, pralidoxime
Snake venom	Crotalidae polyvalent immune fab
Sulfonylurea	Octreotide
Tricyclic antidepressants	Sodium bicarbonate
Warfarin	Vitamin K

REFERENCES

1. Mowrey JB, Spyker DA, Brooks DE, McMillan N, Jay L, et al. 2014 Annual Report of the American Association of Poison Control Centers' National Poison Data System (NPDS): 32nd Annual Report. *Clini Toxicology*. 2004:53(10):962-1147.
2. Grunau BE, Wiens MO, Greidanus M. Dantrolene for the treatment of MDMA toxicity. *CJEM*. 2010;12(5):457-459.

Burns and Smoke Inhalation 69

INTRODUCTION

This chapter will describe the acute evaluation and management of pediatric patients who experience severe burns and/or smoke inhalation.

BURNS

- Burns are a common phenomenon in the pediatric population, but when severe, can be responsible for over 2,500 deaths annually.
- The most common type of burn in children less than age 5 is scald burns, whereas older children experience flame burns more often.

INITIAL EVALUATION

- All burn patients should receive a full trauma evaluation in the emergency department.
- The patient's airway, breathing, and circulation (ABCs) should be evaluated as per normal protocol.
- The extent of burn injury should be determined. This is done by quantifying the percentage body surface area involved, as well as the depth of the burn injury.
- Total body surface area involvement:
  - See Figure 69-1 for approximations for quantifying total body surface area involved in infants and children (do not count erythema).
  - The Lund and Browder Chart or Berkow Formula are recommended resources for accurately quantifying the extent of body surface area involvement.
  - Rule of Nines is employed for adults: 9% total body surface area involved for each upper extremity, 18% for the head, and 14% for each lower extremity.
  - For smaller areas involved, may use the patient's hand size to equal approximately 1% of total body surface area.

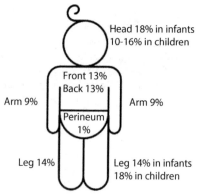

Head 18% in infants
10-16% in children

Front 13%
Back 13%

Arm 9%

Arm 9%

Perineum 1%

Leg 14%

Leg 14% in infants
18% in children

FIGURE 69-1 **Quantifying percentage body surface area involvement.**

- Depth of burn estimation:
  - First-degree burn: erythematous, painful, dry; only epidermis involved
  - Second-degree burn: erythematous, very painful, moist, blistering present; epidermis and dermis involved
  - Third-degree burn: full-thickness burn, not painful, dry; epidermis, dermis, and subcutaneous involvement
- Criteria for transfer to burn center for pediatric patients:
  - Greater than 10% total body surface area involved if second-degree burns
  - Greater than 5% total body surface area involved if third-degree burns
  - Second- or third-degree burns involving face, hands, feet, genitalia, perineum, and major joints
  - Electrical burns, including lightning injury
  - Chemical burns
  - Inhalational injury
  - Burn injury in patients with preexisting medical disorders that may complicate management, prolong recovery, or affect mortality
  - If concomitant trauma, consider transfer if burn injury reflects greatest risk of morbidity or mortality; consider initial treatment in a trauma center if the trauma represents the greatest risk of morbidity or mortality (as determined by physician judgement and hospital/local policy)
  - If the hospital lacks the necessary equipment or expertise in care of burn patients
  - Burn injury in patients with special emotional/social/rehabilitative needs (such as cases involving child abuse)

MANAGEMENT

- Initial resuscitation
  - There are local and systemic responses to burns that result in direct tissue coagulation, dermal destruction/loss of barrier integrity, and release of vasoactive and inflammatory mediators. Secondary organ injury and shock can occur from interstitial edema (from increased capillary permeability and increased hydrostatic pressure), increased systemic vascular resistance, reduced cardiac output, and hypovolemia from fluid losses. This occurs especially when >20% of total body surface area is involved.
  - Fluid resuscitation:
    - The greatest fluid losses occur within the first 24 hours of injury.
    - Fluid resuscitation should begin within 2 hours of the burn for the highest chance of good outcomes.
    - The goal of fluid resuscitation is to maintain good cardiac output and good organ perfusion.
    - Fluid should be titrated to heart rate, blood pressure, and hourly urine output.
    - Various formulas are used to determine how much fluid to administer. One commonly used formula is the Parkland formula which recommends Ringer's lactate for the first 24 hours.
    - The total volume recommended is 4 mL/Kg × % body surface area involved + maintenance fluids
    - Half is given over the first 8 hours, the remaining half over the next 16 hours. This is adjusted to achieve goal urine output.
    - Maintenance fluids are not included if the patient weighs >40 kg.
    - Over-resuscitation should be avoided, as excess fluid can worsen pulmonary edema and subeschar pressures in the lower extremities and abdomen, leading to compartment syndrome.

○ Wound care
  ▪ Large blisters and full-thickness (third-degree) burns are often debrided and grafted.
  ▪ Superficial burns will often heal within several weeks without the need for surgical intervention.
  ▪ Topical agents are applied to prevent infection, control pain, and prevent fluid losses. These agents often contain silver, which has antimicrobial properties.
  ▪ Ensure tetanus vaccination.
○ Nutrition
  ▪ Burn patients often experience a hypermetabolic, hypercatabolic state. Early initiation of nutrition (within the first 24–48 hours) is recommended. Enteral route is preferred. Caloric requirements may be higher than normal.
  ▪ Maintaining normoglycemia (often with the use of insulin) is associated with improved morbidity and mortality.
○ Infection
  ▪ Infections are the most common cause of death following burn injury.
  ▪ Excellent wound care with topical antimicrobial agents has reduced the incidence of wound infections and resulted in decreased mortality.
  ▪ Prophylactic administration of systemic antibiotics is not indicated.

INHALATIONAL INJURIES

- Inhalation injury occurs secondary to inhalation of products of combustion and is the leading cause of death due to fires.
- Inhalational injuries such as those acquired from house fires may not have as many outward physical manifestations as burn injuries.
- Initial evaluation: The same initial evaluation principles apply here as earlier, including evaluation of the patient's airway, breathing, and circulation (ABCs).
  ○ Close evaluation of the airway is key. There may be evidence of facial burn, singed nasal hairs, or soot in the mouth. These patients should be admitted for monitoring.
  ○ The gold standard for diagnosing inhalational injury is with fiber-optic bronchoscopy.
  ○ Intubation should be considered in the setting of inhalation injury with respiratory distress, evidence of upper airway obstruction, upper airway edema, facial burns, singed nasal hairs, or evidence of soot in the mouth.
  ○ Initial diagnostic evaluation should also include an arterial blood gas, co-oximetry, carboxyhemoglobin level, pulse oximetry, CBC, and chest X-ray.
  ○ Management of inhalational injury is usually supportive and may require intubation/mechanical ventilation, bronchodilator therapy, and airway clearance therapies.

CARBON MONOXIDE (CO) POISONING

- CO poisoning is one of the more severe consequences of smoke inhalation.
- Suspect if altered mental status or decreased level of consciousness in a patient with exposure to smoke or fire.
- PaO_2 on an ABG and oxygen saturation on a pulse oximeter will likely remain normal unless other lung injury.
- Carboxyhemoglobin should be measured. Symptoms appear usually once the carboxyhemoglobin level exceeds 15%.
- Oxygen should be applied and will decrease the half-life of CO from 2 to 7 hours in room air to 20 to 30 minutes at 100% FiO_2 administered by a non-rebreathing mask.
- Hyperbaric oxygen therapy is used in some centers to more rapidly reduce high levels of CO by receiving 100% oxygen therapy at greater than atmospheric pressure. A Cochrane

review found no benefit to hyperbaric oxygen therapy; however, it is often used in patients with severe toxicity, neurologic symptoms, and pregnant women.

- Mechanism of CO toxicity
  - CO binds readily to hemoglobin $\rightarrow$ carboxyhemoglobin (COHb).
  - COHb is red, which is why patients with CO toxicity are often described as having "cherry red cyanosis."
  - COHb reduces the oxygen-carrying capacity of the blood $\rightarrow$ tissue hypoxia.
  - CO is also directly toxic to the cytochromes within the electron transport chain.
  - CO binds intracellular myoglobin in the heart, reducing mitochondrial oxygen delivery, interrupting oxidative phosphorylation, and resulting in myocardial injury.
  - All of these processes ultimately result in tissue hypoxia and affect multiple organs including the brain.

CYANIDE TOXICITY

- Cyanide (CN) toxicity is another potential consequence of smoke inhalation (though it is more common in other circumstances such as environmental exposures).
- Diagnosis is often difficult and requires a high level of suspicion. Severe toxicity can lead to blurry vision, respiratory distress, seizures, and unconsciousness.
- Laboratory findings (which are late) include a severe metabolic acidosis with elevated lactate. PaO_2 may be normal, but oxygen saturations will likely be low.
- CN impairs oxygen utilization through binding of cytochromes in the electron transport chain resulting in disruption of oxidative phosphorylation $\rightarrow$ tissue hypoxia, cellular death, and end-organ dysfunction.
- CN may also directly or indirectly interrupt neurotransmitter pathways.
- Treatment primarily focuses on conversion of CN to thiocyanate, which is excreted by the kidneys. Multiple antidote kits are available in the United States:
- Example of one cyanide antidote kit:
  - Amyl nitrite pearls – crushed for inhalation
  - Sodium nitrite – administered intravenously
    - Together, these two components $\rightarrow$ iron to convert to its ferric form on hemoglobin $\rightarrow$ methemoglobin. CN preferentially binds to the ferric form of iron on methemoglobin compared to the ferric form of iron within the cytochrome.
    - CN + methemoglobin $\rightarrow$ cyanomethemoglobin
    - Note: Nitrites may result in hypotension, and the formation of methemoglobin may worsen hypoxia in lung-injured patients.
  - Sodium thiosulfate – administered last and promotes excretion of CN by serving as a sulfur donor to which CN can bind. Rhodanese catalyzes the reaction in the liver by which sulfur is added to CN $\rightarrow$ thiocyanate, which can be excreted by the kidneys.
    - Slow onset of action and can cause nausea/vomiting/hypersensitivity reactions. Thiocyanate accumulation can lead to kidney injury. It is not recommended for use alone.
- More commonly used, safer option includes:
  - Hydroxycobalamin – is a B_{12} precursor that binds CN $\rightarrow$ cyanocobalamin. This can be excreted by the kidneys.

SUMMARY

Overall burns require immediate attention with a trauma evaluation and early fluid resuscitation. Transfer to a burn center may be indicated for specialty care. Smoke inhalation is a common occurrence from exposure to fires, and toxicity by CO and CN should be considered early in the evaluation. Early recognition and intervention can result in reduced morbidity and mortality for these patients.

SUGGESTED READINGS

Gonzalez R, Shanti CM. Overview of current pediatric burn care. *Semin Pediatr Surg.* 2015;24(1):47-49.

Huzar TF, George T, Cross JM. Carbon monoxide and cyanide toxicity: Etiology, pathophysiology and treatment in inhalation injury. *Expert Rev Respir Med.* 2013;7(2):159-170.

Nichols DG, Rogers MC. Chapter 29. Burns, electrical injuries, and smoke inhalation. In Yurt RW, Howell JD, BM G. In Nichols DG, eds. *Rogers' textbook of pediatric intensive care.* 4th ed. Philadelphia: Lippincott Williams & Wilkins; 2008.

Prockop LD, Chichkova RI. Carbon monoxide intoxication: An updated review. *J Neurol Sci.* 2007;262(1-2):122-130.

Rowan MP, Cancio LC, Elster EA, et al. Burn wound healing and treatment: Review and advancements. *Crit Care.* 2015;19:243.

Sheridan RL. Burns. *Crit Care Med.* 2002;30(11 Suppl):S500-514.

70 Biological/Chemical/Terrorism/ Biohazard

OVERVIEW

SPECIAL CONSIDERATIONS IN CHILDREN

- Developmental immaturity: unable to flee or seek medical attention, unable to describe symptoms or give history
- Increased respiratory exposure: closer to the ground, higher minute ventilation
- Increased dermal exposure: less fat, thinner, more permeable skin, larger body surface area:mass ratio
- Increased risk of dehydration due to toxin-induced vomiting and diarrhea
- Increased risk of hypothermia during decontamination procedures
- Immunologic immaturity, resulting in more virulent disease manifestations, greater permeability of blood–brain barrier
- Increased incidence of head injuries: head is larger proportionally, calvarium is thinner
- Increased incidence of multiple-organ injury
- Provider unfamiliarity with pediatric dosing, lack of pediatric equipment, pediatric-sized antidotes, and vaccines

BLAST INJURIES

Explosive charges can be low order (lower energy, no overpressure wave) or high order (high energy, overpressure wave) such as TNT, C4, or ammonium nitrate. High-order explosives are used in up to 66% of terror attacks.

There are four types of blast injuries. Most victims suffer injuries from multiple mechanisms.

- Primary: direct effect of the overpressure wave moving through tissues
- Secondary: penetrating injuries from fragments
- Tertiary: result from the victim impacting a hard surface (fractures, traumatic brain injury [TBI], abrasions)
- Quaternary: burns and injuries caused by the blast itself

Primary blast injuries (PBIs) may not be immediately visible but can be life threatening. The incidence and mortality of PBI are higher when the blast occurs in enclosed rather than open areas because the overpressure wave bounces off solid walls.

BLAST INJURIES BY SYSTEMS

- Primary blast lung injury (PBLI): 3% to 14% of initial survivors, highest mortality risk
  - *Pathophysiology*: Disruption of capillary-alveolar interface, leading to pulmonary hemorrhage, pulmonary edema, pneumothorax, pulmonary fat or air embolus, and IL-8–mediated inflammatory response
  - *Presentation*: Cough, tachypnea, dyspnea, chest pain, cyanosis, hemoptysis, bilateral opacities on chest x-ray (CXR), hypoxemia
  - *Management*: Supportive care with 100% oxygen and maintaining a patent airway, judicious fluid management (avoid fluid overload), lung-protective ventilator strategy with permissive hypercapnia to minimize risk of pneumothorax
    - Prophylactic chest tubes are recommended prior to anesthesia or transport.

- Maintain high suspicion for air or fat embolus and obtain appropriate imaging (CT, echocardiogram, bronchoscopy). Emboli are likely to be multifocal so thoracotomy may not be feasible; use alternative positioning (e.g., lateral decubitus, prone) to increase venous pressure in the damaged lung and prevent more air from embolizing.
  - Selective ventilation may be necessary for severe pulmonary hemorrhage.
  - Extracorporeal membrane oxygenation support (ECMO) can be considered as a last resort.
- Cardiovascular blast injuries:
  - *Pathophysiology*: Primary blast injury results in bradycardia, hypotension, and apnea immediately after the blast (perhaps through a vagal mechanism). Air emboli can cause coronary vessel obstruction and myocardial ischemia. Secondary and tertiary injury can cause cardiac contusion or tamponade.
  - *Management*: Supportive care. Maintain euvolemia. Atropine may be a helpful adjunct.
- Primary blast gastrointestinal injuries: 3% to 6.7% of initial survivors
  - *Pathophysiology*: Overpressure wave causes microvascular damage and tearing across tissue planes, leading to intestinal perforation, hemorrhage, and occasional solid organ rupture.
  - *Presentation*: Abdominal pain, nausea, emesis, hematemesis, melena, hypotension, peritoneal signs. Can present several hours to days after blast.
  - *Management*: Maintain appropriate level of suspicion, diagnose with serial exams, imaging (abdominal xray or CT scan), bowel rest, surgery consult.
- Blast traumatic brain injury (bTBI): Both primary and tertiary injuries are common and difficult to distinguish
  - *Pathophysiology*: Similar to other types of TBI (e.g., contusion, edema, diffuse axonal injury, hematomas, hemorrhage), but with increased incidence of vasospasm and pseudoaneurysms, earlier onset of cerebral edema.
  - *Management*: See Chapter 41. Early decompressive craniectomy may improve outcomes.
- Other blast injuries:
  - *Ophthalmologic* (10% of blast victims): Ruptured globe, foreign body, air embolism, orbital fractures.
  - *Auditory* (9%–47% of blast victims): Tympanic rupture, ossicular chain disruption and fracture, perilymphatic fistula, conductive and sensory hearing loss, basilar membrane rupture, tinnitus, otalgia, otorrhea.

CHEMICAL AGENTS

GENERAL APPROACH

- Exposure occurs through the respiratory system or skin, with direct and systemic toxicity.
- Skin decontamination is crucial and should be done as quickly as possible by personnel in appropriate personal protective equipment (PPE).
  - Remove all clothing and jewelry.
  - Wash the victim with large amounts of soap and water or a 0.5% hypochlorite solution.
  - Blot dry (don't rub).

NERVE AGENTS: TABUN (GA), SARIN (GB), SOMAN (GD), AND VX

- Exposure/pathophysiology:
  - *Form:* Colorless liquids, odorless and tasteless, can be aerosolized, denser than air
  - *Exposure:* Absorption, ingestion, and inhalation
  - *Organophosphate analogs:* Inhibit acetylcholinesterase → excessive acetylcholine stimulation of nicotinic and muscarinic receptors

- Presentation:
  - *SLUDGE:* Salivation, lacrimation, urination, defecation, GI upset, emesis
  - *Respiratory:* Cough, bronchorrhea/bronchospasm, wheezing, dyspnea, respiratory depression, cyanosis—can cause death within 5 to 10 minutes of lethal dose exposure
  - *Cardiovascular:* Bradycardia, hypotension, AV block
  - *CNS:* Muscle fasciculations, seizures, ataxia, altered mental status, coma, weakness/hypotonia
- Diagnosis: Suspected based on presentation, confirmed by response to antidotes
- Management: Decontamination, antidotes for both muscarinic and nicotinic effects
  - *Atropine:* Muscarinic antidote, should be administered (IM) to *all* patients exhibiting signs/symptoms of nerve agent poisoning
    - 0.05 mg/kg IV or IM (max 5 mg); repeat q2–5min prn persistent/recurrent symptoms
  - *Pralidoxime chloride (2-PAM):* Nicotinic antidote, should be given to patients with severe signs/symptoms
    - 25 mg/kg/dose IV/IM (max 1 gram IV or 2 grams IM); repeat in 1 to 2 hours if muscle weakness has not been relieved, then at 10- to 12-hour intervals if cholinergic signs recur
  - *Benzodiazepines* (midazolam is preferred) should be given to prevent and treat seizures

VESICANTS (SULFUR MUSTARD, LEWISITE)

- Exposure/pathophysiology:
  - Alkylating agents cause damage to rapidly reproducing cells and long-term morbidity with extensive damage to skin, respiratory system, eyes, and bone marrow suppression
- Presentation
  - *Skin:* Blisters occur within minutes of skin contact, resulting in severe, burn-like lesions
  - *GI:* If ingested, extensive intestinal mucosal injury can occur
  - *Respiratory:* Respiratory failure (high mortality)
- Management
  - Rapid decontamination is the most important first step
  - Supportive care, similar to traditional burn care but generally do not require high volume fluid replacement
  - British anti-Lewisite is an antidote for Lewisite (3 mg/kg IM q4–6hr)

PULMONARY AGENTS (CHLORINE, PHOSGENE, METHYL ISOCYANATE)

- Exposure/pathophysiology:
  - Gases typically have an odor of newly cut grass or hay
  - Exposure: Inhalation and absorption
  - Injury to both type I and type II pneumocytes and alveolar macrophages → release of prostaglandins and bradykinin → vasodilation and capillary leak
- Presentation:
  - Skin and eye irritation present first; significant respiratory symptoms can be delayed up to 24 hours
  - Respiratory symptoms include cough, wheezing/stridor from airway irritation, and subsequent pulmonary edema and respiratory failure
- Management:
  - Decontamination by moving to fresh air, supplemental oxygen
  - Supportive care for respiratory failure, treatment of bacterial superinfection (commonly seen several days after exposure), careful attention to fluid management
  - Adjunct therapies include corticosteroids and N-acetylcholine (for phosgene specifically), but definitive evidence is lacking

CYANIDE

- Exposure/pathophysiology:
  - *Exposure:* Inhalation, ingestion, or transdermal absorption of vapor, solid, or liquid forms
  - *Cytochrome oxidase inhibitor:* Disrupts cellular metabolism by interrupting oxidative phosphorylation. Also acts as a direct neurotoxin via glutamate stimulation of NMDA receptors.
- Presentation: Sudden change in mental status, hypoxia without cyanosis, metabolic acidosis
  - *Mild:* Tachypnea, dizziness, nausea, vomiting, headache
  - *Severe:* Seizures, coma, respiratory arrest, cardiac arrest
  - *Labs:* Elevated serum lactate, narrow arterial-venous oxygen saturation difference, elevated serum cyanide level
- Management
  - *Initial:* Decontamination (soap and water), fresh air
  - *Supportive care:* Initial survivors will require intensive care for management of acute respiratory distress syndrome (ARDS), shock, acidosis, and seizures
  - *Antidotes:* Indicated in any patient with severe symptoms
    - Hydroxycobalamin binds with cyanide to form a renally excreted compound and is safer than traditional cyanide antidote kits
    - Traditional cyanide antidote kits contain sodium nitrite and sodium thiosulfate; monitor closely for hypotension and methemoglobinemia

RIOT CONTROL AGENTS (CS, CN)

- Exposure/pathophysiology:
  - Lacrimators ("tear gas") are mild akylating agents that irritate the eyes but can also cause damage to other mucosal surfaces
- Presentation:
  - Eye pain, conjunctival injection, blepharospasm, and lacrimation
  - Respiratory symptoms (laryngospasm and bronchospasm) occur rarely but can be fatal
- Management:
  - Irrigation of skin and eyes
  - Supportive care
  - Bronchodilators for respiratory symptoms

BIOLOGIC AGENTS

GENERAL APPROACH

- Detection: May be difficult to differentiate a bioterrorist attack from a natural outbreak, because symptoms may present days to weeks after the attack
- Hints: A sudden outbreak of an unusual illness, diagnosis of a rare disease
- Three categories defined by Centers for Disease Control (CDC), based on morbidity and mortality
  - Category A: Easily disseminated, high mortality rate, require special action for public health preparedness
  - Category B: Moderately easy to disseminate, high morbidity, low mortality, require enhanced surveillance
  - Category C: Emerging pathogens engineered for mass dissemination in the future

CATEGORY A AGENTS

- Anthrax: Caused by *Bacillus anthracis*, a gram-negative, spore-forming bacteria
  - *Exposure:* Ingested (GI anthrax), absorbed (cutaneous anthrax), inhaled (inhalational anthrax)
  - *Pathophysiology:* Secretion of exotoxins results in massive edema and cytokine storm
  - *Presentation:*
    - Cutaneous: Papules form 1 to 7 days post exposure, then become vesicles that ulcerate and form a black eschar
    - Inhalational: Subtle upper respiratory infection (URI)–like symptoms present 1 to 7 days post-exposure (reported as late as 60 days); without treatment progresses to high fever, shock, and death. Fifty percent of patients develop meningitis.
  - *Diagnosis/management:*
    - Requires special attention to culture (high level of suspicion); enzyme-linked immuno-sorbent assay (ELISA) and polymerase chain reaction (PCR) tests available at national reference laboratories
    - Treatment with ciprofloxacin or doxycycline plus clindamycin plus penicillin
    - Amoxicillin and levofloxacin are second-line therapies
    - Prophylaxis with ciprofloxacin or doxycycline × 60 days
- Plague: Caused by *Yersinia pestis*, a gram-negative bacillus
  - *Exposure:* A bioterrorism attack would most likely present as pneumonic plague from aero-solized bacteria, but naturally occurring plague also occurs in septicemic and bubonic forms
  - *Pathophysiology:* Multilobar, hemorrhagic, necrotizing bronchopneumonia
  - *Presentation:* In a bioterrorism scenario, could expect a large number of previously healthy patients to develop severe pneumonia and sepsis without the development of buboes
    - Fever and cough within 6 days of exposure
    - Rapid progression to severe bronchopneumonia with hemoptysis and sepsis
  - *Diagnosis/management:*
    - Gram stain of blood or sputum may reveal gram negative bacilli 24 to 48 hours after exposure
    - Gentamycin, streptomycin, doxycycline, or ciprofloxacin
    - Chloramphenical or levofloxacin are second-line agents
    - Prophylaxis with trimethoprim/sulfamethoxazole × 5 to 7 days
- Smallpox: Caused by the variola major virus, thought to only exist in samples kept securely at the CDC and in Russia
  - *Exposure:* Highly contagious, only a few viral particles needed to induce disease
  - *Presentation:* Incubation period is from 7 to 19 days
    - Initial symptoms are nonspecific: Fever, malaise, vomiting, headache, backache
    - Within 2 to 3 days an erythematous macular rash appears, progressing to papules and pustules which spread centrifugally
    - Death occurs in the second week with multiorgan failure due to overwhelming viremia
  - *Diagnosis/management:*
    - Initial suspicion should be reported immediately to health department.
    - PCR assays are available at national laboratories.
    - Anyone exposed to a case patient should be monitored for a minimum of 17 days on airborne and contact precautions in the hospital or isolated in their homes.
    - Vaccination 72 to 96 hours after exposure decreases severity and may protect against developing the disease.
    - Antivirals (cidofovir) may be helpful based on animal data.

- Tularemia: Caused by *Francisella tularensis*, a small, aerobic, gram-negative coccobacillus
  - *Exposure:* Naturally occurring throughout North America and Europe, usually transmitted by insect bites, handling infected animal meat, or ingestion of contaminated water or food. A bioterrorism attack would likely be in an aerosolized form.
  - *Presentation*: Patients develop flu-like symptoms and bronchitis 3 to 5 days post exposure and can progress to severe necrotizing hemorrhagic pneumonia, with or without bacteremia and sepsis.
  - *Diagnosis/management:*
    - Rapid tests are available at research and reference laboratoris, and tularemia is rarely isolated from routine cultures. Serum antibody titers take 10 days to become positive.
    - Antibiotics for treatment and prophylaxis are the same as for plague.
    - Standard precautions are appropriate, as tularemia is not spread person to person.
- Botulism: Caused by the toxin produced by *Clostridium botulinum*, an anaerobic bacteria.
  - *Exposure*: When used in bioterrorism, botulinum toxin is most likely to be released and inhaled.
  - *Pathophysiology:* The toxin causes inhibition of the release of acetylcholine at the neuromuscular junction, producing paralysis.
  - *Presentation:* Patients present within 12 to 24 hours of inhalational exposure, with cranial nerve palsies, followed by descending paralysis, progressing to respiratory failure.
    - Symptoms include constipation, ileus, dry mouth, mydriasis
  - *Diagnosis/management:*
    - High level of clinical suspicion is important; diagnostic testing by bioassay is available
    - Supportive care, including close monitoring of respiratory status and ventilatory support
    - Antitoxin should be administered at the first onset of symptoms and only shortens the course of illness
    - Prophylactic vaccination is reserved for at-risk individuals
- Viral hemorrhagic fevers: Caused by viruses from five families, all of which produce fever, shock, and bleeding, with high morbidity and mortality.
  - *Exposure*: Except for dengue, which is blood-borne, all are spread by aerosolized particles.
  - *Presentation*: Nonspecific febrile illness with headache, myalgias, and malaise; progresses to shock and hemorrhage.
  - *Diagnosis/management*:
    - A careful travel history to possible endemic areas, exposure to animals or animal feces
    - Rapid enzyme immunoassays are available to detect most viruses
    - Supportive care, including vigorous fluid resuscitation, replacement of blood products, and coagulation factors

RADIOLOGICAL/NUCLEAR

GENERAL APPROACH

- Immediate injuries result from explosive force of a detonation or from trauma sustained during evacuation due to crowd panic.
- Acute radiation syndrome ("radiation sickness") develops within days to weeks after exposure.
- Decontamination is less time sensitive than in biological and chemical exposures, and treatment of critical or life-threatening conditions should occur before decontamination. Removal of clothing will eliminate 90% of contamination, and simple washing with soap and water, as well as flushing of eyes, is typically sufficient.

CLINICAL SIGNS AND SYMPTOMS

- Pathophysiology: Progenitor and rapidly dividing cells are the most significantly affected (hematopoietic, reproductive, and GI systems)
- Nonspecific prodrome: Hours to days of nausea, vomiting, fatigue
- Latent period
- Acute radiation syndrome:
  - *Hematopoietic*: Pancytopenia, hemorrhage, sepsis
  - *GI*: Mucosal sloughing, hemorrhage, bowel obstruction, sepsis
  - *Pulmonary*: Radiation pneumonitis
  - *CNS*: Microvascular injury; intractable seizures and elevated ICP are associated with high mortality

MANAGEMENT

- Supportive care (fluids, nutrition, antimicrobials, skin care, hematopoietic growth factors)
- Consultation with nuclear medicine physicians to determine specific exposure and prognosis
- Specific antidotes are unlikely to be helpful for critically ill patients, but some chelating agents may have efficacy

SUGGESTED READINGS

Graham PL, Foltin GL, Sonnett FM. Terrorism and mass casualty events. In: Nichols DG, ed. *Roger's Textbook of Pediatric Intensive Care*. 4th ed. Philadelphia, PA: Lippincott Williams & Wilkins; 2008:427-440.

Hamele M, Poss WB, Sweney J. Disaster preparedness, pediatric considerations in primary blast injury, chemical and biological terrorism. *World J Crit Care Med*. 2014;3(1):15-23.

Hyper/Hypothermia and the Febrile State

THERMOREGULATION AND HOMEOSTASIS

As endotherms, we autoregulate body temperature across a range of environmental conditions. Our temperature is intimately linked to our resting energy expenditure, which in turn drives our need for energy intake. Understanding the regulation of body temperature in the context of health and disease contributes to practice in the intensive care unit.

- The hypothalamus is the master thermostat
- Body temperature is maintained between 36°C and 37.5°C
- Patients above 38°C or 38.5°C are generally considered febrile
- Fever is a regulated process in response to inflammatory cytokines and pyrogens
- Temperatures above 41°C are considered hyperthermic
- Temperatures below 36°C are considered hypothermic

COOLING DOWN

Core temperature is greater than the set point.

- Sweating and peripheral vasomotor dilatation increase evaporative and radiant heat losses

WARMING UP

Core temperature is less than the set point.

- Peripheral vasoconstriction to limit radiant losses
- Shivering to stimulate heat production
- Increase in metabolic rate to generate cellular heat

CELLULAR HEAT

Intramolecular reactions, such as the generation or cleavage of adenosine triphosphate (ATP), release a small amount of energy as heat. In addition, metabolic uncoupling at the level of the mitochondria drives excess heat production. Some tissues, brown fat and skeletal muscle, specialize in cellular heat generation. The cumulative action of cellular metabolism drives heat generation.

CARDIAC OUTPUT AND THE FEBRILE STATE

- Metabolism increases oxygen consumption (VO_2)
- Oxygen delivery (DO_2) matches demand via neurohormonal feedback mechanisms
  - Febrile patients are tachycardiac to increase cardiac output/DO_2
  - Patients with limitation to cardiac output, such as critical heart failure or shock, are unable to further increase their cardiac output, and decompensated shock may result during fever
- CO_2 production (VCO_2) increases with increased oxygen consumption
  - Minute ventilation increases with VCO_2
  - Febrile patients are tachypneic
  - Febrile patients unable to increase their minute ventilation, such as those with respiratory failure or chemical paralysis, may develop respiratory acidosis with fever.

TREATMENT OF FEVER

- Reduce the production of pyrogens and inflammatory cytokines
  - Address sources of inflammation, infection, or tissue injury
- Lower the thermostat set point using cyclooxygenase-2 inhibitors
  - Nonsteroidal anti-inflammatory agents such as ibuprofen or acetaminophen
- Environmental cooling: Although commonly employed, increasing the rate of heat loss through surface cooling, administration of cold fluids, tepid baths, and ambient temperature reduction may drive the demand for cardiac output
  - Uncontrolled cooling of the critically ill patient may contribute to shock if cardiac output is limited

THERMOCOUPLE

To enable safe environmental cooling, the hypothalamus should be sufficiently anesthetized to minimize the feedback mechanisms increasing the demand for cardiac output.

- Sufficient sedation will allow cooling without driving the demand for cardiac output
- Therapeutic hypermagnesemia targeting >3 mg/dL can reduce muscle shivering
- Skin counter warming provides negative feedback to the hypothalamus during core temperature cooling and may minimize the shivering response

HYPERTHERMIA

A state of dysregulated heat production or insufficient heat loss leading to a rise in core temperature in excess of 41°C not governed by the hypothalamic set point. As temperature rises, tissue injury, rhabdomyolysis, seizures, coma, and death may result.

- Heat stroke occurs when the heat exchange mechanisms have failed due to excessively hot conditions, overexertion, and/or dehydration leading to a rise in core temperature. If untreated, tissue injury and death will occur within hours.
  - Following ABCDE evaluation, initiate cooling by removing inciting factors, then initiate surface evaporative cooling with cool water, circulating air, ice packs, and partial immersion. Ensure adequate hydration and restoration of circulating volume with crystalloid resuscitation (normal saline or lactated Ringer's IV).
- Hyperthermia syndromes: Malignant hyperthermia (MH), malignant hyperthermia–like syndrome (MHLS), neuroleptic malignant syndrome, and serotonin syndrome. Mortality is high with these syndromes, and rapid recognition is essential.
  - Malignant hyperthermia occurs when a genetically susceptible individual is exposed to select anesthetics or succinylcholine leading to excessive calcium release. Sustained muscle contraction drives a hypermetabolic state and rhabdomyolysis. Treatment is removal of the inciting agent, dantrolene to inhibit calcium release from intracellular stores, supportive care, and patient cooling.
  - Malignant hyperthermia–like syndrome resembles MH, yet in the context of hyperglycemic, hyperosmolar non-ketotic states or type II diabetic coma. Treatment is similar to MH with close attention to fluids and electrolytes.
  - Neuroleptic malignant syndrome occurs with administration of dopamine D2 receptor agonists such as select antipsychotic drugs, promethazine, and metoclopramide. In addition to hyperthermia, the canonical syndrome involves muscle rigidity, mental status changes (mild to severe), and autonomic instability (diaphoresis, episodic hypertension, and tachycardia). Treatment is to discontinue the offending agent, initiate cooling, dantrolene, and benzodiazepines if agitation present.

○ Serotonin syndrome caused by exposure to serotonin agonists such as drugs of abuse, herbal remedies, diet pills, or antidepressant medications. This syndrome involves autonomic dysregulation (hyperthermia, diaphoresis, tachycardia, hypertension), mental status changes (mild to severe), and muscle excitation (hyperreflexia, hyperkinesia, and clonus). Treatment is to remove the offending agent, supportive care and patient cooling, and cyproheptadine, a mixed antihistamine/antiserotonin receptor antagonistic.

HYPOTHERMIA

Occurs when core temperature falls below 35° to 36°C, generally from environmental factors, such as water immersion or cold weather exposure, and is compounded in younger children secondary to a high surface area/mass ratio and limited fat stores. Patients with central nervous dysfunction often have a dysregulated thermostat, and exposure to anesthesia blunts the thermoregulatory response. All organ systems are affected by hypothermia, especially the heart and the brain. Autoregulatory mechanisms will drive metabolic demand for cardiac output until heat generation is insufficient and core temperature falls.

- Mild hypothermia (32°–35°C): show initial compensation, with a hypermetabolic state, vasoconstriction, tachycardia, tachypnea, and shivering. Confusion, psychomotor retardation, and mental status changes are common.
- Moderate hypothermia (28°–32°C): results in bradycardia, unconsciousness, hypoventilation, and muscle rigidity.
- Severe hypothermia (<28°C): results in bradycardia, ventricular fibrillation, hypotension, coma, and death.
- Treat hypothermia using supportive care, passive and active external warming, and selective internal rewarming such as warmed humidified air through the ventilator, warm IV fluids, gastric or colonic lavage, or extracorporeal device such as ECMO or cardiac bypass if the patient presents with severe hypothermia in cardiac collapse.

ACTIVE TEMPERATURE CONTROL IN THE INTENSIVE CARE UNIT

Therapeutic mild hypothermia improves outcome in selected populations, such as adults with out-of-hospital cardiac arrest, traumatic brain injury with elevated intracranial pressure, or perinatal asphyxia in the neonate. Attempts to apply mild hypothermia across other disease states and patient populations have met with mixed success, especially in pediatric cardiac arrest or brain injury. Thus, targeted hypothermia should only be applied in consultation with disease specialists rather than implemented as first-line therapy. Controlled cooling leading to moderate-severe hypothermia are widely used during cardiopulmonary bypass whereby cardiac output, oxygenation, and acid/base status are precisely regulated during core cooling with excellent outcomes.

- The case for normothermia: Given the mixed success of therapeutic hypothermia, studies are now focused on the application of active normothermia, recognizing that the absence of fever is protective. Using a variety of pharmacologic means (anti-pyretics, CNS depressants) and external cooling devices (e.g., Artic Sun), febrile patients with low cardiac output states, multisystem organ failure, sepsis, neurologic ischemic injuries, intracranial hypertension, or malignant arrhythmias are being subjected to active normothermia to reduce tissue injury.

SUGGESTED READING

Bakar AM, Schleien CL. Chapter 36: Thermoregulation. In: Shaffner DH, Nichols DG, eds. *Roger's Handbook of Pediatric Critical Care*. 5th ed. Philadelphia: Lippincott Williams & Wilkins; 2016.

Allergy/Immunology/
Genetics

72 Anaphylaxis

DEFINTION

- Etiology: An acute multisystem response caused by a severe reaction to any antigen, such as a drug, vaccine, food, toxin, plant, or venom
- Clinical Presentation:
  - *Systemic vasodilation:*
    - Hypotension
    - Tachycardia
  - *Increased capillary permeability:*
    - Angioedema – may lead to partial or complete airway obstruction
    - Worsens hypotension
  - *Pulmonary vasoconstriction:*
    - Decreased pulmonary blood flow
    - Increased right ventricular afterload
    - Decreased left ventricular preload
  - *Bronchoconstriction/bronchospasm*
    - Respiratory distress $+/-$ stridor, wheezing, or both
  - *Histamine release:*
    - Urticaria
    - Nausea and vomiting

MANAGEMENT

REMOVE/DISCONTINUE OFFENDING AGENT

- Example: Discontinue medication infusion

INITIATE SUPPORTIVE CARE

- ABCs:
  - Administer 100% oxygen
  - Maintain airway:
    - Positioning: place patient supine
    - Stabilization (i.e., bag-mask ventilation and/or endotracheal intubation [ETT] if necessary)
  - Suction as needed
  - Pulse oximetry
  - Obtain intravenous/intraosseous (IV/IO) access
  - EKG monitoring

INITIATE MEDICATION ADMINISTRATION

- Epinephrine:
  - *Intramuscular (IM):*
    - 0.01 mg/kg/dose = 0.01 mL/kg/dose q10–15min prn
    - Max single dose 0.3 mg
    - 1 mg/mL; 1:1000 concentration
  - *IM autoinjector:*
    - Weight 10 to 30 kg = 0.15 mg
    - Weight $\geq$30 kg = 0.3 mg

- ○ *IV/IO bolus dose*:
  - 0.01 mg/kg/dose = 0.1 mL/kg/dose IV/IO q3–5min prn
  - Max single dose 1 mg
  - 0.1 mg/mL; 1:10,000 concentration
- ○ *IV/IO continuous infusion*:
  - 0.1 to 1 mcg/kg/min IV/IO infusion
  - If hypotension persists despite fluids and IM injection
- • Albuterol:
  - ○ *Nebulizer*:
    - Weight <20 kg: 2.5 mg/dose via inhalation q20min prn
    - Weight >20 kg: 5 mg/dose via inhalation q20min prn
  - ○ *Continuous nebulizer*:
    - 0.5 mg/kg per hour via continuous inhalation
    - Max dose 20 mg/hr
    - Indicated for severe bronchospasm
  - ○ *Metered dose inhaler (MDI: 90 mcg/puff)*:
    - 4 to 8 puffs via inhalation q20min prn with spacer (or ETT if intubated)
- • Corticosteroids:
  - ○ *Methylprednisolone* (reduces late-phase reaction):
    - Load 2 mg/kg IV/IM/IO (max 60 mg); use only acetate salt IM
    - Maintenance: 0.5 mg/kg IV/IO q6hr or 1 mg/kg q12hr (max 120 mg/day)
- • Antihistamine:
  - ○ *H_1-receptor antagonist*: diphenhydramine
    - 1 to 2 mg/kg/dose IM/IV/IO over 5 min q4–6hr
    - Maximum *single* dose 50 mg
  - ○ *H_2-receptor antagonist*: ranitidine or famotidine
    - Ranitidine: 1 mg/kg/dose IV
      - Maximum *single* dose of 50 mg
    - Famotidine: 0.25 mg/kg/dose IV
      - Maximum daily dose of 40 mg
  - ○ *The combination of both H_1 and H_2 blocker may be more effective than giving either alone.*
- • Hypotension:
  - ○ *Isotonic crystalloid infusion*:
    - Rapid infusion 20 mL/kg – repeat as needed
    - Normal saline or lactated Ringer's
  - ○ *Epinephrine infusion* (see earlier):
    - Initiate for hypotension that is unresponsive to fluid and IM epinephrine administration
    - Titrate to achieve normal blood pressure for the patient's age

SUGGESTED READINGS

American Heart Association. *Pediatric Advanced Life Support Provider Manual*. Dallas, TX: First American Heart Association Printing; 2016.

American Heart Association. *Pediatric Advanced Life Support Reference Card*. Dallas, TX: American Heart Association; 2016.

American Heart Association. *2015 Handbook of Emergency Cardiovascular Care for Healthcare Providers*. Dallas, TX: First American Heart Association Printing; 2015.

73 Immune Dysfunction and Dysregulation

BALANCED INFLAMMATORY RESPONSE

Immune system components: balanced response by these components ensures elimination of threat with minimal damage to surrounding tissues (Table 73-1).

- Innate immunity:
  - *Pattern recognition receptors (PRRs)* = present on most cells, recognize pathogen-associated molecular patterns (PAMPs) or damage-associated molecular patterns (DAMPs). Lead to the production of cytokines and chemokines to contain threat and recruit cellular components of the immune system. Include the toll-like receptors (Table 73-2), Toll-like and Nod-like receptors, RIG-like receptors, and C-type lectin receptors.
  - *Opsonins* = mark pathogens or cells for clearance by phagocytes.

TABLE 73-1	Examples of Key Effector Molecules of the Innate Immune System		
Effector Molecules		**Primary Source**	**Critical Function**
Pro-inflammatory cytokines	IL-1β	Macrophages, endothelial and epithelial cells	Fever, induces other cytokines, stimulates bone marrow to release neutrophils and platelets, inhibited by anakinra (IL-1 receptor antagonist)
	TNF-α	Macrophages	Fever, induces other cytokines, recruits neutrophils and monocytes, inhibited by infliximab and etanercept
	IL-2	T cells	Induces T-cell proliferation, activates B cells
	IL-6	Macrophages, endothelial and epithelial cells	Mediator of the acute phase response, inhibited by tocilizumab
	IL-12	Macrophages and dendritic cells	Stimulates production of interferons (IFNs)
Chemokines	C-X-C family	Many cells	Chemotactic to neutrophils
	C-C family	Many cells	Chemotactic to monocytes and T cells
Anti-inflammatory cytokines	IL-4	T cells	Inhibits T cells, macrophages, IFN, and IL-12
	IL-10	Monocytes	Suppresses pro-inflammatory cytokines
	TGF-β	Macrophages, many cells	Inhibits phagocytosis, induces inflammatory cell apoptosis
Antiviral interferons	Type I interferon (IFN-α and IFN-β)	Most cell types	Inhibit viral replication through transcription of IFN-regulated genes
	Type II interferon (IFN-γ)	T cells (Th1), NK cells	Inhibits viral replication directly, supports Th1 response, promotes cellular immunity

TABLE 73-2	Key Pattern Recognition Receptors from the Toll-Like Receptor Family	
Toll-like Receptor	**Classic Ligand(s)**	**Source of Ligand**
TLR1	Lipopeptides	Bacteria
TLR2	Lipoteichoic acid	Gram-positive bacteria
TLR3	Double-stranded RNA	RNA viruses
TLR4	Lipopolysaccharide (LPS)	Gram-negative bacteria
TLR5	Flagellin	Bacteria
TLR6	Diacyl lipopeptides	Mycoplasma
TLR7	Single-stranded RNA	RNA viruses
TLR8	Single-stranded RNA	RNA viruses
TLR9	Unmethylated CpG DNA	Bacteria, DNA viruses

- ○ *Complement* = opsonize or directly lyse pathogens via assembly of the membrane attack complex.
- ○ *Cells* = including neutrophils, monocytes/macrophages, dendritic cells, and natural killer cells.
- Adaptive immunity:
  - ○ *T cells.*
    - CD4+ helper T cells:
      - Th1: Triggered by bacteria and viruses. Primary cytokines include IL-2, IFN-γ, TNF.
      - Th2: Triggered by parasites and allergic reactions. Primary cytokines include IL-4, IL-5, IL-10.
      - Th17: Very inflammatory. Primary cytokine is IL-17.
    - CD8+ cytotoxic T cells: Kill infected cells.
  - ○ *B cells.*
    - Plasma B cells: Antibody factories.
    - Memory B cells: Provide long-term protection.

SYSTEMIC INFLAMMATORY RESPONSE SYNDROME (SIRS)

Excessive inflammation: can cause collateral damage to tissues.

- Symptoms: fever or hypothermia, tachycardia, tachypnea, abnormally high or low WBC.
- Secondary to: trauma, post-operative state, infection (= sepsis).
- Treatment: supportive care aimed at avoiding or reversing shock. Experimental therapies directed at PRRs, cytokines, or coagulation cascade have yet to show improvement in mortality.

COMPENSATORY ANTI-INFLAMMATORY RESPONSE SYNDROME (CARS)

Excessive anti-inflammatory response: can lead to immunoparalysis.

- Symptoms: usually asymptomatic until acquire secondary infection.
- Secondary to: inflammatory state. Begins during inflammation, but can persist after resolution and leave patients susceptible to secondary infections.
- Treatment: supportive care. Experimental therapies include immune modulators, including GM-CSF.

MACROPHAGE ACTIVATION SYNDROME (MAS) AND HEMOPHAGOCYTIC LYMPHOHISTIOCYTOSIS (HLH)

Exaggerated activation of phagocytes: often life threatening, can cause significant end-organ damage.

- Hemophagocytic lymphohistiocytosis (HLH): primary forms due to genetic defect in genes encoding perforin or involved in cytolytic granule formation and release. Secondary forms seen with infection (especially viral), malignancies, or immunodeficiency syndromes.
  - *2004 diagnostic criteria* = five of the following eight findings:
    - Fever ≥38.5°C.
    - Splenomegaly.
    - Peripheral blood cytopenia, with at least two of the following: hemoglobin < 9 g/dL (for infants <4 weeks, hemoglobin <10 g/dL); platelets <100,000/µL; absolute neutrophil count < 1000/µL.
    - Triglyceride >265 mg/dL and/or fibrinogen <150 mg/dL.
    - Hemophagocytosis in bone marrow, spleen, lymph node, or liver.
    - Low or absent natural killer (NK) cell activity.
    - Ferritin >500 ng/mL.
    - Elevated soluble CD25 (soluble IL-2 receptor α) two standard deviations above age-adjusted laboratory-specific norms.
  - *Additional tests to consider:* perforin surface expression, quantitative immunoglobulins, lymphocyte subsets, bone marrow biopsy, head imaging, lumbar puncture.
  - *Treatment* = immunosuppression in discussion with hematologist. Typically includes corticosteroids and etoposide. Consider intrathecal methotrexate for CNS involvement. Stem cell transplant for primary HLH.
  - *Differential diagnosis* = sepsis, multiorgan dysfunction syndrome (MODS), drug reaction with eosinophilia and systemic symptoms (DRESS), etc.
- Macrophage activation syndrome (MAS): similar to acquired HLH, but secondary to rheumatologic condition, especially juvenile idiopathic arthritis (JIA).
  - *2016 diagnostic criteria* = in a febrile patient with known/suspected JIA.
    - Ferritin >684 ng/mL AND two of the following:
      - Platelet <181,000/µL.
      - AST >48 units/mL.
      - Triglycerides >146 mg/dL.
      - Fibrinogen <360 mg/dL.
  - *Treatment:* immunosuppression in discussion with rheumatologist.

SUGGESTED READINGS

Coates BM, Staricha KL, Wiese KM, et al. Influenza A virus infection, innate immunity, and childhood. *JAMA Pediatr.* 2015;169:956-963.

Dinarello CA. The IL-1 family and inflammatory diseases. *Clin Exp Rheumatol.* 2002;20: S1-13.

Janeway C. *Immunobiology 5: The Immune System in Health and Disease.* New York: Garland Publishers; 2001.

Takeuchi O, Akira S. Pattern recognition receptors and inflammation. *Cell.* 2010;140:805-820.

van der Poll T, Opal SM. Host-pathogen interactions in sepsis. *Lancet Infect Dis.* 2008;8:32-43.

74

Inborn Errors of Metabolism and Metabolic Emergencies

Inborn errors of metabolism (IEMs), although rare, are becoming more recognized in pediatrics.

Common examples of inborn errors of metabolism are shown in Table 74-1.

Newborn screening tests have aided clinicians in diagnosing most of these disorders shortly after birth. However, some infants and children will present later in life, and it is crucial for pediatric ICU providers to recognize these disorders quickly so treatment can be initiated.

Children with undiagnosed metabolic disorders oftentimes present with:

- Varying states of shock
- Cardiac insufficiency and/or cardiomyopathies
- Feeding intolerance, failure to thrive, vomiting, and lethargy
- Profound dehydration with or without metabolic acidosis
- Altered mental status with or without hyperammonemia
- Intractable seizures
- Developmental delay

TABLE 74-1	Common Examples of Inborn Errors of Metabolism
Type of Metabolic Derangement	**Commonly Seen Disorders**
Urea cycle defects	Ornithine transcarbamylase deficiency
	Citrullinemia
	Argininosuccinic aciduria
Organic acidemias	Maple syrup urine disease
	Proprionic acidemia
	Methylmalonic acidemia
	Isovaleric acidemia
Aminoacidopathies	Phenylketonuria
	Tyrosinemia
	Homocystinuria
Fatty-acid oxidation disorders	Carnitine transport deficiency
	Carnitine palmitoyl transferase deficiency
	Long chain 3-hydroxyacyl-coenzyme A dehydrogenase deficiency (LCHAD)
Glycogen storage disorders	Von Gierke's disease
	Pompe's disease
	McArdle's disease
Mucopolysaccharidoses	Hurler syndrome
	Hunter syndrome
	Sanfilippo syndromes A–D

These predominately autosomal-recessive disorders often result in significant enzyme deficiencies impairing mitochondrial function. Mitochondria therefore:

- Cannot break down proper by-products of certain metabolic pathways, which impairs their function on the cellular level
- Accumulate dysfunctional upstream metabolites, which becomes toxic to the cell and patient
- Shunt metabolites into other pathways, which get overloaded or are unable to process these metabolites

WORKING UP A METABOLIC DISORDER

Physicians who suspect an underlying metabolic disorder or a patient in metabolic crisis should immediately evaluate the following on physical exam:

- Vital signs: Assess for fever or hypothermia, abnormal changes in blood pressure and pulse pressure, alterations in heart rate and rhythm, and variations in respiratory effort (irregular breathing or large Kussmaul breaths)
- General appearance: Observation of coarsened facial features, body odor/smell
- Ophthalmologic exam: Consider a distinct eye exam to evaluate for cataracts, changes in retinal pigmentation
- Cardiovascular exam: Evaluate for signs of cardiogenic shock; assess for brisk or delayed capillary refill, bounding pulses, displaced point of maximal impulse (PMI), murmurs
- Abdominal exam: Direct palpation for hepatosplenomegaly
- Neurologic exam: Note baseline Glasgow Coma Score (GCS) for encephalopathy, hypotonia or hypertonia, brisk tendon reflexes, pupillary irregularities, or cranial nerve deficits

Initial laboratory studies should include the following:

- Arterial blood gas to evaluate for changes in blood pH and the presence of metabolic acidosis and lactate production
- Rapid blood glucose to evaluate for hypoglycemia
- Rapidly run iced ammonia levels on free-flowing blood samples
- Basic metabolic panels to assess bicarbonate levels and electrolyte derangements
- Pyruvate levels
- Blood and urine ketones/β-hydroxybutyrate
- Liver function tests to assess for elevated transaminases
- Coagulation profile to evaluate for disseminated intravascular coagulopathy (DIC)
- Creatinine kinase to assess for rhabdomyolysis
- Plasma amino acids, plasma acylcarnitine profile, carnitine level, urine organic acids

After obtaining these laboratory results, Figure 74-1 can help aid in diagnosing the underlying cause.

ACUTE CLINICAL MANAGEMENT OF INBORN ERRORS OF METABOLISM AND METABOLIC CRISES

1. Assess the ABCs (airway/breathing/circulation) and stabilize the patient:
   - Ensure the patient is receiving adequate respiratory and circulatory support
   - Apply oxygen and noninvasive pressure if indicated
   - Consider intubation if necessary, but recognize that children may often be compensating for an underlying acidosis by breathing quickly or with large tidal volumes, and neuromuscular blockade may acutely worsen their acidosis

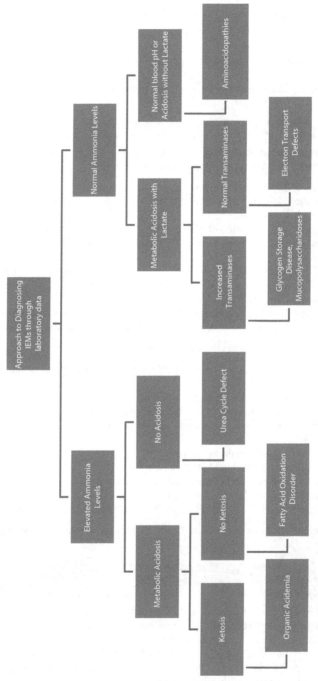

FIGURE 74-1 **Approach to diagnosing inborn errors of metabolism through laboratory data.**

- Frequent neurologic checks to ensure the patient is protecting their airway
- Evaluate patient's hydration status and resuscitate with IV fluids as indicated, but be mindful of:
  - Electrolyte derangements (e.g., correct hypoglycemia rapidly with 2–4 mL/kg of 25% dextrose, correct hyponatremia slowly with 0.9 normal saline)
  - Possible presence of underlying cardiac insufficiency or cardiomyopathy that may worsen with large volume fluid resuscitation
  - Signs and symptoms concerning for cerebral edema (altered mental status with a low GCS <8, abnormal pupils, Cushing's triad: hypertension, irregular respirations, bradycardia)
- Support the child with vasoactive medications/vasopressors if necessary for cardiac insufficiency or shock

2. Initiate disease-specific therapies:
   - Hyperammonemia that occurs acutely or subacutely directly insults the blood–brain barrier and predisposes patients to cerebral edema. This frequently occurs in urea cycle defects, and removal of elevated ammonia levels should occur immediately:
     - Consider lactulose to acidify the intestinal lumen and promote ammonia removal through the stool if the patient is stable for PO or an intragastric infusion
     - Initiate L-arginine infusions of 600 mg/kg over the first few hours, then continue between 200 and 600 mg/kg/day to restore this essential amino acid
     - Enhance nitrogen excretion through the kidneys with an Ammonul infusion (sodium benzoate 250 mg/kg/day and sodium phenylacetate 250 mg/kg/day)
     - Utilize mannitol (1 g/kg) if there is concern for cerebral edema
     - Consider exchange transfusion if not within a dialysis center
     - Placement of an emergent dialysis catheter to initiate continuous venovenous hemodialysis and filtration (CVVHDF) to quickly and safely remove ammonia in consultation with a pediatric nephrologist
   - Hypoglycemia occurs frequently in fatty-acid oxidation defects, and glycogen storage diseases and should be promptly treated after the initial stabilization with D25 boluses. Rebound hypoglycemia occurs more frequently in IEMS, and plasma glucose levels should be checked hourly and slowly spaced.
     - Continuous dextrose infusions with elevated dextrose content (D10 or higher) should be continued in the ICU setting to prevent further mitochondrial catabolism and recurrence of hypoglycemia (3–5mg/kg/min in children, 5–10 mg/kg/min in neonates)
   - Carnitine supplementation should be used for organic acidurias and fatty-acid oxidation disorders to replace the losses of carnitine associated with a metabolic crisis.
     - Give L-carnitine 50 to 100 mg/day bid
   - Liver failure can be a serious presentation of IEMs (mainly urea cycle defects and aminoacidopathies) and can present as altered mental status, uremia, hyperbilirubinemia, jaundice, disseminated intravascular coagulation (DIC), or shock.
     - Treatment of liver failure is mainly supportive but may require invasive monitoring or emergent dialysis
     - Pediatric gastroenterologists should be consulted early to aid in the work up and management since occasionally transplantation is necessary
     - Rapid correction of coagulation abnormalities with fresh frozen plasma (FFP) and vitamin K supplementation may be needed
     - Reduction in peripheral edema with continuous albumin infusions and diuretics may also be of benefit
     - Phototherapy for elevated bilirubin

AFTER STABILIZING A PATIENT IN ACUTE CRISIS FROM AN INBORN ERROR OF METABOLISM

- Consult a pediatric geneticist to aid in managing the patient while inpatient and to establish appropriate treatment options, follow-ups, and referrals for all subspecialists needed as an outpatient
- Provide counseling with a genetics counselor to review dietary restrictions, medication supplementation instruction, and concerning signs and symptoms for repeat crises

SUGGESTED READINGS

Barness LA. An approach to the diagnosis of metabolic disease. *Fetal Pediat Pathol.* 2004;23:3-10.

Garganta CL, Smith WE. Metabolic evaluation of the sick neonate. *Semin Perinatol.* 2005;29:164-172.

Nichols DG; section editors, Alice D. Ackerman, Andrew C. Argent, et al. *Rogers Textbook of Pediatric Intensive Care*, 4th ed. Philadelphia, PA: Lippincott Williams & Wilkins; 2008.

Index

Note: Page numbers with an f and/or t indicate a figure or table on the designated page.

A

Abdominal compartment syndrome, 433
Abusive head trauma (AHT), 105
Acapella, 163
Acetaminophen, 128t–129t
    poisoning, 454–455, 455t, 457t
Acetazolamide, 119, 360t
Acetylcysteine, 113
Acidosis, 181, 183t
Acute appendicitis, 428–429
Acute cellular rejection (ACR), 373
Acute flaccid paralysis, 321–322
Acute hemolytic transfusion reaction, 380t
Acute kidney injury (AKI), 356–361
    causes, 356
    definitions and staging criteria, 357, 358t
    diagnosing, 357–359, 358t
    management, 359–360, 360t
    outcomes, 362
    postoperative, 265
Acute liver failure, 436–438
Acute lung injury, 185
Acute respiratory distress syndrome (ARDS), 185–187
Acyclovir, 143t
Adaptive immunity, 219, 478
Adenosine, 122, 239t
    for cardiac arrest, 50f, 51t
Adenotonsillar disease, 167
Adrenal insufficiency, 409–411
Advanced Trauma Life Support (ATLS), 102
Aerobes, 138t
AHT (abusive head trauma), 105
Airway clearance, 162–165
    chest physical therapy (CPT) or bronchial drainage (BD), 162
    cough assist, 164–165
    high-frequency assisted airway clearance, 163–164
    indications, 162
    intrapulmonary oscillations, 164
    intrapulmonary percussive ventilation (IPV), 164
    positive expiratory pressure (PEP) devices, 162–163
Airway obstruction, 166–174
    lesions and treatments by subsite, 167–173
    managing airway emergencies, 173–174
    nasal obstruction, 167
    pharyngeal obstruction, 167–168
    supraglottic obstruction, 168–173
    symptoms by subsite, 166t
    upper airway obstruction, 166
AKI (acute kidney injury). *See* Acute kidney injury (AKI)
AKIN (Acute Kidney Injury Network) criteria for diagnosing and staging AKI, 357, 358t
Alanine aminotransferase (ALT), 107
Albumin, 115
Albuterol, 113
    for anaphylaxis, 476

Alemtuzumab, for immunosuppression in kidney transplant, 371
Alkali (lye) ingestion, 431, 431t
Alkalosis, 181, 183, 183t
Allen test, 62–63, 64f
Alprostadil, 122
    for postoperative liver transplantation, 442t
Alveolar-arterial gradient, 154
Alveolar gas equation, 154
Alveolar ventilation (VA), 153
Amikacin, 142t
Aminoacidopathies, 480t
Aminoglycosides, 142t
Aminophylline, for asthma, 178
Amiodarone, 122, 238t
    for cardiac arrest, 48f, 50f, 51t
Amphotericin, 143t
Ampicillin, 141t
    for meningitis/encephalitis, 317
    for postoperative liver transplantation, 442t
AMR (antibody-mediated rejection), 373
Amyl nitrate, as antidote for cyanide, 457t
Anabolic flow phase, 417–418
Anaerobes, 138t
Analgesia. *See* Sedation, analgesia, neuromuscular blockade and withdrawal
Anaphylaxis, 215, 475–476
Andersen tube, 95
Anesthesia risk, 326
Anion gap, 6, 181, 181f
Anterior horn cell disorder, 324–325
Anterior spinal artery infarction, 321
Anthrax, 467
Antiarrhythmic medications, 121–122
Antibiogram, 140
Antibiotic resistance, 146
Antibody-mediated rejection (AMR), 373
Anticholinergics
    for asthma, 177
    poisoning, 457t
Anticholinergic toxidrome, 452t
Antidotes, 457t
Antifungals, spectra of, 143t
Antihistimines, for anaphylaxis, 476
Antihypertensive medications, 124–125
Anti-infective agents, 138–148
    antibiogram, 140
    antifungals, spectra of, 143t
    antivirals, 143t
    Gram stain evaluation, 138, 138t
    initial empiric therapy for common clinical presentations in the PICU, 143t–145t
    IV antibiotics, spectra of, 141t–142t
    microbiology, 138–139
    minimum inhibitory concentration (MIC), 139–140, 139f

Index

Index

Index

Index

CPSIA information can be obtained
at www.ICGtesting.com
Printed in the USA
LVHW081137021221
705030LV00009B/94